Brady *Tri-Township Ems*

BASIC TRAUMA LIFE SUPPORT
ADVANCED PREHOSPITAL CARE

Second Edition

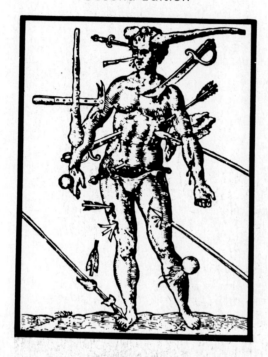

Edited by

John Emory Campbell, M.D.

Alabama Chapter
American College of Emergency Physicians

D1540727

BRADY
A Prentice Hall Division
Englewood Cliffs, New Jersey 07632

Library of Congress Cataloging-in-Publication Data

Campbell, John E., 1943-
    Basic trauma life support : advanced prehospital care / edited by

John E. Campbell. — 2nd ed.
    p.   cm.
    "A Brady book."
    Includes index.
    1. Traumatology.   2. Medical emergencies.   I. Title.
    RC86.7.C34 1988   617´.1026—dc19   88-9900
    ISBN 0-89303-088-0

Editorial/production supervision and
    interior design: Eileen M. O'Sullivan
Manufacturing buyer: Bob Anderson
Page layout: Lorraine Mullaney

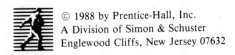 © 1988 by Prentice-Hall, Inc.
A Division of Simon & Schuster
Englewood Cliffs, New Jersey 07632

Printed in the United States of America

10 9 8 7 6 5

ISBN   0-89303-088-0

PRENTICE-HALL INTERNATIONAL (UK) LIMITED, *London*
PRENTICE-HALL OF AUSTRALIA PTY. LIMITED, *Sydney*
PRENTICE-HALL CANADA INC., *Toronto*
PRENTICE-HALL HISPANOAMERICANA, S.A., *Mexico*
PRENTICE-HALL OF INDIA PRIVATE LIMITED, *New Delhi*
PRENTICE-HALL OF JAPAN, INC., *Tokyo*
SIMON & SCHUSTER ASIA PTE. LTD., *Singapore*
EDITORA PRENTICE-HALL DO BRASIL, LTDA., *Rio de Janeiro*

This book is dedicated to Jackie, and all the other BTLS spouses. The only thing better than the experience of saving a life is sharing that experience with someone who understands.

Contents

CHAPTERS

BASIC SKILL STATIONS

ADVANCED SKILL STATIONS

Introduction

The first prehospital trauma course ever developed, *Basic Trauma Life Support* was introduced in August of 1982. BTLS began as a local project of the Alabama Chapter of the American College of Emergency Physicians. After five years of dedicated work by volunteer instructors from every level of emergency medicine, BTLS has become internationally accepted as the training course for prehospital trauma care. The original BTLS course was modeled after the *Advanced Trauma Life Support* course (for physicians) so that the surgeon, emergency physician, trauma nurse, and EMT would think and act along similar lines. The courses differ in many respects because the prehospital situation differs markedly from the hospital. The term "basic trauma life support" is not to suggest that advanced life support procedures are not used in the field, but rather to distinguish the support in the field from the advanced surgical procedures used in the hospital care of the trauma victim.

Basic Trauma Life Support is endorsed by the American College of Emergency Physicians and the National Association of EMS Physicians. The National Registry of Emergency Medical Technicians recognizes the course for 16 hours credit for continuing education for all levels of EMTs. More than this, BTLS has become an international organization of instructors of prehospital trauma care. Each state or province is represented at national meetings. The purpose of the organization is to foster trauma training and maintain up-to-date high standards for the BTLS course.

The BTLS organization with the experience of training over 10,000 students over the last five years is responsible for the second edition of BTLS. Authors include distinguished trauma surgeons, emergency physicians, trauma nurses, and paramedics. We have attempted to make changes that are more practical to the real environment of the prehospital situation. Because EMS varies widely over the world, we have added some basic skill stations and some optional advanced skill stations. There are several new chapters that are pertinent to trauma care but are not included in the course itself.

This course is designed for the advanced EMT, paramedic, and trauma nurse who must initially evaluate and stabilize the trauma patient. Since this is a critical time in the management of these patients, this course is intended to teach the skills necessary for rapid assessment, resuscitation, packaging, and transport. It also stresses those conditions which cannot be stabilized in the field and thus require immediate transport. It is recognized that there is more than one acceptable way to manage most situations, and the ones described here are not the only way. You should have your Medical Control physician go over the material and give you advice as to how the procedures are to be done in your area. Modification of technique is allowed in the teaching of this course.

The primary objectives of the course are to teach you the correct sequence of evaluation and the techniques of resuscitation and packaging of the patient. You will be given enough practical training to perform these drills rapidly and efficiently, thus giving your patient the greatest chance of arriving at the emergency department in time for definitive care to be lifesaving.

Notes for Students

The two-day BTLS course is an intensive, demanding experience that requires preparation in advance of the actual course. You should begin studying the book no less than two weeks before the course. The actual course is designed not to tell you, but rather to show you and allow you to practice managing trauma patients. If properly prepared, you will find this course to be the most enjoyable you have ever taken.

The first 15 chapters are essential and should be studied thoroughly in the weeks preceeding the course. You will be tested on this material. The appendix contains important chapters, but due to time constraints they are not included in the course. You will *not* be tested on the chapters in the appendix.

Many of the skill stations are optional. You should receive a list of those that will be taught in your course.

Notes for Teachers

Though suitable as a reference text about prehospital trauma care, this book is designed to be part of an organized 2-day, hands-on course for advanced EMTs and emergency nurses. An instructor's Guide and slides are available to be used in teaching the BTLS course. This course is monitored and certified in each state, usually by the state chapter of American College of Emergency Physicians in conjunction with a regional state EMS agency. If you need assistance in arranging a certified course in your state, you may write or call:

Pat Gandy, R.N.
Executive Director
Basic Trauma Life Support
P.O. Box 210727
Montgomery, Alabama 36121-0727
(205) 567-2000

Authors

Larry Alred, R.N., C.E.N., EMT-P
Chief Flight Paramedic
SOUTHFLITE-USA
University of South Alabama Medical Center
Mobile, Alabama

Gail V. Anderson, Jr. M.D.
Assistant Professor
Division of Emergency Medicine
Emory University School of Medicine

Director
Surgical Emergency Clinic
Grady Memorial Hospital

Paul S. Auerbach, M.D.
Associate Professor of Surgery & Medicine
Director, Emergency Department
Vanderbilt University Medical Center

Medical Director
Division of Emergency Medical Services
Tennessee Department of Health & Environment

James J. Augustine, M.D.
Clinical Instructor
Department of Emergency Medicine
Wright State University

EMS Director
Miami Valley Hospital
Dayton, Ohio

Jere Baldwin, M.D.
Vice-chief, Emergency Services
Mercy Hospital
Port Huron, Michigan

John E. Campbell, M.D.
Assistant Professor of Surgery
Division of Emergency Services
Department of Surgery
University of Alabama at Birmingham

Daniel L. Cavallaro, NREMT
Clinical Instructor of Medicine
University of South Florida
College of Medicine

James H. Creel, Jr., M.D., FACEP
Chairman, Curriculum Committee
National BTLS

Raymond L. Fowler, M.D., FACEP
President, Georgia Chapter
American College of Emergency Physicians
Vice-President, National BTLS

Director of Emergency Medicine
HCA Parkway Medical Center
Lithia Springs, Georgia

Carden Johnston, M.D., FAAP
Medical Director, Emergency Medicine
The Children's Hospital
Associate Professor of Pediatrics
University of Alabama at Birmingham

Ron W. Lee, M.D.
Director, Division of Emergency Medicine
Saint Mary of Nazareth Hospital Center
Chicago, Illinois

Richard N. Nelson, M.D., FACEP
Assistant Professor
Associate Director
Emergency Medicine Residency Program
Ohio State University

Paul Paris, M.D.
Associate Professor of Medicine
Chief, Division of Emergency Medicine
University of Pittsburgh School of Medicine

Andrew B. Peitzman, M.D.
Assistant Professor of Surgery
University of Pittsburgh School of Medicine

Marlon L. Priest, M.D., FACEP
Associate Professor of Surgery
Medical Director
Emergency Department
University of Alabama Hospitals

Daniel G. Sayers, M.D.
Assistant Professor
Department of Surgery
Section of Emergency Medicine
Bowman Gray School of Medicine

Corey M. Slovis, M.D., FACP, FACEP
Associate Professor of Medicine
Director, Emergency Medicine
Emory University School of Medicine

Medical Director
Emergency Medical Services
Grady Memorial Hospital
Atlanta, Georgia

Steve Smit, EMT-P, I/C
Regional Coordinator
SWM Systems Inc.
Kalamazoo, Michigan

Ronald D. Stewart, M.D., FACEP
Professor and Chief
Division of Emergency Medicine
University of Pittsburgh School of Medicine

Medical Director
Department of Public Safety
City of Pittsburgh

Ronald B. Taylor, M.D.
Instructor
Department of Emergency Medicine
Medical College of Georgia

Diane Threadgill, R.N., B.S.N., C.E.N., E.M.T.
Pediatric Trauma Nurse Coordinator
University of South Alabama College of Medicine
Division of Pediatric Surgery
Mobile, Alabama

Richard C. Treat, M.D.
Associate Professor of Surgery
Trauma–Surgical Critical Care
Department of Surgery
Medical College of Georgia
Augusta, Georgia

Arlo F. Weltge, M.D., FACEP
Director
Southeast Texas Emergency Physicians

Director
Emergency Services
West Houston Medical Center

Howard A. Werman, M.D.
Assistant Professor
Division of Emergency Medicine
Ohio State University

This book is designed to be part of an organized 2-day, hands-on course. There are slides and an Instructor's Guide to be used with this book. This course is monitored and certified in each state, usually by the state chapter of American College of Emergency Physicians in conjunction with a regional state EMS agency. If you do not know who to contact in your state to arrange a certified course, you may obtain this information from:

National Basic Trauma Life Support, Inc.
P.O. Box 210727
Montgomery, Alabama 36121-0727

PART I

— Chapter 1 —

Mechanisms of Injuries Due to Motion

James H. Creel, Jr., M.D., F.A.C.E.P.

Trauma, which accounts for approximately 7% of deaths annually, continues to be a major health care problem in the United States. It is the leading cause of death in Americans ages 1 through 44. The monetary cost for trauma is extremely high. In 1983 the estimated cost for vehicular trauma alone was $36 billion. Even more importantly, trauma was responsible for 45,000 deaths. Trauma is a disease process and the mechanisms of injury must be considered as a part of its etiology. Paramedics must ask themselves two important questions. What happened? How was the patient injured? To give care without appreciation of the mechanisms that produced the injuries and thus not be able to predict what possible pathology might exist is less than optimal trauma care. If one understands the mechanisms of injury and maintains a high degree of suspicion, one may well be able to predict the occult injuries and save precious time in preparing for their treatment. This is extremely useful in assessing what may be a potentially unstable patient: for example, a victim who has been in a head-on collision and has slight upper abdominal tenderness, a heart rate of 110, a narrow pulse pressure of 120/90, and delayed capillary refill. Do you take your time with this patient or transport immediately?

Although there are many mechanisms of injury (burns, drowning, toxic inhalations, etc.), the most common are injuries due to movement. Motion injuries are by and large responsible for the majority of the mortality in the United States. In this chapter we review the most common mechanisms of motion injuries and stress the potential injuries that may be associated with these mechanisms. It is essential to develop an awareness of mechanisms of injury and thus have a high index of suspicion for occult injuries. Always consider the potential injury to be present until it is ruled out in a hospital setting.

There are three basic mechanisms of motion injury:

1. Rapid forward deceleration
2. Rapid vertical deceleration
3. Projectile penetration

Motor Vehicle Accidents

Various injury patterns are discussed in the following examples, which relate to automobiles, motorcycles, all-terrain vehicles, and tractors. The important concept to appreciate is that the kinetic energy of motion must be absorbed, and that absorption of energy is the basic component in producing injury. Motion injury may be blunt or penetrating. Generally, blunt trauma is more common in a rural setting, and penetrating trauma is more common in the urban setting. Rapid forward deceleration is usually blunt but may be penetrating. The most common example of rapid forward deceleration is the motor vehicle accident (MVA). A paramedic should consider all MVAs as occurring in three separate events:

1. Machine collision
2. Body collision
3. Organ collision

Consider approaching a MVA in which an automobile has hit a tree head-on at 40 mph. Appreciation of the rapid forward decelerating mechanism, coupled with a high degree of suspicion should make you concerned that the victim may have possible head injury, cervical spine injury, myocardial contusion, any of the "deadly dozen" chest injuries, intraabdominal injuries, and musculoskeletal injuries (especially fracture or dislocation of the hip). To explain the forces involved here, you must consider Sir Issac Newton's second law of motion: "A body in motion remains in motion in a straight line unless acted upon by an outside force." This law is well exemplified in the automobile accident. The kinetic energy of the vehicle's forward motion is absorbed as each part of the vehicle is brought to a sudden halt by the im-

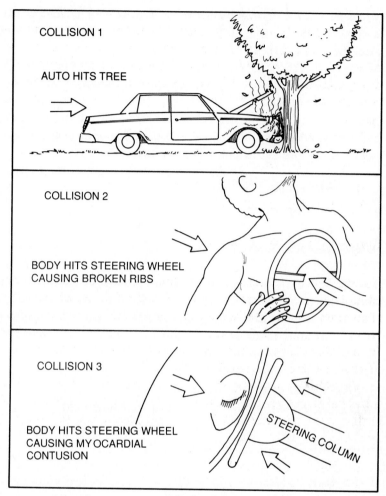

COLLISION 1

AUTO HITS TREE

COLLISION 2

BODY HITS STEERING WHEEL
CAUSING BROKEN RIBS

COLLISION 3

BODY HITS STEERING WHEEL
CAUSING MYOCARDIAL
CONTUSION

STEERING COLUMN

Figure 1–1.

pact. Remember that the body of the occupant is also traveling at 40 mph, until impacted by a structure within the car, such as the steering wheel, dashboard, or windshield. With awareness of this mechanism, one can see the multitude of potential injuries that may occur. The clues you should be aware of are:

1. Deformity of the vehicle (indication of forces involved)
2. Deformity of interior structures (indication of the point of victim impact)
3. Deformity (injury patterns) of the victim (indication of what parts of the body may have been involved in the impact)

There are four common forms of automobile accidents: (1) head-on collision, (2) T-bone or lateral impact collision, (3) rear-end collision, and (4) rollover collision.

Head-On Collision

The energy of an unrestrained body being brought to a sudden halt in this type of MVA is capable of producing multiple injuries. There are four basic weapons of the car which inflict injuries:

1. Windshield
2. Steering wheel
3. Dashboard
4. Miscellaneous

Windshield injuries occur in rapid forward decelerating events, where the unrestrained occupant impacts forcefully with the windshield. The possibility for injury is great under these conditions. Of utmost concern is the potential for airway and serious cervical spine (C-spine) injury. Remembering the three separate collision events, the paramedic notes the following:

Machine collision: deformed front end
Body collision: spiderweb pattern of windshield
Organ collision: coup/contracoup brain, soft tissue injury (scalp, face, neck), hyperextension/flexion of C-spine

From the spiderweb appearance of the windshield and appreciation of the mechanism of injury, the paramedic should maintain a high degree of suspicion of possible occult injuries of the C-spine. The head usually strikes the windshield, resulting in direct trauma to that structure. External signs of trauma include cuts, abrasions, and contusions. These may be quite dramatic in appearance; however, the key concern is airway maintenance with C-spine immobilization and evaluation of level of consciousness.

Steering wheel injuries occur most often to an unrestrained driver of a vehicle in a head-on collision. The driver may subsequently also impact with the windshield. The steering wheel is the vehicle's most lethal weapon for an unrestrained driver, and any degree of steering wheel deformity must be treated with a high degree of suspicion for face, neck, thoracic, or abdominal injury. The two components of this weapon are the ring and the column. The ring is a semirigid plastic-covered metal ring attached to a fixed inflexible post—in this author's view, a twentieth-century battering ram. Utilizing the three-collision concept, check for the presence of the following:

Machine collision: front-end deformity
Body collision: ring fracture/deformity, column normal/displaced
Organ collision: traumatic tattooing of skin

The "ring of injuries" illustration should be etched in the minds of all trauma care providers. The type of injury depends entirely on the area of the body that impacts with the steering wheel. These may be readily visible by means of direct trauma, such as lacerations of the mouth and chin, contusion/bruises of the anterior neck, traumatic tattoos of the chest wall, and bruising of the abdomen. These external signs may be subtle or dramatic in appearance—but more important, they may represent only the tip of the iceberg. Deeper structures and organs may harbor occult injuries due to shearing forces,

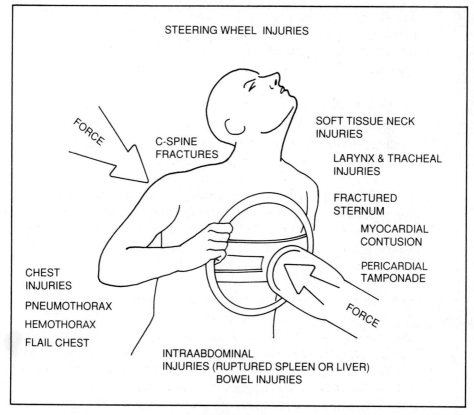

Figure 1–2.

compression forces, and displacement of kinetic energy. Organs that are susceptible to shearing injuries due to their ligamentous attachments are the aortic arch, liver, spleen, kidneys, and bowel. With the exception of small-bowel tears, these injuries are sources for occult bleeds and hemorrhagic shock. Compression injuries are common with the lung, heart, diaphragm, and urinary bladder. Manifestations include respiratory distress, which may be due to pulmonary contusions, pnemothorax, diaphragmatic hernia (bowel sounds in chest), or flail chest. Consider a bruised chest wall as a myocardial contusion that requires ECG monitoring.

In summary, the steering wheel is a very lethal weapon that is capable of producing devastating injuries, many of which are occult. Steering wheel deformity is a cause for alarm and must heighten your degree of suspicion. This information must be relayed to medical control.

An unrestrained occupant who strikes the dashboard has the possibility of receiving a variety of injuries depending upon the area of the body that hits the dashboard. Most commonly, this involves the face and knees; however, many types of injuries have occurred (see Figure 1–3). Applying the three-event concept of collision, you will note:

Machine collision: deformity of the car
Body collision: fracture/deformity of the dash
Organ collision: facial trauma, coup/contracoup brain, hyperextension/flexion C-spine, knee trauma

Facial, brain, and C-spine injuries have already been discussed. Like chest contusion, knee trauma may represent only the tip of the iceberg. Knees commonly impact with the dashboard. This may range from simple contusion noted about the patella to severe compound fracture of the patella. Frank dislocation of the knees can occur. In addition, this kinetic energy may be transmitted proximally and result in fracture of the femur or fracture/dislocated hips. On occasion the pelvis can strike the dashboard, resulting in acetabulum fractures as well as pelvic fractures. These injuries are associated with hemorrhage that may lead to shock. Maintain a high degree of suspicion and always palpate the femurs as well as gently rocking the pelvis and palpating the symphysis pubis.

Miscellaneous Weapons: Unrestrained objects in the vehicle (e.g., luggage, groceries, books, and most important, passengers) may become deadly missiles in a rapid forward decelerating type of event. Restrained occupants are much more likely to survive than unrestrained occupants because they are protected from much of the impact inside the auto and are restrained from being ejected

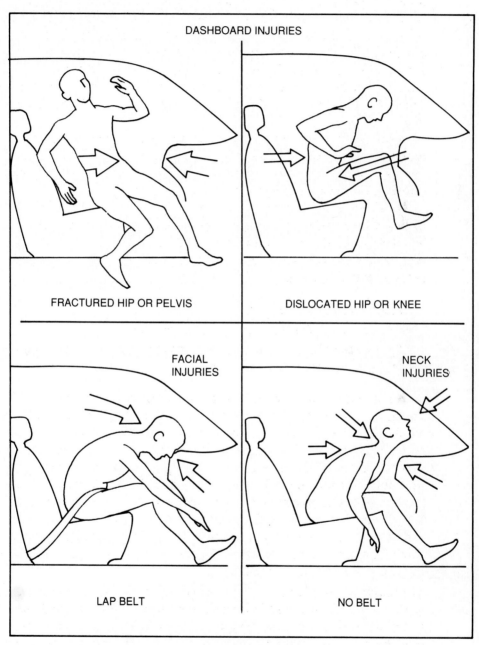

Figure 1–3.

from the auto. These occupants are, however, still susceptible to certain injuries. A lap belt is intended to go across the pelvis (iliac crests), not across the abdomen. If the belt is in place and the victim is subjected to a frontal deceleration accident, his or her body will tend to fold together like a clasp knife. The head may be thrown forward into the steering wheel or dashboard. Facial, head, and/or neck injuries are common. Abdominal injuries occur if the lap belt is positioned improperly. The compression forces that are produced when a body is suddenly folded about the waist may injure the abdomen or the lumbar spine.

The three-point restraint or cross-chest lap belt secures the body much better than does a lap belt alone. The chest and pelvis are restrained, so life-threatening injuries are much less common. The head is not restrained, and therefore the neck is still subjected to stresses that may cause fractures, dislocations, or spinal cord injuries. Clavicular fractures (where the chest strap crosses) are common. Internal organ damage may still occur due to organ movement inside the body.

Air bags are designed to inflate from the center of the steering wheel and the dashboard to protect front-seat occupants in case of a frontal deceleration accident. If these function properly, they cushion the head and chest at the instant of impact. This is very effective in decreasing injury to the face, neck, and chest. You should still immobilize the neck until it has been thoroughly examined. Air bags deflate immediately, so they protect against

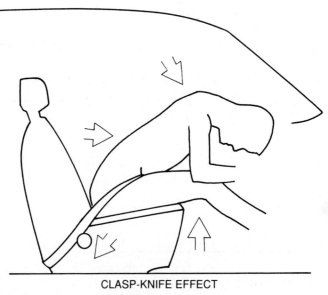

CLASP-KNIFE EFFECT

Figure 1–4.

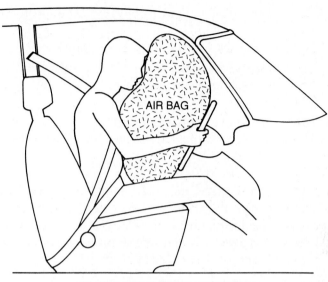

AIR BAG AND 3-POINT RESTRAINT
Figure 1–5.

only one impact. A driver whose car hits more than one object is unprotected after the initial collision. They also do not prevent "down and under" movement, so drivers who are extended (tall drivers and drivers of small, low-slung autos) may still impact with their legs and suffer leg, pelvis, or abdominal injuries. It is important for occupants to wear chest and lap belts even when a car is equipped with air bags.

T-bone or Lateral Impact Collision

The mechanism of the T-bone collision is similar to that of the head-on collision, with the addition of lateral energy displacement. Common areas of anatomical injury are the following:

1. Head
2. Neck
3. Thorax
4. Abdomen
5. Pelvis
6. Upper arms/shoulder

Machine collision: primary deformity of the car, check the impact side (driver/passenger)

Body collision: degree of door deformity (i.e., arm rest bent, outward or inward bowing of door)

Organ collision: includes multiple possibilities:

   Head: coup/contracoup due to lateral displacement

   Neck: lateral displacement injuries range from cervical muscle strain to subluxation with neurological deficit

   Thorax/abdomen: injury due to direct force either from inward bowing of door or unrestrained passenger being propelled across seat

Injuries of the thorax range from soft tissue to flail chest, lung contusion, pneumothorax, or hemothorax. Abdominal injuries include those of both solid and hollow organs. Pelvic injuries may include fracture/dislocation, bladder rupture, and urethral injuries. Shoulder girdle or lower-extremity injuries are common, depending on where the impact occurs.

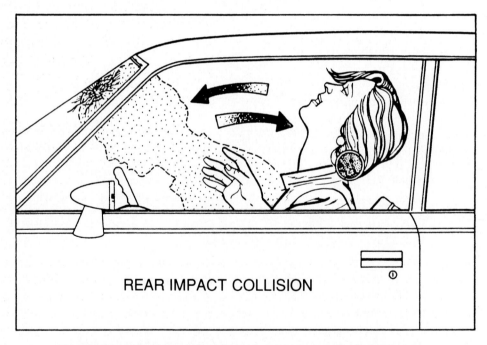

REAR IMPACT COLLISION

Figure 1–6. Cervical strain. Severe strain is usually evident from the history of the accident. Hyperextension or hyperflexion is often the mechanism of injury, which may involve either stretching or tearing of ligaments. Symptoms include neck immobility (caused by pain) and spasm of injured muscles.

Rear-End Collision

In the most common form of rear-end collision, a stationary car is struck from the rear by a moving vehicle. Also, a slower-moving car may be impacted from the rear by a faster-moving car. The sudden increase in acceleration produces posterior displacement of the occupants and possible hyperextension of the spine if the headrest is not properly adjusted. There may also be rapid forward deceleration if the car suddenly strikes something in the front or if the driver applies the brakes suddenly. The paramedic should check for deformity of the auto anterior and posterior, as well as interior deformity and headrest position. The potential for C-spine injuries is great. Also be alert for associated deceleration injuries.

Rollover Collision

This form of accident has a great potential to be lethal to the occupant in that the likelihood of being ejected is very great. Occupants ejected from the car are 25 times as likely to be killed than those who aren't ejected. The potential for injuries is great, encompassing all the injuries previously mentioned. The chance for axial loading injuries of the spine is increased in this form of MVA. Paramedics must be alert for clues that imply that the car turned over (i.e., roof dents, scratches, debris, and deformity of roof posts).

In summary, the paramedic must note the type of MVA and the clues that are implicit in the exterior/interior deformities of the vehicle. Maintain a high degree of suspicion of occult injuries and thus keep scene time to a minimum. These observations and clues are essential to good-quality patient care and must be relayed to medical control and the receiving physician.

Tractor Accidents

Another large motorized vehicle with which the paramedic must be familiar is the tractor. The National Safety Council reports that one-third of all farm accident fatalities involve tractors. There are basically two types of tractors: two-wheel drive and four-wheel drive. In both the center of gravity is high, and thus the tractors are easily turned over. The majority of fatal accidents are due to the tractor turning over and crushing the driver. Most overturns (85%) are to the side; these are less likely to pin the driver because he or she has a chance to jump or be thrown clear. Rear overturns, although less frequent, are more likely to entrap and crush the driver because he or she has almost no opportunity to jump free. The primary mechanism is the crush in-

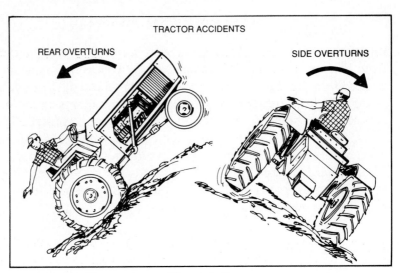

Figure 1–7.

jury, and the severity depends on the part of the anatomy that is involved. Additional mechanisms are chemical burns from gasoline, diesel fuel, hydraulic fluid, or even battery acid. Thermal burns from hot engine parts or ignited fuel are common.

Management consists of scene stabilization, followed quickly by primary survey and resuscitation. The following check list is used in scene stabilization:

1. Engine off
2. Rear wheels locked
3. Fuel situation and fire hazard addressed

While the victim is being surveyed, other rescuers must stabilize the tractor. The center of gravity must be identified before an attempt is made to lift the tractor. The center of gravity of a two-wheel-drive tractor is located approximately 10 inches above and 24 inches in front of the rear axle. The center of gravity of a four-wheel-drive tractor is closer to the midline of the machine. Because tractors usually overturn on soft ground and their centers of gravity are tricky to determine, great care must be taken during lifting to avoid a second crush injury. Because of the weight of the tractor and the length of time (usually prolonged) pinned, anticipate serious injuries. Often, the patient will go into profound shock as the compressing weight of the tractor is removed—similar to what happens when antishock trousers are suddenly deflated. Rapid, safe management of tractor accidents requires special exercises in lifting heavy machinery as well as good basic trauma life support (BTLS) management.

Small-Vehicle Accidents

Other small vehicles that fall into the motion injury category include the motorcycle, all-terrain vehicle (ATV), and the snowmobile. The operators of these machines are not encased within them and, of course, there are no restraining devices. When the operator is subjected to the classic head-on, lateral impact, rear-end, or rollover collisions, his or her only form of protection is:

1. Evasive maneuvering
2. Helmet usage
3. Protective clothing (e.g., leather clothes, helmet, boots)
4. Use of the vehicle to absorb kinetic energy (e.g., bike slide)

Motorcycles: It is important to wear helmets, but they are only marginally effective. Seventy-five percent of motorcycle deaths are attributed to head injury. The operator of a motorcycle involved in an accident is much like an ejected automobile occupant. Injuries depend on the part of the anatomy subjected to kinetic energy. Because of the lack of protective incasement, there is a higher frequency of head, neck, or extremity injury. Important clues include deformity of the motorcycle, the distance of skid, and deformity of stationary objects or cars. Again, a high degree of suspicion, appreciation of environmental clues (skid marks, vehicular deformity), identification of "load and go," and strict BTLS protocols constitute the optimal standard of prehospital care.

All-Terrain Vehicles: The ATV is one of the newer additions to the arsenal of trauma weapons. The ATV was designed as a vehicle to traverse rough terrain, used initially by ranchers, hunters, and farmers. Unfortunately, some people view the ATV as a fast toy. Careless misuse has resulted in ever-increasing morbidity and mortality from accidents—sadly, frequently among the very young. The two basic designs are either three-wheeled or four-wheeled. The four-wheel design affords reasonable stability and handling, but the three-wheeled ATV has a high center of gravity and is very prone to rollover when turned sharply. The three most common mechanisms are:

1. Vehicle rollover
2. Fall-off of rider
3. Forward deceleration of rider from vehicle impact with stationary object

The injuries produced depend on the mechanism and the part of the anatomy that is impacted. The most frequent injuries are fractures, about half of which are above and half below the diaphragm. The major bony injuries involves the clavicles, sternum, and ribs. Be very suspicious of head or spinal injury.

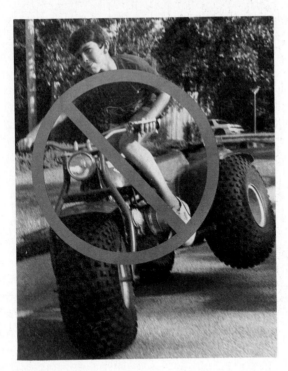

Figure 1–8. ATVs—Not for children.

Snowmobiles: Snowmobiles are used as both recreational and utility vehicles. The snowmobile has a low clearance and a low center of gravity. The injuries common to the use of this vehicle are very similar to those that occur with the ATV. Turnovers are somewhat more common, however, and since the vehicle is usually heavier than an ATV, crush injuries are seen more frequently. Again, the injury pattern depends on the part of the anatomy that is directly involved. Be alert for possible coexisting hypothermia. A common injury with the snowmobile is the "hangman" or "clothesline" injury that results from running under wire fences. Be very alert for occult cervical spine injuries and potential airway compromise.

Pedestrian Injuries: The pedestrian struck by a car almost always suffers severe internal injuries as well as fractures. This is true even if the vehicle is traveling at low speed. The mass of the auto is so large that high speed is not necessary to impart high energy transfer. When high speed is involved the results are disastrous. There are two mechanisms of injury. The first is when the bumper of the auto strikes the body, and the second is when the body, accelerated by the transfer of forces strikes the ground or some other object. An adult usually has bilateral lower leg or knee fractures plus whatever secondary injuries occur when his body strikes the hood of the car and then later the ground. Children are shorter so the bumper is more likely to hit them in the pelvis or torso. They usually land on their heads in the secondary impact. When answering a call to an auto-pedestrian accident, be prepared for broken bones, internal injuries, and head injuries.

Rapid Vertical Deceleration

The mechanism for falls is vertical deceleration. The types of injuries sustained depend on three factors which the paramedic must identify and relay to medical control:

1. Distance of fall
2. Anatomical area impacted
3. Surface struck

The primary groups involved in vertical falls are adults, and children under the age of 5. In children, the falls most commonly involve males and occur mostly in the summer months in urban high-rise multiple-occupant dwellings. Predisposing factors include poor supervision, defective railings, and the curiosity associated with that age group. Head injuries are common in falls by children because the head is the heaviest part of the body and thus impacts first. Adult falls are generally occupational or due to the influence of alcohol or drugs. It is not uncommon for falls to occur during attempts to escape from fire or criminal activity. Generally, adults attempt to land on their feet; thus their falls are more controlled. In this landing form, the victim usually impacts initially on the feet and then tilts backward landing on the buttocks and outstretched hands. Classically, this "lover's leap" fall may result in the following potential injuries:

Fractures of the feet or legs
Hip injuries/pelvic injury
Axial loading to the lumbar and cervical spine
Vertical deceleration forces to the organs
Colles' fractures of the wrists

The greater the height, the greater the potential for injury. However, do not be deceived into believing that there is little risk for serious injury in a short-distance fall. Surface density (concrete versus sawdust) and irregularity (gym floor versus staircase) also influence the potential for severity of injury. This information must be relayed to medical control together with other pertinent information.

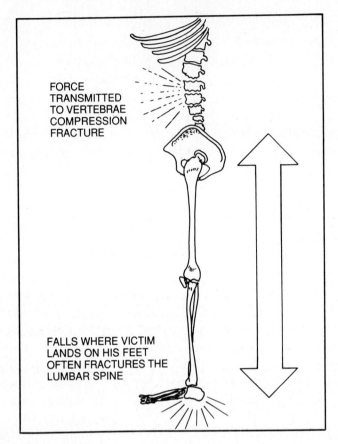

FORCE
TRANSMITTED
TO VERTEBRAE
COMPRESSION
FRACTURE

FALLS WHERE VICTIM
LANDS ON HIS FEET
OFTEN FRACTURES THE
LUMBAR SPINE

Figure 1–9.

Projectile Penetration

Numerous objects are capable of producing penetration injuries. These range from the industrial saw blade that breaks at an extremely high rpm rate to the foreign body hurled by a lawn mower, most of which are capable of penetrating the thorax or abdomen. However, the most common forms of penetrating wounds in our society come from knives and guns.

Knife wound severity depends on the anatomical area insulted, blade length, and angle of penetration. Remember, an upper abdominal stab wound may cause intrathoracic organ injury, and stab wounds below the fourth intercostal space may have penetrated the abdomen. The golden rule with knife wounds that still have the blade inside is: Do not remove the knife.

Most penetration wounds inflicted by firearms in our society are due to handguns, rifles, and shotguns. Important facts to obtain, if possible, are the type of weapon, caliber, and distance from which the weapon was fired.

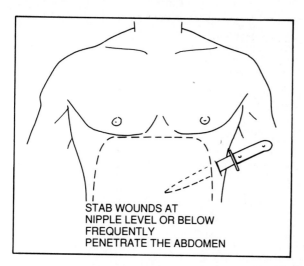

STAB WOUNDS AT
NIPPLE LEVEL OR BELOW
FREQUENTLY
PENETRATE THE ABDOMEN

Figure 1–10.

Useful Ballistics Information

Caliber: refers to the internal diameter of the barrel, and this correponds to the ammunition used for the particular weapon.

Rifling: refers to a series of spiral grooves in the interior surface of the barrel of some weapons which impart a stabilizing spin to the missile.

Ammunition: case, primer, powder, and slug.

Bullet construction: usually solid lead alloy and may have a full or partial copper or steel jacket. The shape may be rounded, flat, conical, or pointed. The bullet nose may be soft or hollow (for expansion or fragmentation).

Wound Ballistics

Because of the popularity of the kinetic energy theory,

$$\text{kinetic energy} = \tfrac{1}{2}\text{mass} \times \text{velocity}^2$$

which is heavily weighted toward velocity, weapons are classified as high velocity or low velocity. Weapons with velocities below 2000 ft/sec are considered low velocity and include essentially all handguns and some rifles. Injuries from these weapons are much less destructive than from missiles that exceed that level. These weapons are certainly capable of inflicting lethal injuries, depending on the body area struck. All wounds inflicted by high-velocity weapons carry the additional factor of hydrostatic pressure. This factor alone can increase the injury.

Factors that contribute to tissue damage include:

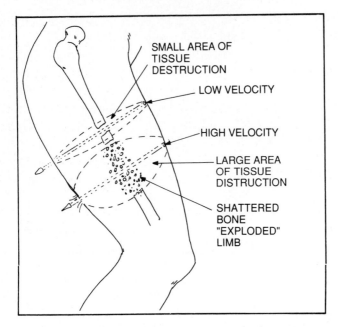

Figure 1–11.

1. *Missile size.* The larger the bullet, the more resistance and the larger the permanent track.
2. *Missile deformity.* Hollow point and soft nose flatten out on impact, resulting in a larger surface area involved.
3. *Semijacket.* The jacket expands and adds to the surface area.
4. *Tumbling.* Tumbling of the missile causes a wider path of destruction.
5. *Yaw.* The missile can oscillate vertically and horizontally about its axis, resulting in a larger surface area presenting to the tissue.

The wounds consist of three parts:

1. *Entry wound.*
2. *Exit wound.* Not all entry wounds will have exit wounds, and on occasion there may be multiple exits due to fragmentation of bone and missile; generally, the exit wound is larger than the entry wound and has ragged edges.
3. *Internal wound.* Low velocity inflicts damage primarily by damaging tissue that the missile contacts. High velocity inflicts damage by tissue contacted and transfer of kinetic energy to surrounding tissues. Damage is related to:
    a. Shock waves
    b. Temporary cavity, which is 30 to 40 times the bullet's diameter and creates immense tissue pressures

    c.   Pulsation of the temporary cavity, which creates pressure changes in the adjacent tissue

Generally, the damage done is proportional to the tissue density. Highly dense organs such as bone, muscle, and liver sustain more damage than do less dense organs such as lungs. A key factor to remember is that when a bullet enters a body, its trajectory will not always be a straight line. Any patient with missile penetration of the head, thorax, or abdomen should be transported immediately. Persons who have been shot while wearing a flak vest should be managed with caution; be alert for possible cardiac and other organ contusion.

In shotgun wounds, injury is determined by the kinetic energy at impact, which is influenced by:

1. Powder
2. Size of pellets
3. Choke of muzzle
4. Distance to target

Velocity and kinetic energy dissipate rapidly with distance. At 40 yards the velocity is one-half of the initial muzzle velocity.

Blast Injuries

Blast injuries occur primarily in industrial settings, such as grain elevator and gas fume explosions. However, as threat of terrorist activity can no longer be considered remote, blast injury management must be added to BTLS training and knowledge. The mechanism of injury by blast/explosion is due to three factors:

1. *Primary:* initial air blast
2. *Secondary:* victim being struck by material propelled by the blast force
3. *Tertiary:* total body displacement and impact

Injuries due to the primary air blast are almost exclusive to air-containing organs.

Auditory system injuries usually involve ruptured tympanic membranes. Lung injuries may include pneumothorax, parenchymal hemorrhage, and especially, alveolar rupture. Alveolar rupture may cause air embolus, which may be manifested by bizarre central nervous system symptoms.

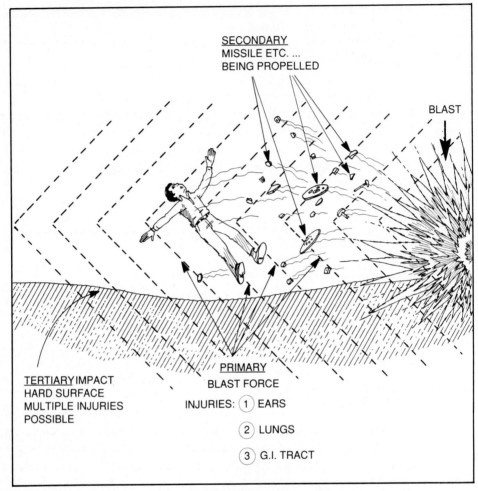

Figure 1–12.

Gastrointestinal tract injuries may vary from mild intestinal and stomach contusions to frank rupture.

Injuries sustained via secondary factors are similar to those discussed previously. Tertiary injuries are much the same as would be expected from ejection from an automobile. With a blast victim, always suspect lung injuries.

In summary, the mechanism of injury must be identified and appreciated as part of the overall management of a trauma patient. What happened? What type of energy was applied? What part of the body was affected? What was the distance from the blast? With this knowledge and the high degree of suspicion, trauma care will be delivered to the best of the paramedic's ability.

Chapter 2

Field Evaluation and Management of the Trauma Patient

John E. Campbell, M.D.

It is heartbreaking to see a life lost, especially if it happens because treatment is instituted too little and too late. For a severely injured patient, time is of the essence. The direct relationship between definitive (surgical) treatment and survival of trauma patients was first discovered by Dr. R. Adams Cowley of the famous Shock-Trauma Unit in Baltimore, Maryland. He found that if the seriously injured patient was in the operating room within an hour of the time of injury the highest survival rate was obtained (about 85 percent). He calls this the "golden hour". Every action in the field must have a lifesaving purpose because you are trading minutes of the "golden hour" for every action done before transport. Evaluation and resuscitation must be reduced to the most efficient and critical steps. The habit of assessing and treating every trauma patient in a preplanned logical and sequential manner must be developed.

There are certain concepts that you must always keep in mind when you approach patients who are injured:

1. Trauma patients are not "treated" in the field. They are treated in the emergency department or operating room. Only critical interventions are made in the field.

2. Most trauma fatalities are due to the patient not arriving in the operating room soon enough to be saved.

3. All trauma care revolves around making the most efficient use of time so that the patient is transported to the *appropriate* hospital as soon as possible.

As the first person to treat the patient, you are a *critical* member of the EMS system. The trauma victim's fate depends on the speed, judgment, and skill of your actions.

The "golden hour" begins when the victim is injured, not when you begin your evaluation. Minutes lost before you arrive are just as important as minutes lost because of disorganized actions at the scene. You must learn to squeeze the most out of *every* minute of the rescue process. Rapid management does not mean simply racing down the highway at breakneck speed, throwing the victim into the back of the ambulance, and racing to the nearest emergency department. You can maximize the patient's chance of survival if you perform your duties properly during the six stages of an ambulance call. These are outlined below.

1. *Predispatch.* This is the first (and often ignored) stage of prehospital care. You cannot give lifesaving care if you cannot find the accident, if you do not know the shortest route, or if your ambulance or rescue vehicle is not ready to respond. Before you begin taking ambulance calls, you must learn the area that you serve. You should know the streets and highways well enough to pick the shortest route immediately. You should know an alternate route in case traffic, weather, or other conditions make it unwise to take the shortest route. Fast driving will not make up for the lack of map training. Between runs the vehicle must be checked, fueled, and restocked immediately.

2. *Dispatch.* The rescue crew must have the proper information to respond rapidly to a call:
    a. *Exact nature of the call.* What happened? How many victims? Are there dangers at the scene? Will special equipment be needed?
    b. *Exact location of the call.* This cannot be overemphasized. If an exact address cannot be given, get directions that are as precise as possible.
    c. *Callback number.* This can be invaluable if you have trouble locating the scene of the accident. Units equipped with a Radio Telephone Switch Station (RTSS) or cellular telephone can call back for more information about the accident while they are responding.

3. *Travel to the scene.* Make a rapid, yet careful response using your best

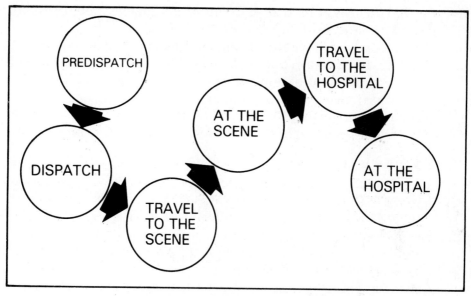

Figure 2-1. Six stages of an ambulance call.

judgment concerning the fastest route. Obtain the necessary information from the dispatcher (or from a callback to the scene) so that you can make decisions about backup help and equipment needed.

4. *Actions at the scene.* You must make a quick assessment of the overall situation. Park the ambulance as close as possible, keeping in mind the dangers (i.e., traffic, fire, explosion, power lines) of the scene. Quickly note the apparent mechanisms of injury. Be aware of the number of victims and call for help if needed. As a general rule, one ambulance is needed for every seriously injured victim. Evaluate the most seriously injured victim first (unless you have a disaster, in which case use disaster protocols). Evaluate, resuscitate, and package the patients using the priority plan. Be rapid but careful and *gentle.* Rough handling aggravates injuries.

5. *Travel to the hospital.* Select the most suitable route and hospital according to your local protocols. The most experienced EMT should remain at the patient's side and provide continuous monitoring. Notify medical control if the patient's condition deteriorates during transport. Notify the receiving facility of your estimated time of arrival and any special needs. It is important to report to medical control as early as possible. Frequently, critical members of the trauma team (surgeons, operating room crew, etc.) must be called to the hospital. Minutes lost waiting for the proper physician to arrive can be just as fatal as minutes lost waiting for the EMT to arrive.

6. *Actions at the hospital.* You should continue your care until you are relieved by the emergency department staff; never leave a patient unattended. Report pertinent information about the victim to the nurse or physician in charge. This should include a description of the scene, mechanisms of injuries, observed and suspected injuries, procedures performed, and changes in condition. Remain as long as you are needed. When no longer required, you should complete your run report and immediately prepare your vehicle for return to service.

Trauma Assessment

On-scene trauma assessment begins with certain actions *before* you approach the victim. Failure to perform preliminary actions may jeopardize your life as well as that of your patient.

Preliminary Actions at the Scene

A. *Scene survey*
   1. Assess the scene for hazards.
      a. Is the ambulance or rescue vehicle parked in the nearest safe place?
      b. Is it safe to approach the victim?
      c. Do you need special equipment (turnout gear, breathing equipment) to approach the victim? **Do not become a victim!**
      d. Does the victim require immediate movement because of hazards?
   2. Does the victim require extrication? Is special equipment needed?
   3. Note mechanisms of injury.
   4. Note the number of victims.
      a. If more than one victim, call for more ambulances now. Usually, one ambulance is needed for each seriously injured victim. If there are many victims, notify medical control to initiate the disaster protocol.
      b. Are all victims accounted for? If no conscious victims, look for schoolbooks or diaper bag in car, passenger list, or other clues.
B. *Equipment.* If possible, carry all essential equipment to the scene as you go. This prevents loss of time running back and forth to the rescue vehicle. You will almost always need:
   1. Long backboard with attached head-immobilization device
   2. Cervical-immobilization device
   3. Oxygen and airway equipment
   4. Antishock garment
   5. Trauma box (bandage material, BP cuff, stethoscope)

Patient Assessment and Management

There are four steps in management of the trauma victim:

1. *Primary survey.* Find all immediate threats to life.
2. *Transport decision and critical interventions.* Decide if a life threat exists ("load and go" situation) and if a lifesaving intervention must be done before or during transport.
3. *Secondary survey.* Reassess for change and do a rapid, complete head-to-toe exam, and communicate these to medical control.
4. *Definitive care.* The final stabilization, often requiring surgery and blood, usually takes place in the operating room, and hopefully, takes place within the first hour after injury.

To make the most efficient use of time, patient assessment is broken down as follows:

1. *Primary survey.* This is a rapid exam to determine life-threatening conditions. The information that you gather here is used to make decisions about critical interventions and time of transport. This exam should not take over $1\frac{1}{2}$ to 2 minutes. This exam is so important that nothing is allowed to interrupt it except airway obstruction or cardiac arrest. Respiratory distress (other than airway obstruction) is not an indication to interrupt the primary survey because the cause of respiratory distress is frequently found during examination of the chest. Major bleeding is also controlled at this time.
2. *Transport decision and critical interventions.* When you finish the primary survey, you have enough information to decide if a critical situation is present. Patients with critical trauma situations are immediately transported. Almost all treatment will be done during transport. Certain interventions will have to be done on the scene (attempt removal of airway obstruction, stop major bleeding, seal sucking chest wounds, hyperventilate, decompress tension pneumothorax, etc.), but most treatment must wait until the patient is in the ambulance and transport is begun. You must spend your patient's minutes wisely—the critical patient has none to spare!
3. *Secondary survey.* Critical patients always have the secondary exam done during transport. If the primary survey has revealed no critical condition, you perform this exam on the scene. The secondary survey is a rapid, detailed exam to pick up all injuries, both obvious and potential. This exam also establishes the baseline from which many treatment decisions will eventually be made. It is important to record this

exam. Critical interventions and the secondary survey should be kept to under 5 minutes if possible (even in patients that appear to be stable).

4. *Communications with medical control.* This is a trauma skill that is often performed poorly. Critical patients require early contact with medical control so that the hospital is prepared for your arrival and appropriate personnel are notified. Most patients are not critical and in such cases, communications can wait until you are ready to transport. All communications should be concise and to the point.

Assessment Priorities

A. *Primary survey*
    1. Evaluate **airway,** C-spine control, and initial level of consciousness.
    2. Evaluate **breathing.**
    3. Evaluate **circulation.**
    4. Stop major **bleeding.**
B. *Transport decision and critical interventions*
C. *Secondary survey*
    1. Vital signs
    2. History of patient and trauma event
    3. Head-to-toe exam (including neurological)
    4. Further bandaging and splinting
    5. Monitor continually

These steps must be memorized until you can perform them in the correct sequence without stopping to think about what comes next. They are the ABCs of basic trauma life support.

Patient Assessment Using the Priority Plan

Once you approach the victim, your exam should proceed quickly and smoothly. Unless held up by extrication, total on-scene time should be under 10 minutes. *Critical victims should have on-scene times of 5 minutes or less.* Nothing interrupts the primary survey except treatment of airway obstruction or cardiac arrest.

A. *Evaluate airway, C-spine control, intial LOC (level of consciousness).* Assessment begins immediately, even if the victim is being extricated. Extrication should not interfere with patient care. The same priorities apply continually before, during, and after extrication. The team leader should approach the victim from the front (face to face—so the victim does not have to turn his head to see you). A second EMT immediately, gently but firmly, stabilizes the neck in a neutral position. There are times when the team leader may need to stabilize the neck initially. The EMT stabilizing the neck must not release his hold until someone relieves him or a suitable stabilization device is applied. The team leader should say to the patient: "We are EMTs here to help you. What happened? The patient's reply gives immediate information about both the airway and the level of consciousness. If the patient responds appropriately to your question, you have established that he has an open airway and that his level of consciousness is normal. If the patient cannot speak or is unconscious, you must evaluate the airway further. Look, listen, and feel for the movement of air. Be sure that both rate and tidal volume are adequate. Open the mouth and clear the airway if necessary. If the airway is obstructed, use an appropriate method to open *before* finishing the primary survey. Because of the ever-present danger of spinal injury, you must never extend the neck to open the airway of a trauma patient. Patients with airway difficulty or decreased level of consciousness are in the "load and go" category. All patients with decreased LOC should be hyperventilated (24 breaths per minute) if they will allow you to do so. Your partner may use his knees to maintain immobilization of the neck, freeing his hands to apply oxygen or use a bag–valve–mask to assist ventilation. This is another reason that all equipment should be within immediate reach. If you assist or control ventilation, be sure that the patient gets not only adequate ventilatory rate, but also an adequate volume with each breath. *All* victims of multiple trauma should receive oxygen.

B.   *Assess breathing and circulation.* It is impractical to separate evaluation of breathing and circulation, since you must check both as you quickly look, listen, and feel the neck and chest. There is much information to be gained when this examination is performed correctly. (Remember: If the patient is not breathing, you must immediately give two full breaths and then check for a carotid pulse. If there is no pulse, you must begin cardiopulmonary resuscitation.) After your partner has immobilized the neck and (if necessary) opened the airway with a modified jaw thrust, you should proceed with evaluation of breathing and circulation in the following manner.

1.   Place your face over the patient's mouth so that you can judge both the rate and quality of breathing. Is breathing too fast (>24/breaths per minute) or too slow (<12 breaths per minute)? Is the victim mov-

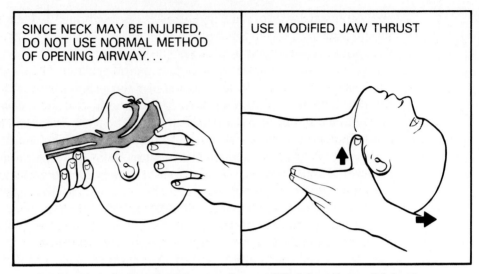

Figure 2–2. Opening airway using modified jaw thrust. Maintain in-line stabilization while pushing up on the angles of the jaw with your thumbs.

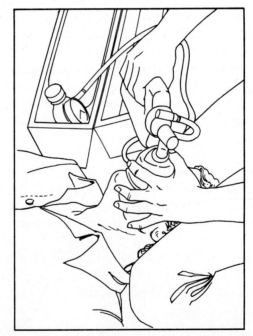

Figure 2–3. Using your knees to maintain immobilization of the neck will free your hands to assist ventilation.

ing an adequate volume of air when he breathes? Any abnormality of breathing signals a search for the cause as well as administration of oxygen and possibly breathing assistance. Your partner can apply the non-rebreather oxygen mask or bag–valve device (while stabilizing the neck with his knees) without interrupting your survey.

2. As your partner holds the neck stable, he will find that it is simple to feel the carotid pulse with his index finger. He should note rate and quality, then compare with your evaluation of the pulse at the wrist. Also evaluate skin color/condition and capillary refill. This information, combined with LOC, is the best early assessment of circulatory status and the presence of shock. If the pulse is present at the neck and the wrist, the blood pressure is greater than 80 mmHg. (It may be normal; judge by the strength of the pulse—it is not yet time to use the blood pressure cuff. If a pulse is present at the neck but not at the wrist, the blood pressure is between 60 and 80 mmHg; this means *late* shock. Even if the pulse is present and strong at the neck and wrist, you may be able to diagnose *early* shock by other signs. Other signs of shock include slow capillary refill, rapid heart rate (>100 beats per minute), cold sweaty skin, pale appearance, confusion, weakness, or thirst. Remember, the patient with spinal shock may not be pale, cold, or sweaty and will not have a rapid pulse. He will have low blood pressure and paralysis.

3. As soon as you have noted the breathing and pulse, quickly *look and feel* the neck to see if the trachea is in the midline, if the neck

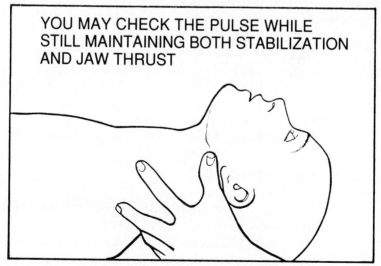

YOU MAY CHECK THE PULSE WHILE STILL MAINTAINING BOTH STABILIZATION AND JAW THRUST

Figure 2–4. Checking carotid pulse.

veins are flat or distended, and if there is discoloration, swelling, or subcutaneous emphysema. You may apply a rigid extrication collar at this time. (*Note:* If the team leader is stabilizing the neck, he should transfer this duty to another EMT at this time.)

4.   Now look, feel, and listen to the chest. If there is any difficulty with respiration, the chest must be bared for examination: This is no time for modesty; chest injuries often kill quickly. Look for sucking chest wounds, flail segments, contusions, or deformities. Note if the ribs rise with respiration or if there is only diaphragmatic breathing. Feel for instability, tenderness, or crepitation. Listen for breath sounds. Listen with the stethoscope over the lateral chest about the fourth interspace in the midaxillary line on one side, then immediately compare with the other side. You may also listen to the anterior chest about the second interspace on both sides. The important determination is whether breath sounds are *present and equal* on both sides. If breath sounds are not equal (decreased or absent on one side), you should percuss the chest to determine if it is tympanic (pneumothorax) or dull (hemothorax). If abnormalities are found during the chest exam (open chest wound, flail chest, respiratory difficulty), you should make the appropriate intervention (seal open wound, *hand stabilize* flail, give oxygen, assist ventilation, decompress tension pneumothorax).

5.   Stop active bleeding. Your other partner should have already done this, or at least begun to do this. Almost all bleeding can be stopped by direct pressure; use gauze pads and bandage or elastic wraps. You may use air splints or antishock garment to tamponade bleeding. Tourniquets may be needed in *rare* situations. If a dressing becomes blood soaked, you may remove the dressing and redress *once* to be sure you are getting pressure on the bleeding area. It is important that you report such excessive bleeding to the receiving physician. Do not use clamps or stop bleeders; you may cause injuries to other structures (nerves are present alongside arteries).

6.   Perform a MAST survey. If your primary survey identified the presence of a critical trauma situation, you should modify the primary survey by adding the MAST survey. Critical conditions require transport before performing the secondary survey. Since you will apply the antishock garment (MAST or PASG) before you do the secondary survey, you need to check quickly the areas of the body that will be hidden by the garment. *You must expose the body to do this.* Quickly cut off the clothes, maintaining body warmth and

modesty with a sheet or blanket. The MAST survey consists of a quick examination of the abdomen, pelvis, and legs.

At this point you have enough information to determine critical trauma situations that should be treated by "load and go."

Critical Injuries/Conditions

1. Airway obstruction unrelieved by mechanical methods (i.e., suction, forceps)
2. Conditions resulting in possible inadequate breathing
    a. Large open chest wound (sucking chest wound)
    b. Large flail chest
    c. Tension pneumothorax
    d. Major blunt chest injury
3. Traumatic cardiopulmonary arrest
4. Shock
    a. Hemorrhagic
    b. Spinal
    c. Mycardial contusion
    d. Pericardial tamponade
5. Head injury with decreased level of consciousness.

Critical injuries can be further simplified into three conditions based on signs and symptoms:

1. Difficulty with respiration
2. Difficulty with circulation (shock)
3. Decreased level of consciousness

Any trauma patient with one or more of these conditions falls into the "load and go" category. When you finish the primary survey, you have enough information to decide if the patient is critical or stable. If the patient has one of the critical conditions, you should immediately transfer him to a long backboard (check his back as you log-roll him), apply MAST and oxygen, load him into an ambulance (if available), and transport rapidly to the nearest appropriate emergency facility. Lifesaving procedures may be needed but should not hold up transport. There are a few brief procedures that are done while at the scene (appropriate airway management, stop major bleeding, seal sucking chest wound, hand stabilize flail, hyperventilate, decompress tension pneumothorax, begin CPR), but most are reserved for transport. *You must weigh every field procedure against the time it will take to perform.* You are spending minutes of the patient's golden hour; be sure the procedure is worth the cost. Non-lifesaving procedures (splinting and bandaging) must not hold up transport. Be sure to call medical control early so that the hospital is prepared for your arrival.

If the primary survey fails to identify a critical trauma situation, you should transfer the victim to the backboard (check the back) and proceed with the secondary survey. (*Note:* You should think of the antishock trousers as a part of the backboard. The trousers are always unfolded on the backboard, ready to be applied if needed.)

Secondary Survey

This exam is to provide an orderly head-to-toes survey to assess for other injuries. The critical patient has this exam performed during transport to the hospital. The patient who appears stable should have this exam done at the scene. Even if the patient appears stable and you elect to perform this exam at the scene, keep the time under 5 minutes. "Stable" patients may become "unstable" quite rapidly.

1. *Vital signs.* Record pulse, respiration, and blood pressure (obtain accurate recordings and use the BP cuff now).
2. *History.* Obtain a history of the injury (your partner may already have done this) via:
    a. Personal observation.
    b. Bystanders.
    c. Victim. In unconscious patients, look for a medic alert tag. Take an *ample* history from conscious patients:
        A   allergies
        M   medications
        P   past medical history (other illnesses)
        L   last meal (when was it eaten)
        E   events preceding the injury
3. *Head-to-toes exam*
    a. Begin at the head examining for contusions, lacerations, raccoon eyes, Battle's sign, and drainage of blood or fluid from the ears or nose. Assess the airway again.
    b. Check the neck again. Look for lacerations, contusions, tenderness, distended neck veins, or deviated trachea. Check the pulse

again. If not already done, apply a cervical immobilization device at this time.

c. Recheck the chest. Be sure that breath sounds are still present and equal on each side. Recheck seals over open wounds. Make sure that flails are well stabilized (hand stabilization is adequate until you are in the ambulance).

d. Examine the abdomen. Look for signs of blunt or penetrating trauma. Feel for tenderness. Do not waste time listening for bowel sounds. If the abdomen is painful to gentle pressure during examination, you can expect the patient to be bleeding internally. If the abdomen is both distended and painful, you can expect hemorrhagic shock very quickly.

e. Assess pelvis and extremities. Be sure to check and record distal sensation and pulses on all fractures. Do this before and after straightening any fracture. Angulated fractures of the upper extremities are usually best splinted as found. Most fractures of the lower extremities are *gently* straightened by using traction splints or air splints. *Critical patients have all splints applied during transport.*

Transport immediately if your secondary survey reveals any of the following:

1. Tender, distended abdomen.

2. Pelvic instability

3. Bilateral femur fractures

Even though the patient may appear stable at this time, he will probably soon develop shock because of the large blood loss that is associated with these injuries.

4. *Brief neurological exam*
   a. *Level of consciousness*
      A   alert
      V   responds to verbal stimuli
      P   responds to pain
      U   unresponsive
   b. *Motor.* Can he move fingers and toes?
   c. *Sensation.* Can he feel you when you touch his fingers and toes? Does the unconscious patient respond when you pinch his fingers and toes?

    d. *Pupils.* Are they equal or unequal? Do they respond to light?

The neurological exam is very simple but is frequently forgotten. It gives important baseline information that is used in later treatment decisions. Perform and record this exam.

    5. If necessary, finish bandaging and splinting.

    6. Continually monitor and reevaluate the patient.

If the patient's condition worsens, repeat every step of the primary survey.

    Accurately record what you see and what you do. Record changes in the patient's condition during transport. Record the time the antishock garment or tourniquet is applied. Extenuating circumstances or significant details should be recorded in the comments or remarks section of the run report. (Review the documentation in Appendix B.)

Contacting Medical Control

This is important so that the emergency department can be prepared for the arrival of the patient. It is extremely important to do this as early as possible when you have a patient with a critical condition. It takes time to get the appropriate surgeon and the operating room team called in. The critical victim has no time to wait. (Review communications in Appendix A.) The procedure to communicate with medical control is given below.

Phase I: Establishing Contact

    1. Initiation of call
        EMS service
        Level of function (basic, paramedic, etc.)
        Unit number
        Medical control facility being contacted
    2. Receiving facility response
        Name of facility
        Name and title of radio operator
        Renaming of calling EMS service

Phase II: In-the-Field Report

    3. Re-identification
        EMS Service
        Level of function
        Unit number

   4. Chief complaint/on-scene report
      One brief sentence
      Include age, sex, complaint, and/or mechanism of injury
   5. Lifesaving resuscitation
      Patient's response to lifesaving interventions
   6. Vital signs/primary survey abnormalities
      Vital signs in stable patient or primary survey in unstable patient
   7. ETA
   8. Request for orders
      State what is desired or state "no orders requested"

Phase III: Hospital-Controlled Activity

   9. Physician response
      Physician will agree, deny, or state desired orders
      Physician may request additional history and/or information
   10. EMT response
      Clarification or response to requested intervention or therapy

Phase IV: Sign-Off

   11. EMS unit sign-off
   12. Base station sign-off

   Transport the patient to the facility named by medical control. Notify the facility of the estimated time of arrival (ETA), the condition of the patient, and any special needs on arrival.

Summary

This is the content of the course in one chapter: a rapid, orderly, thorough examination of the trauma patient with priorities of examination and treatment always in mind. The continuous practice of approaching the patient in this way will allow you to concentrate on the patient rather than trying to figure out what to do next. Optimum speed is achieved by teamwork. *Teamwork* is achieved by practice. During the predispatch stage, you should plan regular exercises in patient evaluation in order to perfect each team member's role in the priority plan. The following pages contain a brief outline of the primary and secondary survey as well as the thoughts that should go through your mind as you perform the survey.

THE BASIC TRAUMA LIFE SUPPORT PRIMARY SURVEY

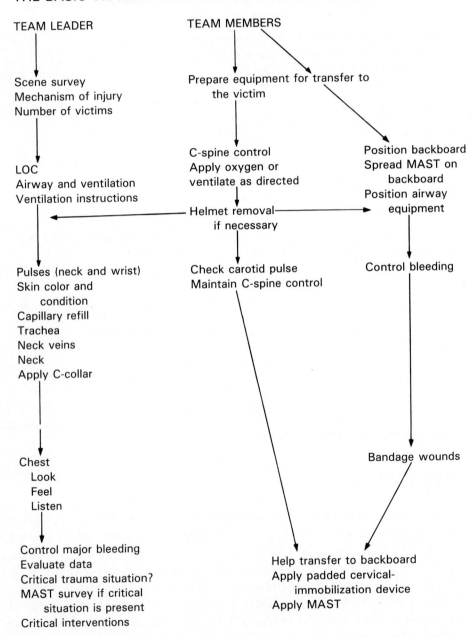

TEAM LEADER

Scene survey
Mechanism of injury
Number of victims

LOC
Airway and ventilation
Ventilation instructions

Pulses (neck and wrist)
Skin color and
    condition
Capillary refill
Trachea
Neck veins
Neck
Apply C-collar

Chest
    Look
    Feel
    Listen

Control major bleeding
Evaluate data
Critical trauma situation?
MAST survey if critical
    situation is present
Critical interventions

TEAM MEMBERS

Prepare equipment for transfer to
    the victim

C-spine control
Apply oxygen or
ventilate as directed

Helmet removal
if necessary

Check carotid pulse
Maintain C-spine control

Position backboard
Spread MAST on
    backboard
Position airway
    equipment

Control bleeding

Bandage wounds

Help transfer to backboard
Apply padded cervical-
    immobilization device
Apply MAST

This is what should be going through your mind as you perform each step of the survey. They are also the phrases you should repeat (like a parrot) to the instructor as you are being tested on patient evaluation.

SCENE SURVEY

I am surveying the scene: Are there any dangers?
I am surveying the mechanisms of injury.
Are there any other victims?

LEVEL OF CONSCIOUSNESS

We are EMTs here to help you. What happened?
Please do not move until we have checked you for injuries.

AIRWAY

Is the airway clear?
What is the rate and quality of respiration?

VENTILATION INSTRUCTIONS

Order oxygen for any airway difficulty, head injury, or shock.
Assist ventilation if hypoventilating.
Hyperventilate altered level of consciousness.

PULSES

What is the rate and quality of the pulse at the neck and the wrist?

SKIN COLOR AND CONDITION

What is the skin color and condition?

CAPILLARY REFILL

Is the capillary refill normal or delayed?

TRACHEA

Is the trachea midline or deviated?

NECK VEINS

Are the neck veins flat or distended?

NECK

Are there signs of trauma to the neck?

CHEST

I am looking at the chest: Are there any penetrations, contusions, deformities, or paradoxical motions?

I am feeling the chest: Is there any crepitation, tenderness, or instability?

I am listening to the chest: Are the breath sounds present and equal?

IF BREATH SOUNDS ARE NOT EQUAL:

I am percussing the chest: Is there tympany (hyperresonance) or dullness on either side?

BLEEDING

Is there any significant bleeding?

MAST SURVEY

ABDOMEN

Are there any contusions, penetrations, distention, or tenderness of the abdomen?

PELVIS

Is the pelvis tender or unstable?

LOWER EXTREMITIES

Is there any sign of trauma to the legs?

EXAM OF THE BACK
(Done during transfer to the backboard)

Is there any sign of trauma to the back?

THE BASIC TRAUMA LIFE SUPPORT SECONDARY SURVEY

When performing the secondary survey, you must visualize and palpate from head to toes. Everyone gets a secondary survey: stable patients while at the scene, critical patients during transport. If other team members are available, the blood pressure and accurate pulse and respiratory rates may be taken by one of them.

HEAD

1. Palpate
   Entire scalp for lacerations or contusions
   Face for tenderness or fractures
2. Look
   For Battle's sign
   For blood or fluid in ears
   For raccoon eyes
   For blood or fluid from nose
   For pupil size, equality, reaction to light
   For burns of face, nose hairs, mouth

For skin changes
   Pallor
   Cyanosis
   Diaphoresis
   Bruising
3. Reassess
  a. Airway
    Recheck patency.
    If burn victim, assess for signs of inhalation injury.
  b. Breathing
    Rate (accurately and record)
    Quality

NECK (If collar has been applied, remove the front)

Reassess circulation
   Pulse Rate (accurately and record)
   Pulse quality
   Blood pressure (done by partner if possible)
Signs of trauma?
JVD?
Tracheal deviation?

CHEST

Look for penetrations, contusions, deformities, or paradoxical motions.
Feel for instability, tenderness, crepitation.
Listen for breath sounds in all lung fields; if breath sounds unequal:
1. Evaluate for tension pneumothorax and hemothorax.
2. If intubated, check ET tube placement.

ABDOMEN (If MAST has been applied, this has been completed)

Look for penetrations, contusions, distention.
Palpate all four quadrants for tenderness.

PELVIS (If MAST has been applied, this has been completed)

Compress laterally and over symphysis for tenderness or instability.

LOWER EXTREMITIES (If MAST applied, do pulses, neuro, cap refill)

Visualize and palpate for signs of trauma.
Check distal pulses.
Do neurological
   sensory (pinch toes)
   motor (move toes)
Check range of motion.
Repeat capillary refill.

UPPER EXTREMITIES

Visualize and palpate for signs of trauma.
Begin at the midline, checking clavicles, shoulders, arms, and hands.
Check distal pulses.
Do neurological
    sensory (pinch fingers)
    motor (move fingers)
Check range of motion.
Repeat capillary refill (unless you have already made the diagnosis of shock).

PARROT PHRASES—SECONDARY SURVEY

HEAD

I am feeling the scalp: Are there lacerations, contusions, or deformity?
I am feeling the face: Are there contusions or deformity?
Are Battle's sign or raccoon eyes present?
Is blood or fluid draining from the ears or nose?
What is pupil size? Are the pupils equal? Do they react to light?
Is there pallor, cyanosis, diaphoresis, or bruising?
Are there burns of the face, nose hairs, or inside the mouth?

AIRWAY

Is the airway clear?
What is the rate and quality of respiration?
Are there signs of burns in the mouth or nose (if a burn victim)?

CIRCULATION

What is the rate and quality of the pulse?
What is the blood pressure?
Is the capillary refill normal or delayed? (Not done if a diagnosis of shock has already been made.)

NECK

Are there signs of trauma to the neck?
Are the neck veins flat or distended?
Is the trachea midline or deviated?

CHEST

I am looking at the chest: Are there any penetrations, contusions, deformities, or paradoxical motion?
I am feeling the chest: Is there any crepitation, tenderness, or instability?
I am listening to the chest: Are the breath sounds present and equal?
I am percussing the chest: Is it hyperresonant or dull? (Do only if breath sounds are unequal.)

ABDOMEN (If MAST has been applied, this has been completed)

I am looking at the abdomen: Are there penetrations, contusions, or distention?
I am feeling the abdomen: Is there any tenderness?

PELVIS (If MAST has been applied, this has been completed)

Is the pelvis tender or unstable?

LOWER EXTREMITIES (If MAST has been applied, do pulses, neuro, and capillary refill)

Are there any signs of trauma to the legs?
Are pulses present?
Can he feel me touch his toes?
Can he move his toes?
Is range of motion normal?
Is capillary refill normal or delayed? (Not done if a diagnosis of shock has already been made.)

UPPER EXTREMITIES

Is there any sign of trauma to the arms?
Are pulses present?
Can he feel me touch his fingers?
Can he move his fingers?
Is range of motion normal?
Is capillary refill normal or delayed? (Not done if a diagnosis of shock has already been made.)

Chapter 3

Field Airway Control
for the Trauma Patient

Ronald D. Stewart, M.D., F.A.C.E.P.

Of all the tasks expected of field teams caring for the trauma patient, none is more important than that of airway control. Maintaining an open airway and adequate ventilation in the trauma patient can be a challenge in any setting, but it can be almost impossible in the adverse environment of the field, with its poor lighting, the oft-present chaos surrounding an accident, the position of the patient, and perhaps hostile onlookers.

Airway control is a task that needs to be mastered, but it cannot wait until we get to the hospital. Patients who are hypoxic or underventilated, or both, are in need of immediate help—help that only we can give them in the initial stages of their care. It falls to us, then, to be fully versed in the basic structure and function of the airway, in how to achieve and maintain a patent airway, and in how to oxygenate and ventilate a patient.

Because of the unpredictable nature of the field environment, we will be called on to manage patients' airways in almost every conceivable situation; in wrecked cars, dangling above rivers, in the middle of a shopping center, at the side of a busy highway. We therefore need *options* and alternatives from which to choose. What will work for one patient may not work for another. One patient may require a simple jaw thrust to open an airway, while another may require a surgical procedure to prevent impending death.

Whatever the methods required, we must always start with the basics. It is of little value—and in some cases downright dangerous—to apply "advanced" techniques of airway control before beginning basic maneuvers. Our discussion of airway control in the trauma patient will be rooted in several fundamental truths: Air should go in and out, oxygen is good, and blue is bad. Everything else follows from this.

Anatomy

The airway begins at the tip of the nose and the lips and ends at the *alveolar-capillary membrane,* through which gas exchange takes place between the air sacs of the lung (the *alveoli*) and the lung's capillary network. The airway consists of chambers and pipes that conduct air and its 21% oxygen content to the alveoli during inspiration and carry away the waste *carbon dioxide* that diffuses from the blood into the alveoli.

The beginning of the respiratory tract, the *nasal cavity* and *oropharynx,* perform important functions (Figure 3–1). Lined with moist *mucous membranes,* these areas serve to warm and filter inhaled gases. They are highly vascular and contain protective lymphoid tissue. Bypassing this portion of the respiratory tract through the use of an endotracheal tube will reduce the natural protection for the vulnerable lung, and we will have to assume some of those tasks. That is why suctioning of the airway becomes of such importance in intubated patients, in addition to the warming and humidification of gases.

The lining of the respiratory tract is delicate and highly vascular. It deserves every bit of respect we can give it, and that means preventing undue trauma, using liberally lubricated tubes, and avoiding unnecessary poking about. The *nasal cavity* is divided by a very vascular midline *septum;* on the lateral walls of the nose are "shelves" called the *turbinates.* These projections, which increase the surface area of the mucosa, can get in the way of tubes or other devices being introduced into the nostrils. Careful sliding of a well-lubricated tube's bevel along the floor or the septum of the nasal cavity will usually prevent getting "hooked up" in the turbinates.

The teeth are the first obstruction we meet in the oral part of the airway. They may be more obstructive in some patients than in others. In any case, the same general principle always applies: Patients should have the same number of teeth at the end of an airway procedure as they had at the beginning.

The tongue is a large chunk of muscle and represents the next potential obstruction. These muscles are attached to the jaw anteriorly and through a series of muscles and ligaments to the *hyoid bone,* a "wishbone-like" structure just under the chin from which the cartilage skeleton (the *larynx*) of the upper airway is suspended. The *epiglottis* is also connected to the hyoid, and

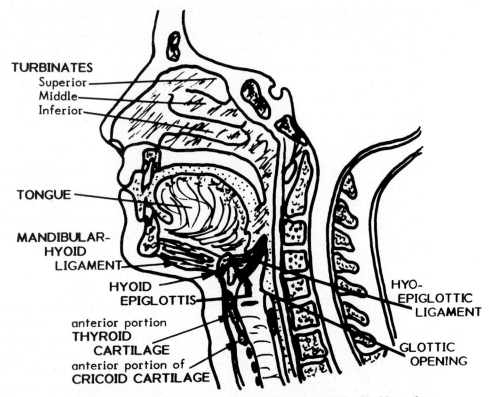

Figure 3–1. ANATOMY OF THE UPPER AIRWAY: Note that
the tongue, hyoid bone and epiglottis are attached to the
mandible by a series of ligaments. Lifting forward on the jaw
will therefore displace all of these structures.

elevating the hyoid will lift upward on the epiglottis and open the airway
further.

The epiglottis is one of the main anatomic landmarks in the airway. We
must be familiar with it and be able to identify it by sight as well as by touch.
It looks like a floppy piece of cartilage covered by mucosa—which is exactly
what it is—and it feels like the tragus, the cartilage at the opening of the ear
canal. Its function is unclear; it may be a "leftover" (i.e., vestigial) piece of
anatomy. But it is important to those of us charged with airway control. The
epiglottis is attached to the hyoid and thence to the mandible by a series of
ligaments and muscles. In the unconscious patient the tongue can produce
some airway obstruction by falling back against the soft palate and even the
posterior pharyngeal wall. However, it is the epiglottis that will produce complete airway obstruction in the supine unconscious patient whose jaw is relaxed
and whose head and neck are in the neutral position [1]. In such patients it
will fall down against the glottic opening and prevent ventilation.

It is essential to understand this crucial fact in the management of the airway. To ensure a patent airway in a patient, the hyoid must be displaced anteriorly by lifting forward on the jaw ("chin lift," "jaw thrust"), or by pulling on the tongue (Figure 3–2). These maneuvers lift the tongue out of the way, and keep the epiglottis elevated away from the posterior pharyngeal wall and glottic opening. Both naso- and orotracheal intubation will require elevation of the epiglottis by a laryngoscope or the fingers, by pulling on the tongue, or by lifting forward on the jaw.

On either side of the epiglottis is a recess called the *pyriform fossa*. An endotracheal tube can "catch up" in either one, the left or right, and such a situation can be dangerous if the tube is forced and thus perforates the mucosa—a disastrous complication of a careless intubation attempt. Pyriform fossa placement of an endotracheal tube can be identified easily by "tenting" of the skin on either side of the superior aspect of the *laryngeal promi-*

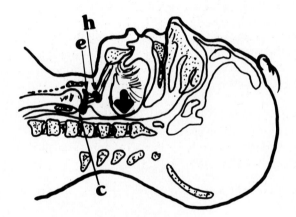

Figure 3–2(a). The epiglottis (e) is attached to the hyoid (h) and thence to the mandible. When the mandible is relaxed and falls back, the tongue falls upward against the soft palate and the posterior pharyngeal wall, while the epiglottis falls over the glottic opening (c).

Figure 3–2(b). Extension of the head and lifting the chin will pull the tongue and the epiglottis upward and forward, exposing the glottic opening (o) and ensuring a patent airway. In the trauma patient, only the jaw, or chin and jaw, should be displaced forward while the head and neck should be kept in alignment.

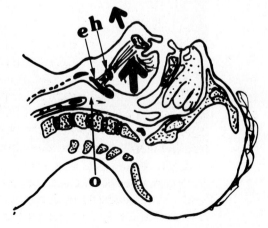

nence ("Adam's apple"), or by transillumination if a lighted stylet is being used to intubate (Figure 3–3).

The *vocal cords* are protected by the *thyroid cartilage,* a boxlike structure shaped like a "C," with the open part of the C representing its posterior wall, which is covered with muscle. When the cords vibrate, sound is produced. In some patients they can close entirely in *laryngospasm,* producing complete airway obstruction. The thyroid cartilage can easily be seen in most people on the anterior surface of the neck as the laryngeal prominence (Figure 3–4a).

Inferior to the thyroid cartilage is another part of the larynx, the *cricoid,* a cartilage shaped like a signet ring with the ring in front and the signet behind. It can be palpated as a small bump on the anterior surface of the neck inferior to the laryngeal prominence (Figure 3–4). Just behind the posterior wall of the cricoid cartilage lies the esophagus. Pressure on the cricoid at the front of the neck will close off the esophagus to pressures as high as 100 cmH$_2$O [2]. This maneuver (*Sellick's maneuver*) will reduce the risk of gastric regurgitation during the process of intubation and should prevent insufflation of air

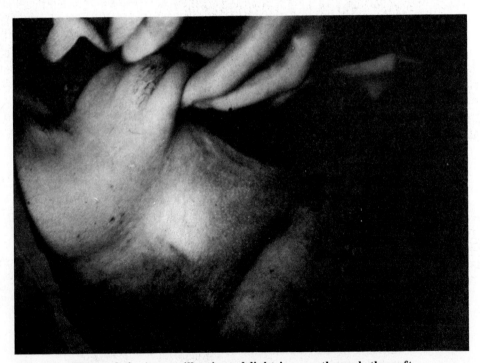

Figure 3–3. A transilluminated light is seen through the soft tissues of the neck when the lighted stylet is placed in the pyriform fossa.

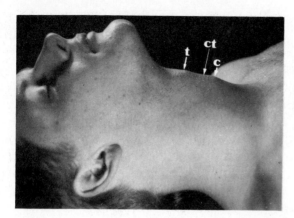

Figure 3–4(a). External view of the anterior neck, showing the surface landmarks for: t—the thyroid cartilage (laryngeal) prominence; ct—cricothyroid membrane; c—cricoid cartilage.

Figure 3–4(b). Cut-away view showing the important landmarks of the larynx and upper airway: h—hyoid; t—thyroid cartilage; ct—cricothyroid membrane; c—cricoid cartilage.

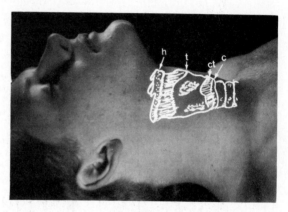

during positive pressure ventilation by mouth-to-mouth, mouth-to-mask, bag-valve-mask, or demand-valve.

Connecting the inferior border of the thyroid cartilage with the superior aspect of the cricoid is the *cricothyroid membrane,* a very important landmark through which direct access can be gained to the airway below the cords. It can be readily palpated on most patients by finding the most prominent part of the thyroid cartilage and then sliding the palpating index finger down until there is felt a second "bump" just before the finger palpates a last depression before the *sternal notch.* That final "bump" is the *cricoid cartilage,* and at the upper edge of this is the cricothyroid *membrane* (Figure 3–4). The sternal notch is, itself, an important landmark, for this is the point at which the cuff of a properly placed endotracheal tube should lie. The sternal notch is readily palpated at the junction of the clavicles with the upper edge of the sternum.

The *tracheal rings,* C-shaped cartilagenous supports for the trachea, continue beyond the cricoid cartilage, and the trachea soon divides into the *left* and *right mainstem bronchus.* The open part of the C-shaped rings lies posterior against the esophagus. An impacted swallowed foreign body that remains in the esophagus, or a misplaced esophageal airway or endotracheal tube cuff, can create tracheal obstruction by pressing against the soft posterior tracheal wall and narrowing the tracheal lumen. The point at which the trachea divides is called the *carina.* It is important to note that the right mainstem bronchus takes off at an angle that is slightly more in line with the trachea (Figure 3–5). As a result, tubes or other foreign bodies that are poked or that trickle down the airway usually end up in the right mainstem bronchus. Avoiding a right mainstem bronchus intubation should be one of the goals of a properly performed intubation.

It is important to know how far some of these major anatomic landmarks are from the teeth. Not only will a knowledge of these help in placing an endotracheal tube at the correct level, but remembering only three numbers will allow us to detect a tube that is too far into the airway, or not in far enough. The three numbers to remember are: 15, 20, and 25. *Fifteen* is the distance (in centimeters) from the teeth of the vocal cords of the average adult; *twenty* (5 cm farther down the airway) is the *sternal notch;* and 5 cm farther again, at *twenty-five,* is the *carina* (Figure 3–6). These are average distances and can vary within a few centimeters. In an intubated patient, flexion or extension

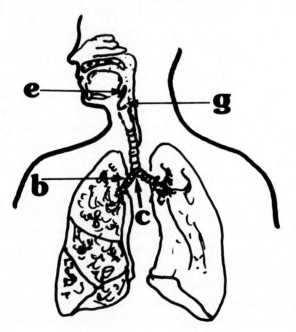

Figure 3–5. The sternal notch, at which point the clavicles join the sternum, marks the position of the tip of a well-placed endotracheal tube. Note that the left mainstem bronchus curves off at the carina at an angle slightly more in line with the trachea. e—epiglottis; g—glottic opening; b—right mainstem bronchus; c— carnia.

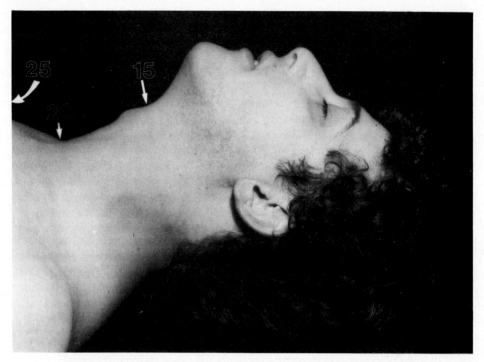

Figure 3-6. Major airway landmarks and distances from the teeth. 15 = 15cm from teeth to cords, 20 = 20 cms from sternal notch; 25 = teeth to carnia. Note prominence of thyroid cartilage.

of the head will move the endotracheal tube down as much as 2 to 2.5 cm farther into the airway with flexion, or upward to the same extent with extension. Tubes can easily become dislodged in a field setting, and detection of misplacement can be very difficult. Taping the head down or guarding against movement will not only lessen the risk of tube displacement but will also reduce trauma to the tracheal mucosa. Less movement of the tube will cause less stimulation to the patient's airway reflexes and may result in a more stable cardiovascular system and intracranial pressure in the patient.

To help protect the airway from becoming blocked and to reduce the risk of aspiration, the body has developed brisk reflexes that, when activated, will attempt to expel any offending foreign material from the oropharynx, from around the glottic opening, or from the trachea. These areas are well supplied by sensitive nerves that can activate the swallowing, gag, and cough reflex. Activation of swallowing, gagging, or coughing by stimulation of the upper airway can cause significant cardiovascular stimulation as well as elevation in intracranial pressure. Patients can be protected from such unwanted effects by suppressing the reflexes through the use of topical or intravenous lidocaine.

The *lungs* are the organs through which this gas exchange takes place. They are contained within a "cage" formed by the ribs, and usually fill up the *pleural space*—the *potential* space between the internal chest wall and the lung surface. The lungs have only one opening to the outside, the *glottic opening,* the space between the vocal cords. Expansion of the chest wall (the cage) and movement of the diaphragm downward cause the lungs to expand (since the pleural space is airtight), and air rushes in through the *glottis,* the only opening to the outside. The air travels down the smaller and smaller tubes to the *alveoli,* where gas exchange takes place.

Normal breathing, then, takes place because of the negative pressure inside the (potential) pleural space that "draws" air in through the upper airway from the outside. In any patient who is unable to do this, or whose airway needs protecting, we may choose to "pump" air or oxygen in through the glottic opening—*intermittent positive pressure ventilation*—and we use various devices to accomplish this. Pumping air into the oropharynx is no guarantee that it will go through the glottic opening and thence to the lungs. The oropharynx also leads to the esophagus, and pressure in the oropharynx of greater than 25 cmH$_2$O will open the esophagus and lead to air being pumped into the stomach (gastric insufflation). Bag–valve–masks can well exceed this pressure, and currently available demand valves can produce pressures as high as 60 cmH$_2$O. This is why *Sellick's maneuver* (posterior pressure on the cricoid cartilage) is so very important as a basic airway procedure.

The movement of air or gases in and out of the lungs is called *ventilation*. At rest, adults normally take in about 450 to 500 cc with each breath. This is called the *tidal volume* and is measured by a respirometer. Multiplying that value by the number of breaths per minute (the respiratory rate) gives the *minute volume,* the amount of air breathed in (or, officially, out) each minute. This is an important value, and is normally 6 to 8 liters per minute (L/min). Anything greater than this resting value could be termed *hyperventilation,* and values lower than this, *hypoventilation.*

When we are obliged to ventilate a patient using intermittent positive pressure ventilation, we should know approximately how much volume we are delivering with each breath we give (*delivered volume*). We can estimate the minute volume by multiplying this volume by the ventilatory rate. A demand valve that delivers oxygen at the rate of 100 L/min will have a delivered volume of 1660 cc each second that the valve is activated. Delivering over a liter of volume at a pressure of 60 cmH$_2$O will almost guarantee gastric insufflation and all the complications resulting from it. Bag–mask breathing may be no better; pressures generated by squeezing the bag may equal or exceed 60 cmH$_2$O.

Delivered volumes are usually less with bag resuscitators than with demand valves. There are two reasons for this. The average resuscitator bag holds only 1800 cc of gas, and that is the absolute limit to the volume that could be delivered were anyone able to squeeze the bag completely. Using one hand, an average adult can squeeze approximately 800 cc of gas from a bag–mask device; a two-handed squeeze will deliver approximately 1200 cc. The other reason for greater delivered volumes with demand valves is that a demand valve allows the rescuer to hold a mask on the face with *both* hands, thus decreasing mask leak. Keep in mind that these volumes, delivered from the ventilating port of these devices, equal the volumes delivered to the patient only if an endotracheal tube is in place. In other words, they do not take into account mask leak (more about mask leak later).

When air, or air containing oxygen, is delivered by positive pressure into the lungs of a patient, the "give" or elasticity of the lungs and chest wall will very much influence how easy it will be for the patient to breathe. If mask ventilation is being performed, a normal elasticity of the lungs and chest wall will allow air to enter the glottic opening and little gastric distension should result. However, if the elasticity is poor, ventilation will be harder to achieve. The ability of the lungs and chest wall to expand and therefore ventilate a patient is known as *compliance*. It is better to speak of "good compliance" or "bad compliance" rather than "high" or "low" compliance, since the latter terms can be somewhat confusing.

Compliance is an important concept, since it governs whether or not we can adequately ventilate a patient. Compliance can become bad (i.e., low) in some disease states of the lung or in patients who have an injury to the chest wall. In cardiac arrest compliance will also become bad, due to poor circulation to the muscles. This makes ventilating the patient all the more difficult. With an endotracheal tube in place the patient's compliance becomes an important clinical sign and may reveal airway problems. A detectable worsening of compliance will occur well before blood pressure changes in tension pneumothorax. Poor compliance will also be felt in right mainstem intubation, and pulling back on the tube will result in an immediate improvement in the ability to ventilate (i.e., better compliance).

Airway Equipment

The most important rule to follow in regard to airway equipment is that it should be in working order and immediately available. It will do the patient no good if you have to run to get a suction. In other words, "be prepared." This is not difficult. Three basic pieces of equipment are necessary for the initial response to "unknown" field calls: a "jump bag," containing materials for bandaging, IVs, and so on; a monitor-defibrillator; and an "airway kit."

The *field airway kit* should be completely self-contained and should contain everything needed to secure an airway in any patient. Equipment now available is lightweight and portable. Oxygen cylinders are aluminum, and newer suction devices are less bulky and lighter. It is no longer acceptable to have suction units that are bulky and stored separate from a source of oxygen. Suction units should be contained in a kit with oxygen and other essential airway tools. A lightweight airway kit should consist of the following (Figure 3–7):

1. Oxygen D cylinder, preferably aluminum
2. Portable, battery-powered suction unit
3. Oxygen cannulae and masks
4. Endotracheal intubation wrap

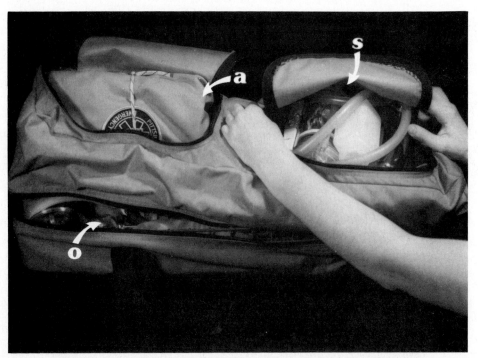

Figure 3–7. An airway kit containing the essentials for airway management. Note that portable suction is included in this design (s). The total weight (with aluminum "D" oxygen cylinder) is approximately 10 kg. (22 lbs), about the same as a steel "E" oxygen cylinder. a = airway wrap; o = oxygen cylinder.

5. Bag–valve–mask ventilating device
6. Pocket mask with supplemental oxygen intake
7. Translaryngeal oxygen cannula and manual ventilator

All equipment should be checked each shift and the kit should have a card attached initialed by the person checking it.

The Patent Airway

One of the first maneuvers essential to caring for a patient is ensuring a *patent* or *open* airway. Without this, all other care is of little use. This must be done quickly, for patients will not tolerate hypoxia for more than a few minutes. The effect of hypoxia on an unconscious injured patient can be devastating, and if hypoxia is compounded by the absence of adequate perfusion, the patient is in even more difficult straits. In patients with head trauma, not only can airway compromise damage an injured brain because of hypoxia, but it can build up high levels of CO_2 that can increase blood flow to the brain and therefore increase intracranial pressure.

Ensuring a patent airway in a patient can be a major challenge in a field setting. Not only can trauma disrupt the anatomy of the face and airway, but resultant bleeding can lead to airflow obstruction as well as to obscuring airway landmarks. Add to this the risk of cervical spine injury, and the challenge is readily apparent. We must also remember that some airway maneuvers, including suction and insertion of naso- and oropharyngeal airways, may stimulate a patient's protective reflexes and increase the likelihood of vomiting and aspiration, cardiovascular stimulation, and increased intracranial pressure.

The first step in providing a patent airway is to ensure that the tongue and epiglottis are lifted forward and maintained in that position. This is done simply by pulling forward on the tongue, the jaw, or both the jaw and tongue. Alternatively, the jaw can be displaced or lifted forward by placing the fingers under the angles of the mandible. Any of these maneuvers will prevent the tongue from falling backward against the soft palate or posterior pharyngeal wall, and will pull forward on the hyoid, lifting the epiglottis up out of the way. These are essential maneuvers for both basic and advanced airway procedures. Done properly, they will result in an open airway without the necessity of tilting backward on the head or moving the neck. Immobilization procedures for the cervical spine can be carried out once the patency of the airway is assured.

Recommending the maneuvers mentioned above assumes that the patient has been placed supine and that there is an ability on the part of either the

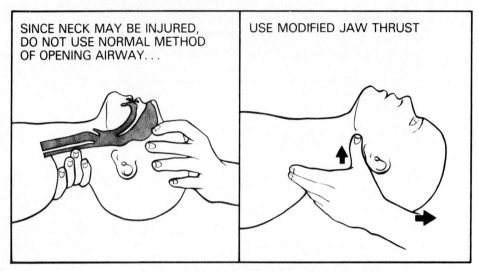

Figure 3-8(a). Modified jaw thrust.

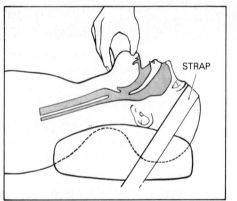

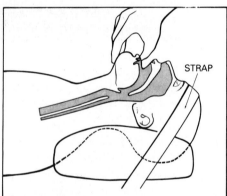

Figure 3-8(b). Chin lift.   Figure 3-8(c). Jaw lift.

patient or the rescuer to clear the airway of blood or secretions. Should the patient be unable to control the airway and should suction not be available, the patient should be placed carefully in the "coma position," or *left semi-prone.* This can be done with a rigid C-collar in place, with several rescuers to keep the vertebral column in alignment and prevent undue movement (Figure 3-9). In this position secretions can drain, the tongue and epiglottis are displaced forward, and the airway should remain patent. The risk of C-spine damage is less than the disaster that would occur should the patient vomit

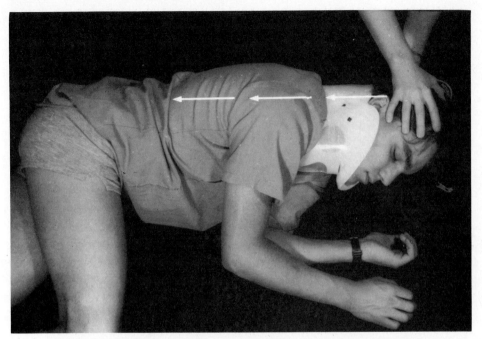

Figure 3–9. THE "COMA" POSITION—In patients suspected of having sustained trauma, and when suction and immobilization devices are not available, this position can be used to prevent aspiration. Sufficient personnel should be available to move the patient carefully, with vertebral column kept in alignment (arrows).

while supine. It is important to keep the head, neck, and vertebral column in alignment, but not to exert traction on head and neck.

Maintaining a patent airway requires constant vigilance and care on the part of the rescuer. There are several essentials for this task: continual observation of the patient, an adequate suction device with large-bore tubing and attachments, and airway adjuncts.

Observation

The patient who is injured is at risk of airway compromise even if completely conscious and awake. This is due, in part, to the fact that many of these patients have full stomachs, are anxious, and are prone to vomiting. We should have no difficulty understanding their plight when we further consider that we poke them with IVs, that we may have a shock suit in place, and that we have bound them down on a hard surface with a rigid collar in place and their head and neck fixed solidly to a board. In addition, some patients will be bleeding into their oropharynx and swallowing blood.

In view of these facts, patients deserve constant observation for airway problems following injury. Any patient who might be in any way at risk of airway compromise must be assigned one team member who must be on the lookout for difficulties in breathing or airway control.

The general appearance of the patient, the respiratory rate, and any complaints must be noted and attended to. In a spontaneously breathing patient, the caregiver must check frequently for the adequacy of tidal volume by feeling over mouth and nose and observing chest wall movements. The supplemental oxygen line is checked periodically to ensure that oxygen is being delivered to the patient at a given flow rate or percentage. Blood and secretions must be cleared. The rescuer must be alert for sounds that indicate trouble. In a few words, *noisy breathing is obstructed breathing,* and one must be alert for this danger sign. Should the patient have an endotracheal tube in place, compliance should be noted and any change must trigger a search for the cause. Combative patients should be considered hypoxic until a systematic but rapid evaluation indicates that this is unlikely.

Suction

All patients who are injured and who have cervical immobilization in place should be considered at high risk for airway compromise. One of the greatest threats to the patent airway is that of vomiting and aspiration, particularly in patients who have recently eaten a large meal washed down with large quantities of alcohol. As a result, portable suction devices should be considered basic equipment for field trauma care and should have the following characteristics:

1. They should be mounted in a kit with an oxygen cylinder and other airway equipment; they should not be separated or stored remote from oxygen; otherwise, they represent an "extra" piece of equipment requiring extra hands.
2. They should be battery powered rather than oxygen driven.
3. They should generate sufficient pressure *and* volume displacement that they can suction pieces of food, clots, and thick secretions from the oropharynx.
4. They should have tubing of sufficient diameter (0.8 to 1 cm) to handle whatever is to be suctioned from the patient.

Suction tips of more recent design are of large bore, particularly the new rigid "tonsil-tip" suckers that can handle most clots and bleeding. In some cases the suction tubing itself can be used to withdraw large amounts of blood or gastric contents. A 6-mm endotracheal tube can be used with a connector as a suction tip. The tube's side hole removes the necessity for a proximal control valve to interrupt suction.

Airway Adjuncts

Equipment to aid in ensuring a patent airway will include various naso- and oropharyngeal airways. Insertion of these devices must be reserved for patients whose protective reflexes are sufficiently depressed to tolerate them. Care must be taken not to provoke vomiting or gagging, since both occurrences are bad for these patients. The nasopharyngeal airway will be better tolerated than will the oropharyngeal. In fact, patients who are easily able to tolerate a proper-size oropharyngeal airway should be considered candidates for intubation because their protective reflexes are so depressed that they accept the airway.

Nasopharyngeal airways should be soft and of appropriate length. They are designed to prevent the tongue and epiglottis from falling against the posterior pharyngeal wall. After liberal lubrication the airway is inserted with the bevel passing along the floor of the nasal cavity or the septum, to avoid the turbinates (Figure 3–10). The distal end should rest posterior to the epiglot-

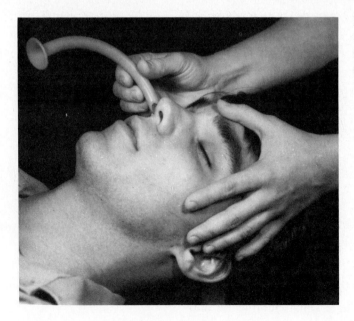

Figure 3–10. The nasopharyngeal airway is inserted with the bevel slid along the septum or floor of the nasal cavity.

tis. In a pinch, a 6- or 6.5-mm endotracheal tube can be cut and serve as a nasopharyngeal airway. With gentle insertion there should be few problems with this airway. However, bleeding and trauma to the nasal mucosa are not infrequent. Mild hemorrhage from the nose after insertion of the airway is not an indication to remove it. In fact, it is probably better to keep it in place so as not to disturb the clot or reactivate the bleeding.

An oropharyngeal airway is designed to keep the tongue off the posterior pharyngeal wall and thereby help maintain a patent airway. It is inserted with the distal end pointing toward the soft palate and then rotated to lie along the tongue, the distal end just posterior to the epiglottis. Special oropharyngeal airways are available. One, the Williams Airway Intubator, has a large circular opening through which an endotracheal tube can be inserted or suctioning can be done. It is designed as an intubator guide. Other varieties of oropharyngeal airways include those with proximal ends that protrude from the lips and are designed to be used with balloon masks that seal the mouth and nose (Figure 3–11).

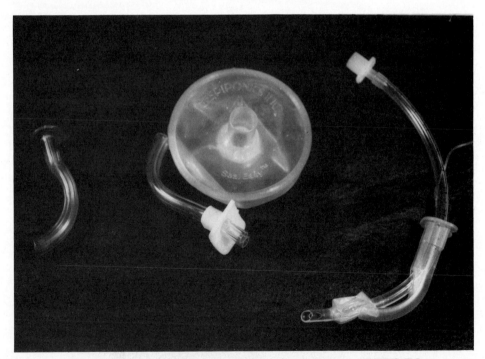

Figure 3–11(a). Samples of oropharyngeal airways. (LEFT TO RIGHT): Guedel; SealEasy^{tm}, used with balloon mask as shown; The Williams' airway intubator, shown accepting a 7mm endotracheal tube.

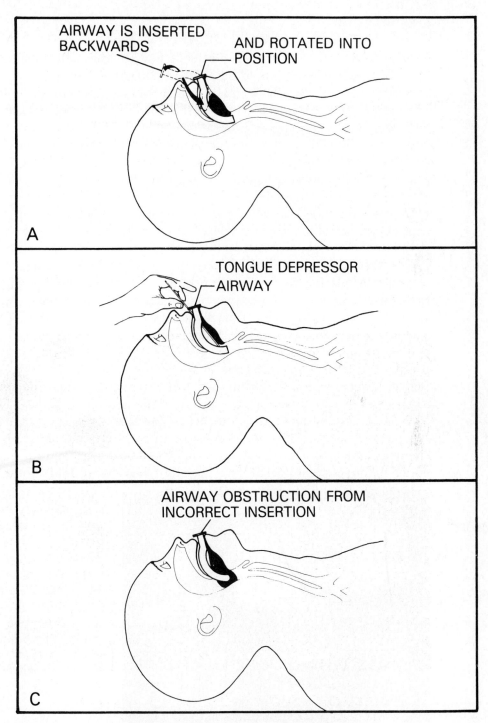

Figure 3–11(b). Insertion of oral airway.

Oxygenation

Patients who are injured need supplemental oxygen, especially if they are unconscious. It is well recognized that patients suffering from head injury are frequently hypoxic. Supplemental oxygen should be supplied by simple face mask run at 10 to 12 L/min. This will provide the patient with about 40 to 50% oxygen. Non-rebreathing masks with a reservoir bag can provide 60 to 90% oxygen with flow rates into the bag of 12 to 15 L/min. Nasal cannulae are well tolerated by most patients, but provide low concentrations of oxygen, about 25 to 30%, depending on the respiratory rate and tidal volume of the patient.

Depending on the method of positive pressure ventilation used in the patient, supplemental oxygen must be used to ensure adequate oxygenation. Oxygenation must be supplemented during mouth-to-mask ventilation by running oxygen at 10 to 12 L/min through the oxygen nipple attached to most masks, or by placing the oxygen tubing under the mask and running it at the same rate. Alternatively, the oxygen percentage of mouth-to-mask breathing can be increased by the rescuer placing a nasal cannula on himself. This increases the delivered oxygen percentage from 17% to about 30%.

Resuscitator bags require an oxygen flow rate of at least 15 L/min to increase the delivered oxygen from 21% (air) to 40 or 50%. The oxygen percentage delivered to the patient with 15 L/min running into the bag will depend on the rate of ventilation and the refilling time of the bag. Higher percentages will be delivered if the rate is slower and the bag is allowed to refill over 3 seconds. The importance of these factors will be reduced or eliminated if a large (2.5 L) bag reservoir is used or if a demand valve is connected to the reservoir port of the resuscitator bag (Figure 3–12). If the latter

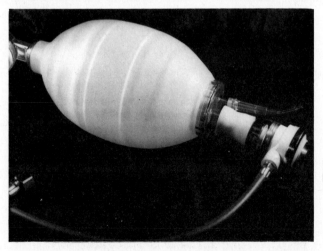

Figure 3–12. Demand-valve used as a reservoir providing 100% oxygen to a standard (Laerdal) ventilating bag. Note the oxygen inlet nipple is sealed with tubing closed at one end. If you use this device, NEVER manually activate the demand value.

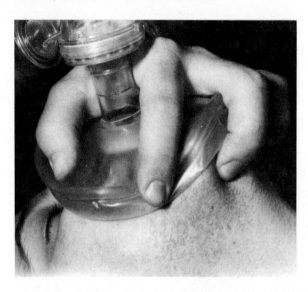

Figure 3-13. The SealEasy^{tm} balloon mask has been shown to reduce mask leak and provide greater volumes during ventilation with bag/mask devices.

method is used, at no time should the demand valve be activated to fill the bag more quickly. This would produce continuous airway pressures that might be as high as 40 cmH$_2$O or more.

Oxygen-powered demand valves have the advantage of delivering 100% oxygen to the patient, but they do so at very high flow rates (100 L/min). Pressures in the oropharynx can be as high as 40 to 60 cmH$_2$O, and the use of these devices can therefore result in gastric distension, with all its risks and potential for complications. Higher delivered volumes can be expected with these devices because it is possible to seal the mask on the face with both hands. However, with the demand valve it is not possible to feel compliance, and overdistension of the lungs may occur as well as further insufflation of oxygen into the stomach. Chest-wall movement, which is recommended as the endpoint of the inspiratory phase with demand valves, is neither an accurate nor an easily appreciated field observation. Because of these great disadvantages, oxygen-powered resuscitator valves are not recommended for use in trauma patients.

Bag–valve–mask devices, or resuscitator bags, are basically fixed-volume ventilators that deliver a volume of about 600 to 800 when squeezed with an adult hand. Several studies have shown that lower volumes are frequently delivered, and a two-person technique is recommended by some to overcome the problem of mask leak. The recent design of a balloon mask (SealEasy) allows for better ventilation with a bag–valve device, and is now becoming standard in some EMS systems (Figure 3-13). Resuscitator bags offer the advantage of a better appreciation of the patient's compliance and should be the only device used if an endotracheal tube is in place.

Esophageal Obturator Airways

The esophageal obturator airway (EOA) is designed to be inserted into the esophagus at a level beyond the carina. A cuff can be inflated to reduce the likelihood of gastric distension or regurgitation during bag–mask or demand valve–mask ventilation. Since its introduction into field medicine in the early 1970s, the EOA was designed to be used in the hands of field personnel who had not been trained to intubate the trachea. Since that time endotracheal intubation by paramedical personnel has become a fairly accepted standard, and use of the device has declined. In addition, controversy surrounding its use surfaced when some studies suggested that it did not provide as adequate ventilation as was originally thought. Although never intended as a replacement for the endotracheal tube, the EOA has frequently been compared to it.

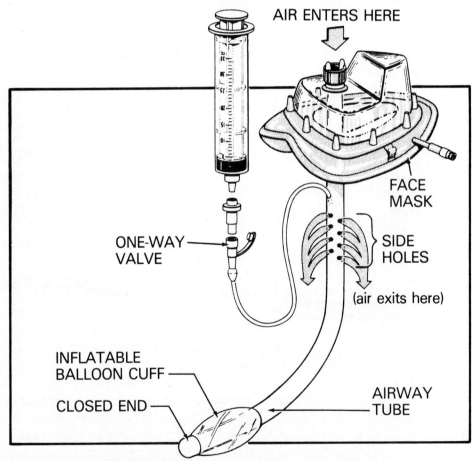

Figure 3–14. Esophageal obturator airway (EOA).

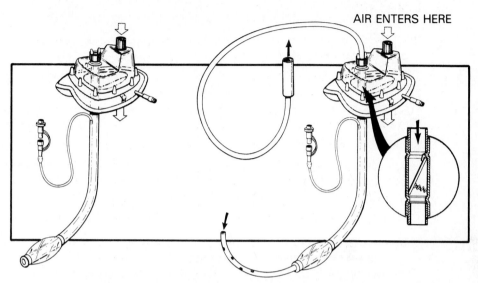

Figure 3–15. Esophageal gastric tube airway (EGTA).

A more recent design, the *esophageal gastric tube airway,* has been introduced and should replace the older versions of the EOA. This design allows for the placement of a nasogastric tube through the lumen of the obturator for decompression of the stomach. In addition, ventilation occurs directly into the oropharynx rather than through the holes of the obturator.

Several essentials must be remembered about the use of the EGTA:

1. It is used only in patients who are unresponsive and without protective reflexes.

2. It should *not* be used in patients with upper airway or facial trauma, where bleeding into the oropharynx is a problem. It must *not* be used in any patient with injury to the esophagus (e.g., caustic ingestions), or in children who are below the age of 15 and are of average height and weight.

3. Adequate mask seal must be ensured; this means appropriate lifting forward of the jaw, with every attempt to avoid movement of the head and neck.

4. Great attention must be paid to proper placement. Unrecognized *intratracheal* placement is a lethal complication that produces complete airway obstruction. Such an occurrence is not always easy to detect, and the results are catastrophic. One of the great disadvantages of this airway is the fact that correct placement can be determined only by

auscultation and observation of chest movement—both may be quite unreliable in a field setting.

5. Insertion must be gentle and without force.

Insertion

The airway is relatively easily inserted and must never be forced. In the supine patient the following procedure is followed:

1. Ventilation should be carried out with mouth-to-mask or bag–valve-mask and suctioning performed prior to insertion of the airway.

2. After liberal lubrication, the airway, with mask attached, is slid into the oropharynx while the tongue and jaw are pulled forward.

3. The airway is advanced along the tongue and into the esophagus. Care should be taken to observe the neck "tenting" of the skin in the area of the pyriform fossae, or anterior displacement of the laryngeal prominence indicates that misplacement has occurred, and repositioning by pulling back on the airway and reinsertion are indicated.

4. Following gentle insertion (without force) so that the mask now rests easily on the face, the mask is sealed firmly on the face as the jaw is pulled forward to ensure a patent airway.

5. Prior to inflating the cuff, ventilation is attempted with a mouth-to-mask or bag–valve device. If the chest is seen to rise, breath sounds are heard, and compliance appears good, the cuff of the airway is inflated with 35 cc of air.

6. Following inflation, the lung fields are auscultated again and the chest wall is *felt* as well as being observed for movement. The epigastrium should not distend. *If there is any doubt about placement of the airway, remove it and reinsert.*

The EGTA is not recommended *in place of* the endotracheal tube, but rather, can be used for patients in whom attempts at endotracheal intubation have been unsuccessful. Even in these, careful attempts at intubation should be continued despite the successful insertion of an EGTA.

Pharyngotracheal Airways

A recent airway device incorporates two tubes and a balloon that can be inflated to fill the oropharynx. This *pharyngotracheal (PTL) airway* is a combination of the EOA and an endotracheal tube and represents an attempt to solve the problem of possible intratracheal placement of the EOA, as well as seeking to provide for tracheal ventilation should blind insertion result in intratracheal positioning. Although preliminary studies appear interesting, particularly in upper airway bleeding, much more work must be done prior to accepting this device for use in the trauma patient.

Positive Pressure Ventilation

Positive pressure ventilation in trauma patients can take various forms, from mouth-to-mouth to bag–endotracheal tube. Most patients able to tolerate an oropharyngeal airway should be considered candidates for the placement of an endotracheal tube. Prior to this procedure being carried out, patients must be oxygenated, usually with some form of positive pressure ventilation. Whatever initial method is chosen, the following essentials must be kept in mind:

1. Supplemental oxygen must be provided for the patient during positive pressure ventilation.
2. Suction must be immediately available.
3. Ventilation must be done carefully to avoid gastric distension and to reduce the risk of regurgitation and possible aspiration. The best insurance against these disasters is Sellick's maneuver, posteriorward pressure over the cricoid cartilage. This should be a routine maneuver in all cases of mask ventilation or in patients undergoing endotracheal intubation.
4. Careful attention must be paid to estimating the minute volume being delivered to the patient; in trauma patients, a minute volume of at least 12 to 15 L should be provided. This is more easily estimated when patients are intubated and being ventilated by resuscitator bag. If an adult's hand will squeeze approximately 700 cc from a bag, "bagging" the patient every 3 or 4 seconds (15 to 20 times/min) would provide a minute volume of from 10.5 to 14 L. This should be enough to provide for the patient's increased ventilatory needs. In the case of bag-mask breathing, up to 40% mask leak can be expected. Recent innovative mask designs can reduce this, and a two-rescuer technique, in which one rescuer holds the mask in place with both hands while a second one squeezes the bag, may better ensure adequate delivered volumes. Field personnel tend to ventilate patients at an increased rate, but delivered volumes are often deficient. Attention must be paid to delivered volumes as well, since rate alone cannot wholly compensate for grossly inadequate ventilatory volumes.

Ventilation Techniques

Mouth-to-Mouth

This is a most reliable and effective method of ventilation, with the advantage of requiring no equipment and a minimum of experience and training. In addition, delivered volumes are consistently adequate since mouth seal is effectively and easily maintained. In addition, compliance can be "felt" more accurately, and high oropharyngeal pressures are therefore less likely. The greatest disadvantage of mouth-to-mouth is the fact that it delivers only 17% oxygen. This can be supplemented by placing a nasal cannula on the rescuer and running it at 6 to 8 L/min, thereby increasing the delivered oxygen percentage to about 30%. Further disadvantages include the fact that many patients have copious secretions, bleeding, gastric regurgitation, or a combination of these. This makes this method of ventilation, however efficient, less attractive. The possibility of disease transmission, although remote, has become a fear among even veteran team members.

Mouth-to-Mask

Most of the disadvantages of mouth-to-mouth ventilation can be overcome by interposing a face mask between the rescuer's mouth and that of the patient. Commercially designed pocket masks are particularly suited for the initial ventilation of many types of patients, and some have a side port for supplemental oxygen. Pocket ventilating masks have consistently been shown to deliver larger volumes than bag–mask devices and with an obviously greater percentage of oxygen than mouth-to-mouth ventilation.

The mask is seated firmly on the face covering the mouth and nose, with the thumbs and index fingers pressing the mask downward against the face. The small, ring, and long fingers are hooked around the angle and body of the mandible and displace the jaw upward, pulling the jaw and therefore the tongue forward. If there is an oxygen inlet, the gas should be turned on and run at about 12 L/min. If there is no inlet but oxygen tubing is available, the oxygen can be run through the tubing slipped under the rim of the mask. Alternatively, the rescuer can place a nasal cannula on himself and run it at 6 L/min.

The rescuer breathes for the patient by blowing into the mask opening and delivering the volume over 2 seconds while watching the chest rise. The patient's compliance can be estimated by the force required to see the chest wall

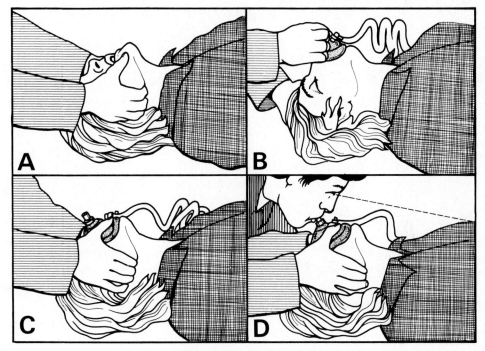

Figure 3–16. Pocket mask.

rise. Between ventilations the mask seal can be relaxed, and by turning his face away from the mask opening the rescuer can feel with the cheek the exhaled volume. Should there be difficulty in ventilation and the chest not rise, the jaw should be repositioned, the mask seal checked, and another ventilation given.

Mouth-to-mask ventilation has significant advantages over other methods, and should be more widely used, as recommended by those who have studied the problem of field ventilation.

Demand Valve — Not trauma

Oxygen-powered resuscitator valves deliver 100% oxygen to the patient under high flow rates that up until recently have exceeded 100 L/min. Recent recommendations have suggested a reduction in these flow rates to only 40 L/min. Because of the difficulty in estimating compliance with these devices, and because of the high intraoral and intrapulmonary pressures possible, they are not to be recommended for trauma patients.

Bag Valve Mask

This descendant of the anesthetic bag is a fixed-volume ventilator with an average delivered volume of about 700 cc. With a two-handed squeeze, over 1 L can be delivered to the patient. Allowing the bag to refill slowly (over 2 to 3 seconds) will substantially increase the percentage of oxygen when no reservoir, or a corrugated tube reservoir, is used. The use of a 2.5 L bag reservoir, or the demand-valve reservoir system, removes the influence of rate or refilling time on the percentage of oxygen delivered to the patient.

The most important problem associated with bag–mask devices is that of volumes delivered. Mask leak is a serious problem, decreasing the volume delivered to the oropharynx by sometimes 40% or more. In addition, masks of conventional design have significant dead space beneath them, thus increasing the challenge to the rescuer to provide an adequate volume to the patient. A recent design of a balloon mask which eliminates dead space beneath the mask and provides an improved seal over the nose and mouth has been shown in mannikin studies to decrease mask leak and improve ventilation. It is recommended particularly for trauma patients (Figure 3–13).

The technique of bag–valve–mask breathing is an art based on several sound physical principles. Some basics must be observed, whether a one-rescuer or two-rescuer technique is used. Oxygen supplementation is essential. The minute volume can be estimated when the person in charge of the airway knows the approximate volume that his hand delivers with one squeeze of the resuscitator bag. By adjusting the ventilatory rate, an adequate minute volume can be delivered appropriate to the patient's size and needs.

Delivering the appropriate volume will depend very much on reducing mask leak. This can be done by using a mask designed to eliminate dead space and provide a better seal of the patient's mouth and nose (the SealEasy mask), or by using two rescuers, one to maintain the seal and the other to compress the bag. The advantage of the balloon mask is that one rescuer can usually ventilate while the other performs Sellick's maneuver. Whether the one- or two-rescuer technique is used, it should be standard practice to perform the maneuver whenever a patient is being ventilated without an endotracheal tube in place.

A better seal can sometimes be obtained, and larger volumes delivered, with either a balloon or a conventional mask by the use of an extension tubing attached to the ventilating port of the bag–valve device (Figure 3–17). This permits the mask to be better seated on the face without a "levering" effect from the rigid ventilating port connector that tends to unseat the mask. With the extension in place, the bag can be more easily compressed, even against the knee or thigh, thus increasing the delivered volume and overcoming any mask leak (Figure 3–17).

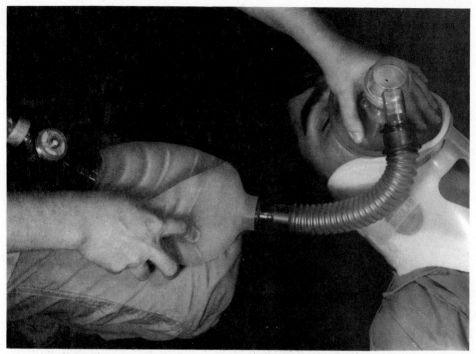

Figure 3–17. A ventilating port extension attached to a
ventilating bag permits a better mask seal and therefore greater
delivered volumes. When the bag is compressed against the
rescuer's thigh as shown, delivered volumes may be
further increased.

Successful ventilation of a patient by bag–valve–mask devices can be
achieved with attention to the following:

1.   Frequent checking to ensure bag and oxygen connections are tight and
     functioning (e.g., the oxygen bag reservoir should remain filled dur-
     ing ventilation)
2.   Proper mask seal, accomplished by using a balloon mask or two-rescuer
     technique with ventilating port extension
3.   Performing Sellick's maneuver
4.   Estimating the minute volume needed for the patient and adjusting
     bag compression and ventilatory rate accordingly

Once an endotracheal tube is in place, ventilation can proceed without regard
to mask leak. The combination of the endotracheal tube and ventilating bag

allows us to detect important information about the compliance and airway pressures of the patient. Several cases of tension pneumothorax and right main-stem bronchus intubations have been detected by rescuers who noted a worsening of compliance during ventilation of trauma patients. It has been shown in animals that in the case of a developing tension pneumothorax, a compliance change can be detected well in advance of a drop in blood pressure. It appears as well that clinicians can readily detect these changes and therefore could conceivably be alerted to a developing tension pneumothorax in patients.

Endotracheal Intubation

The gold standard of airway care in patients who cannot protect their airways or in those needing assistance in breathing is the endotracheal tube. Several problems face use when we decide to intubate a trauma patient. First, it frequently must be done under the most difficult circumstances—on the side of the road, in a crashed vehicle, under a train. In addition, the patient may be immobilized, with cervical collars or other equipment in place. This may so restrict movement and visualization of the airway that alternative methods of intubation have to be considered. Add to this the fact that we must take precautions not to move the head and neck, and our dilemma is readily appreciated.

Although the original method of intubation was clearly tactile or digital, this was later changed by the invention of the laryngoscope, which allowed visualization of the upper airway and placement of the tube under direct vision. The ability to see the actual passage of the tube through the glottic opening rendered tactile orotracheal intubation obsolete, and its practice largely died out until interest in it was recently revived.

Although direct orotracheal intubation should be considered the primary method of placing a tube in the trachea, the procedure is not always easy, nor is it indicated in all patients. In the management of trauma patients particularly, options must be available to permit successful intubation in even the most challenging of situations and patients. There is evidence that the technique of direct-vision orotracheal intubation results in movement of the head and neck. The question therefore arises as to whether the use of this method presents an added risk in possible cervical spine injuries. Controversy exists as to whether such movement is either substantial or of real clinical significance. In short, the method of intubation should be suited to each patient. Those with a low risk of C-spine injury can be intubated in the conventional way, using a laryngoscope. Intubation by the nasotracheal route, the tactile or transillumination methods, or a combination of the two should be reserved for patients with specific indications for alternative techniques.

Preparations

Whatever the method of intubation used, both patients and rescuers should be prepared for the procedure. The following are considered basic to all intubation procedures:

1. *Oxygenation.* All patients should be ventilated, or should breathe high-flow oxygen (12 L/min) for several minutes prior to the attempt.
2. *Gloves.* Rubber examining gloves (not necessarily sterile) should be worn for all intubation procedures.
3. *Equipment.* All equipment should have been checked and should be kept at hand in an organized kit (Figure 3–18). For laryngoscopic

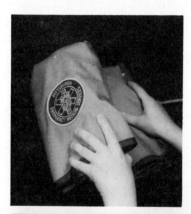

Figure 3–18(a). BTLS AIRWAY CHAPTER

Figure 3–18(b). An "INTUBATION WRAP" contains the essentials for carrying out endotracheal intubation. The kit folds on itself and is compact and portable (a). When opened (b), it provides a clean working surface. Note the transparent pockets.

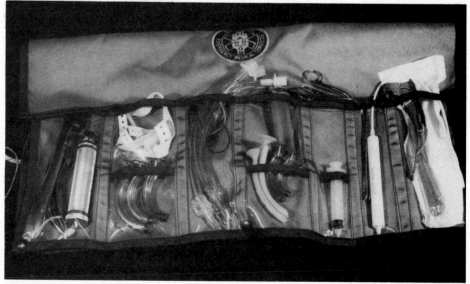

intubation, the endotracheal tube should be held in a "hockey stick" shape by a malleable stylet that is first lubricated and inserted until the distal end is just *proximal* to the side hole of the endotracheal tube. The cuff of the endotracheal tube should be checked by inflating it with 10 cc of air. The air should then be *completely* removed and the syringe filled with air left attached to the pilot tube. The cuff and distal end of the tube is then lubricated.

4. *Suction.* Suction must be immediately at hand.

5. *Assistant.* An assistant should be available to help in the procedure, and Sellick's maneuver should be applied during ventilation and the subsequent intubation attempt. The assistant may also aid in holding the head and neck immobile and counting aloud to 30.

6. *Lidocaine.* Intravenous lidocaine HCl, given 4 to 5 minutes before intubation is attempted has been shown to decrease the adverse cardiovascular and intracranial pressure effects of the intubation procedure. *If time permits,* an IV bolus dose of 100 to 125 mg may be given to all adult patients prior to intubation or suctioning.

Intubation Techniques

Laryngoscopic Orotracheal Method

In this method the upper airway and the glottic opening are visualized and the tube is slipped gently through the cords. Its advantages include the ability to see obstructions and to visualize accurate placement of the tube. It has the disadvantage of requiring a relatively relaxed patient without anatomic distortion, and with minimal bleeding or secretions.

Equipment: Laryngoscopic intubation will require the following:

1. Straight (Miller) or curved (MacIntosh) blade and laryngoscope handle
2. Transparent endotracheal tube, 28 to 33 cm in length and 7, 7.5, or 8.0 mm in internal diameter
3. Stylet to help mold the tube into a "hockey stick" shape
4. Water-soluble lubricant (there is no need for it to contain a local anesthetic)
5. 10- or 12-cc syringe
6. Magill forceps
7. Tape/tincture of benzoin or endotracheal tube holder

Following ventilation and initial preparations, the following steps should be carried out:

1. An assistant holds the head, performs Sellick's maneuver, and counts slowly *aloud* to 30.
2. The intubator pulls down on the chin and slides the blade into the right side of the patient's mouth, pushing the tongue to the left and "inching" the blade down along the tongue in an attempt to see the epiglottis. [*Note:* A key maneuver must be performed here; the blade must pull forward on the tongue to lift up the epiglottis and bring it into view (Figure 3–19).]

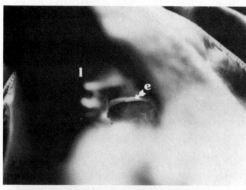

Figure 3–19(a). LANDMARKS DURING INTUBATION—View looking into the oropharynx during the act of direct laryngoscopy. A—the laryngoscope (1) is inserted into the vallecula and the tongue is pulled forward to expose the epiglottis (e).

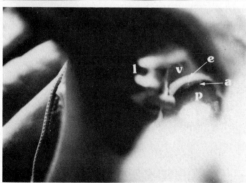

Figure 3–19(b). B—pulling forward further (not *levering*) in a straight line allows the arytenoid cartilages (a) to become into view; l = laryngoscope; p = posterior pharyngeal wall; v = vallecula; e = epiglottis.

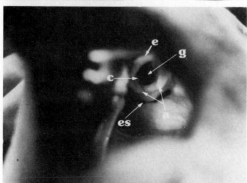

Figure 3–19(c). C—intubator's view of larynx. e—epiglottis; g—glottic opening; c—cords; a—arytenoids; es—esophagus.

3. The laryngoscope blade is used to lift the tongue and epiglottis up and forward in a straight line. "Levering" the blade is a common error with novices and can result in broken teeth and other trauma. The laryngoscope is essentially a "hook" to lift the tongue and epiglottis up and out of the way so that the glottic opening can be identified.

4. The tube is advanced along the right side of the oropharynx once the epiglottis is seen. When the glottic opening (or even just the arytenoid cartilages) is identified, the tube is slipped through to a depth of about 5 cm beyond the cords.

5. Should visualization be difficult, an assistant can put posteriorward pressure on the laryngeal prominence to bring the cords into view.

6. While the tube is still held firmly, the cuff is inflated and ventilation begun.

7. The tube is then checked for placement (see page 80).

Nasotracheal Method

The nasotracheal route of endotracheal intubation in a field setting may be justified when the patient's mouth cannot be opened because of clenched jaws and when the patient cannot be ventilated by other means. The great disadvantage of this method is its relative difficulty, depending as it does on an appreciation of the intensity of the breath sounds of spontaneously breathing patients. It is a blind procedure and as such requires extra effort to demonstrate proper intratracheal placement.

Guidance of the tube through the glottic opening is a question of the intubator perceiving the intensity of the sound of the patient breathing out. The tube can, with some difficulty, be guided toward the point of maximum intensity and slipped through the cords. Breath sounds can be better heard and felt with the ear placed against the proximal opening of the tube or, even better, the bell of a single-tube stethoscope can be removed and the tube inserted into the endotracheal tube (Figure 3–20).

Note: The tube will not fit into anything less than an 8.5-mm tube. It does not have to—wedging the end of it into the adapter is all that is needed for the tube to become an "extension" of the stethoscope.

The success of this method will also depend on an anterior curve to the tube that will prevent its passing into the esophagus. This may better be achieved by preparing two tubes prior to carrying out the intubation attempt. The distal end of the 33-cm tube is inserted into the proximal adapter, thus molding it into a formed circle. Preparing two tubes permits the immediate use of a second, more rigid tube should the first plastic tube become warm

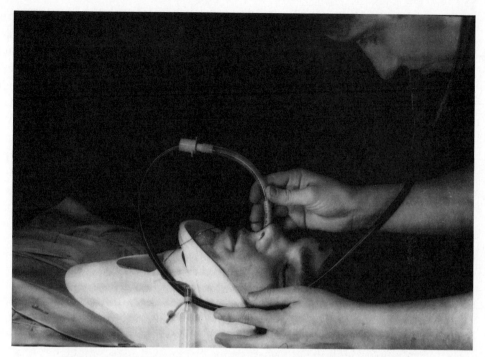

Figure 3–20. Following removal of the stethoscope's diaphragm and bell, the tubing can be squeezed into the adapter of the endotracheal tube as an aid to listening for breath sounds during nasotracheal intubation.

with body temperature, thus losing its anterior curve. The Endotrol, a directional-tip tube, has been introduced to help in achieving an anterior curve, but this has not been shown to be extremely helpful. Displacing the tongue and jaw forward may also be helpful in achieving placement, since this maneuver lifts the epiglottis anteriorly out of the way of the advancing tube.

Following lubrication of its cuff and distal end, a 7- or 7.5-mm endotracheal tube with the bevel placed against the floor or septum of the nasal cavity is slipped distally through the largest naris.

Note: If time permits, a local spray of 4% lidocaine mixed with 0.25% phenylephrine can be applied to the nasal mucosa. This will provide mucosal vasoconstriction and anesthesia, and will help reduce the stimulation caused by the procedure.

When the tube tip reaches the posterior pharyngeal wall, great care must be taken in "rounding the bend" and then directing the tube toward the glottic opening. By watching the neck at the laryngeal prominence the intubator can judge the approximate placement of the tube; tenting of skin on either side of the prominence indicates catching up of the tube in the pyriform fossa, a problem solved by slight withdrawal and rotation of the tube to the midline. Bulging and anterior displacement of the laryngeal prominence usually indicates that the tube has entered the glottic opening and has been correctly placed. At this point the patient, especially if not deeply comatose, will cough, strain, or both. This may be alarming to the novice intubator, who might interpret this as laryngospasm or misplacement of the tube. The temptation may be to pull the tube and ventilate, since the patient may not breathe immediately. Holding the hand or ear over the opening of the tube to detect airflow may reassure the intubator that the tube is correctly placed, and the cuff may be inflated and ventilation begun. A stringent protocol must now be followed to prove intratracheal placement (see page 80).

Digital Method

The original method of endotracheal intubation, quite widely known in the eighteenth century, was the "tactile" or "digital" technique. The intubator merely felt the epiglottis with the fingers and slipped the endotracheal tube distally through the glottic opening. Recently, the technique has been refined and demonstrated to be of use in the field for a wide variety of patients.

Indications: Tactile orotracheal intubation is particularly useful for deeply comatose or cardiac arrest patients, who:

1. Are difficult to position properly
2. Are somewhat inaccessible to the full view of the rescuer
3. May be at risk of cervical spine injury
4. Have facial injuries that distort anatomy
5. Have copious oropharyngeal bleeding or secretions that render visualization difficult

Personnel may prefer to perform tactile intubation when they are more confident in their ability with the technique, or when a laryngoscope fails or is not immediately available. We have found the technique most valuable in those patients in difficult positions (e.g., extrications) and in those who have copious secretions despite adequate attempts at suctioning.

Equipment: This method of intubation requires the following:

1. Endotracheal tube, 7.0-, 7.5-, or 8.0-mm internal diameter

2. Malleable stylet (*Note:* Some prefer to perform the procedure without a stylet)
3. Water-soluble lubricant
4. 12-cc syringe
5. Dental prod, mouth gag, or other device for placing between the teeth
6. Rubber examining gloves

Techniques: Following proper preparation of the patient (oxygenation, suctioning, etc.), the intubation is done with an assistant or an immobilizing device holding the head steady (if head or neck trauma is present). Sellick's maneuver is performed, and an assistant counts aloud to 30.

1. The tube is prepared by inserting the lubricated stylet and bending the tube into an "open-J" configuration. The stylet should *not* protrude beyond the tip of the tube, but it should come to at least the side hole.
2. A water-soluble lubricant is used liberally on the tip and cuff of the tube.
3. Gloves are used for protection.
4. The intubator kneels at the patient's left shoulder facing the patient and places a dental prod or mouth gag between the patient's molars (Figure 3–21a).

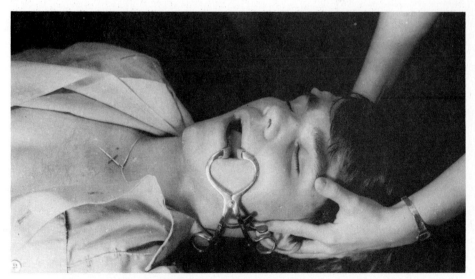

Figure 3–21(a). DIGITAL INTUBATION—A: preparing patient with use of mouth (dental) prod to protect the intubator against being bitten.

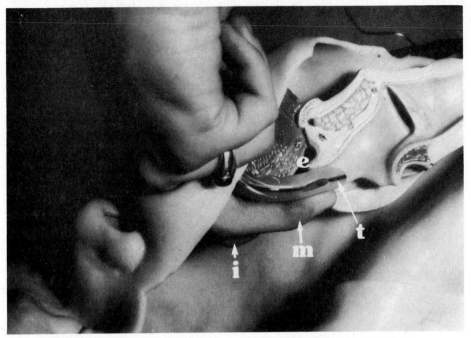

Figure 3–21(b). B: the fingers are slid down the tongue and the
tube guided towards the epiglottis (e) by the long (m) and
index (i) fingers.

5. The intubator then "walks" the index and middle fingers of his left hand down the midline of the tongue, all the while pulling forward on the tongue and jaw. *This is a most important maneuver and serves to lift the epiglottis up within reach of the probing fingers* (Figure 3–21b).

6. The middle finger palpates the epiglottis; it feels much like the tragus of the ear.

7. The epiglottis is pressed forward and the tube is slipped into the mouth at the left labial angle anterior to the palpating fingers (Figure 3–21b). The index finger is used to keep the tube tip against the side of the middle finger (that is still palpating the epiglottis). This guides the tip to the epiglottis. The side hole of the tube can also be used as a landmark to ensure that the intubator is always aware of the position of the tip of the endotracheal tube. *This is a crucial principle of this technique.*

8. The middle and index fingers guide the tube tip to lie against the epiglottis in front and the fingers behind. The right hand then advances the

tube distally through the cords as the index and middle fingers of the left palpating hand press forward to prevent the tube from slipping posteriorward into the esophagus.

Note: At this point the tube–stylet combination may encounter resistance, especially if the distal curve of the tube is sharp. This usually means that the tube tip is impinging on the anterior wall of the thyroid or cricoid cartilage. Pulling back slightly on the stylet will allow the tube to conform to the anatomy, and the tube should slip distally.

Complete the intubation according to protocol, and ensure correct placement (see page 80).

Transillumination (Lighted Stylet) Method

The transillumination or lighted stylet method of endotracheal intubation is based on the fact that a bright light inserted inside the upper airway can be seen through the soft tissues of the neck when inside the larynx or trachea. This permits the intubator to guide the tube tip through the glottic opening without directly visualizing the cords. This has been called the "indirect visual" method, and has been shown in several studies to be reliable, quick, and atraumatic. It is particularly attractive in trauma patients since it appears to move the head and neck less than do conventional orotracheal methods.

Equipment

1.   *Stylet.* The lighted stylet (Figure 3–22a) is a malleable wire connecting

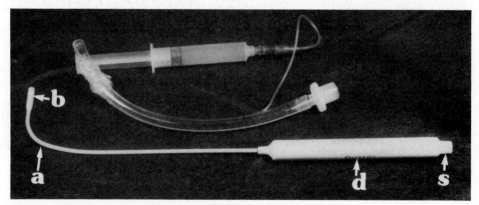

Figure 3–22(a). THE LIGHTED STYLET: A: s—on/off switch; d—battery housing; a—distal bend; b—bulb.

a proximal battery housing to a distal light bulb, covered with a tough plastic coating that prevents the light from being separated from the wire. The wire stylet part is 25 cm in length. An on/off switch is located at the proximal end of the battery housing.

2. *Endotracheal tubes.* All tubes should be 7.5 to 8.5 mm (internal diameter), and should be cut to 25 cm to accommodate the stylet. [*Note:* A longer (33-cm) stylet will soon be commercially available.]

3. Other equipment will be standard to any intubation procedure: suction, oxygen, gloves, lubricant, and so on.

Technique: The success of this method of intubation will depend on several factors:

1. Level of ambient light
2. Pulling forward on the patient's tongue, or tongue and jaw
3. Bend of the stylet/tube

The light should be cut down to about 10% of normal, or the neck should be shielded from direct sun or bright daylight. While the transilluminated light can be perceived in thin patients even in daylight, success will be more likely the darker the surroundings.

Pulling forward on the tongue—or tongue and jaw—lifts the epiglottis up out of the way. This is *essential* to this method (Figure 3–22b).

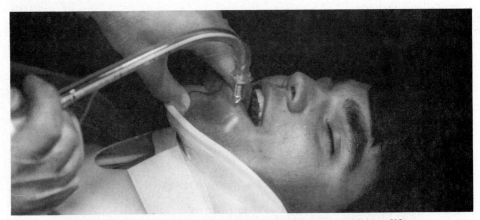

Figure 3–22(b). B: pulling forward on the tongue and jaw lifts
the epiglottis and allows for intubation with the stylet. The bend
in the stylet must not be too far proximal so that it will not
strike against the posterior pharyngeal wall. Note gloves
are worn.

The stylet–tube combination should be bent just proximal to the cuff—a bend that is too far proximal will cause the tube to strike against the posterior pharyngeal wall and prevent the tube from advancing anteriorly through the glottic opening. The lubricated stylet is slipped into the tube and held firmly against the battery housing while the tube–stylet is bent. Bend more sharply if the patient is not in the sniffing position.

Following oxygenation of the patient, the following steps are followed to ensure a successful intubation:

1. The intubator stands or kneels on either side facing the patient's head. Gloves are worn for the procedure. The light is turned on.

2. The patient's tongue—or, more easily, the tongue and jaw—is grasped by the intubator and drawn gently forward while the liberally lubricated tube–stylet combination is slipped down the tongue.

3. Using a "soup-ladle" motion, the epiglottis is "hooked" up to the tube–stylet and the transilluminated light can be seen in the midline. Correct placement at or beyond the cords is indicated by the appearance of a circumscribed, easily perceived light at the level of the laryngeal prominence (Figure 3–23, right). A bright light seen on either side of the upper aspect of the prominence indicates right or left pyriform fossa placement (Figure 3–23, left). A dull glow, diffuse and difficult to see, indicates esophageal placement.

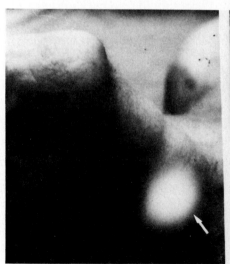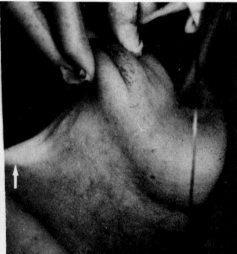

Figure 3–23. (Left)—Clearly-seen light transilluminated from the right pyriform fossa. (Right)—The bright circumscribed glow seen when the tip of the stylet is at or beyond the cprds.

4. When the light is seen, the stylet is held firmly in place and the fingers of the other hand support the tube lying along the tongue as they advance the tube off the stylet more distally into the larynx.

The intubation is completed in the usual way. Again, it is doubly important to prove intratracheal placement because the upper airway was not directly visualized. A strict protocol, outlined below, should be followed.

Confirmation of Tube Placement

One of the greatest challenges of intubation facing prehospital care providers is ensuring correct intratracheal placement of endotracheal tubes. An unrecognized esophageal intubation is a lethal complication of a lifesaving procedure, and is, even in the context of field care, inexcusable. Every effort must be made to avoid this catastrophe, and a strict protocol must be developed and followed to reduce the risk.

Although the most reliable method of ensuring proper placement is actually visualizing the tube passing through the glottic opening, this is often a luxury that we cannot always count on in field care of the trauma patient. Visualization of the arytenoids is perhaps as much as we can expect, especially in a patient whose head and neck are immobilized and at risk if moved.

A simple, yet effective protocol for tube confirmation is possible and practical for the field setting. Such a protocol should recognize the unreliable nature of auscultation as a sole method of confirming intratracheal placement. Correct intratracheal placement should be suspected from the following signs:

1. An anteriorward displacement of the laryngeal prominence as the tube is passed distally.

2. Coughing, bucking, or straining on the part of the patient. [*Note: Phonation* (any noise made with the vocal cords) is *absolute evidence that the tube is in the esophagus and should be removed immediately.*]

3. Breath condensation on the tube with each ventilation—not 100% reliable, but very suggestive of intratracheal placement.

4. Normal compliance with bag ventilation. The bag does not suddenly "collapse," but rather, there is some resilience to it and resistance to lung inflation.

5. No air leak after cuff inflation—persistent leak indicates esophageal intubation until proven otherwise.

The following procedure should then be carried out to prove correct placement:

1. *Auscultation* of six sites:
    a. Right and left apex.
    b. Right and left midaxillary line.
    c. The *epigastrium*—perhaps the most important; it should be silent, with no sounds heard.
    d. The sternal notch—"tracheal" sounds should readily be heard there.

2. *Palpation* of the chest wall to feel the ribs parting and the chest wall moving and gentle palpation of the tube cuff in the sternal notch while the pilot balloon is compressed between the index finger and thumb; a pressure wave should be felt in the pilot balloon.

3. *Inspection* for full movement of the chest with ventilation; watch for any change in the patient's color or in the ECG reading.

4. *Transillumination.* A flexible lighted stylet designed for nasotracheal intubation is available and can readily be passed distally after lubrication into the tube (Figure 3–24a). A bright glow first in the oropharynx,

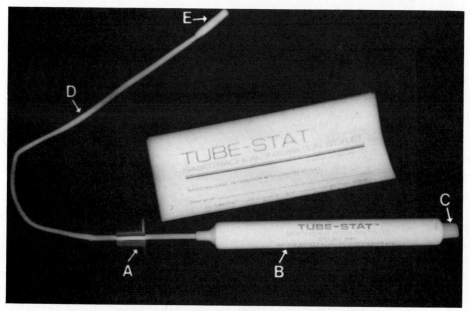

Figure 3–24(a). A: The soft flexible stylet can be slipped distally into an in-place tube to prove intratracheal placement. A—adapter; B—battery housing; C—on/off switch; E—bulb; D—soft wire stylet.

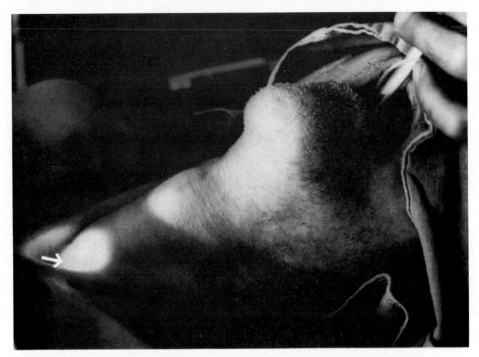

Figure 3–24(b). B: Dim ambient lighting will assist in identifying the bright circumscribed glow of correct intratracheal placement.

then at the laryngeal prominence (the light in the oropharynx disappears as the bulb passes the cords), is almost absolute evidence of intratracheal placement (Figure 3–24b). It is essential that the ambient lighting be as low as possible for this procedure to be successful. Covering the neck to shield it from light will help. In the ambulance, the lights in the patient compartment can be turned out.

The protocol for confirmation of tube placement should be applied following intubation only after several minutes of ventilation. Thereafter the protocol should be followed after movement of the patient from the floor to the stretcher, after loading into the ambulance, and immediately prior to arrival at the hospital. If at any time placement is in doubt, *visualize directly or remove the tube*. Never *assume* that the tube is in the right place—always be *sure* and *record* that the protocol has been carefully followed.

Anchoring the Tube

Anchoring the tube can be a frustrating exercise. Not only does it require some fine movements of the hands when we appear to be all thumbs, but it is difficult to perform this task when ventilation, movement, or extrication is being carried out. There is one thing to keep in mind; there is no substitute for the human anchor. That is, one person should be held responsible for ensuring that the tube is held fast and that it does not migrate in or out of the airway. To lose a tube can be a catastrophe, especially if the patient is rather inaccessible or the intubation was a difficult one to begin with.

Fixing the endotracheal tube in place is important for several reasons. First, movement of the tube in the trachea will produce more mucosal damage and may increase the risk of post-intubation complications. In addition, movement of the tube will stimulate the patient to cough, strain, or both, leading to cardiovascular and intracranial pressure changes that could be detrimental. Most of all, there is a greater risk in the field of dislodging a tube and losing control of the airway if it is not anchored solidly in place.

The endotracheal tube can be secured in place either by tape or by a commercially available holder. Although taping a tube in place is convenient and relatively easily done, it is not always effective, since there is often a problem with the tape sticking to skin, which is often wet with rain, blood, airway secretions, or vomitus. If tape is to be used, several principles should be followed:

1. An oropharyngeal airway should also be in place to prevent the patient from biting down on the tube.
2. The patient's face should be dried off and tincture of benzoin applied to ensure proper adhesion of the tape.
3. The tape should be carried right around the patient's neck in anchoring the tube.
4. The tube should be anchored at the labial angle, not in the midline.

Because of the difficulty of fixing the tube in place with tape, we prefer to use a commercial endotracheal tube holder that uses a small rubber strap to fix the tube in a plastic holder that acts as a bite block (Figure 3–25). A second rubber strap passes round the patient's neck. Although this is not an ideal solution, it is easier to use and more quickly applied. If tube holders with Velcro are used, care must be taken not to get the small hooks embedded in the fingers or in the patient's lips.

Since flexion or extension of the patient's head can move the tube in or

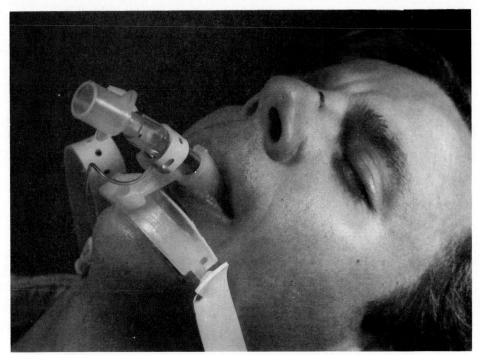

Figure 3–25. A commercial endotracheal tube holder. Note the two separate rubber straps holding the tube around the neck and in a bite block.

out of the airway by 2 or 3 cm, it is a good practice to restrict head and neck movement of any patient who has an endotracheal tube in place. If the patient is immobilized because of the risk of cervical spine injury, we need not worry about this. However, in those who do not have a collar or other device in place, we prefer to tape the head to the longboard or stretcher in order to restrict movement. Failing this, the airway manager is required to ensure that the head and neck are kept in a neutral position.

Although endotracheal intubation may be thought of as the definitive airway control procedure in selected trauma patients, there are some instances in which access below the level of the cords is required and intubation cannot provide that. At other times, for some reason or another, the patient is very difficult to intubate. These cases provide the greatest challenge and require that we have one other option available to use—*translaryngeal jet ventilation.*

Translaryngeal Jet Ventilation

When access below the level of the cords is sought, *translaryngeal jet ventilation* (TLJV) provides a quick, reliable, and relatively safe method of adequate oxygenation and ventilation, especially in the trauma patient. Many misconceptions and erroneous impressions persist about this technique, and the medical literature is in a state of confusion on the subject. Clinical experience and studies done using appropriate equipment in both animals and patients would clearly indicate the following:

1. Patients can be both oxygenated and ventilated with this technique, which delivers 100% oxygen in volumes exceeding 1 L per second.
2. Ventilation can proceed indefinitely, provided that the correct-size cannula is used with the proper driving pressure.
3. Cannulae of 14 gauge or larger, with side holes, must be used.
4. Driving pressures of at least 50 psi must be used to deliver sufficient volumes to ensure adequate ventilation.

Patients cannot be ventilated using small-bore cannulae with continuous-flow oxygen attached; the principles listed above must be adhered to if this technique is to be used safely and effectively.

Equipment: The tools needed for TLJV should be prepared well in advance and stored in a small bag or kit:

1. *14- or 13-gauge cannula, with side holes.* These sizes are the *minimum* necessary for adequate ventilation. Side holes are especially important, since they prevent the cannula from remaining against the tracheal wall and subjecting it to sudden pressures that could rupture it (Figure 3–26).
2. *Manual jet ventilator device.* These are commercially available and are merely valves that allow high-pressure oxygen to flow through them when a button is depressed. They should have high-pressure tubing attached solidly with special fasteners and tape.
3. *Wrench.* A small wrench should be *attached* to the jet ventilator tubing so that no time will be lost looking for a way to tap into the oxygen tank, or turn it on.

A cannula, recently designed especially for TLJV, has proven particularly useful in field practice (Figure 3–26). This 13-gauge ventilating cannula, with side holes and a slight curve that allows for ease of insertion, has as a major feature an around-the-neck tie that fixes it in place very conveniently. A patently unattractive feature of this cannula is the 15-mm connector at the ventilating port, since its presence suggests that the patient could be ventilated through the cannula with demand valve or bag–valve resuscitator bag. It is *absolutely impossible* to ventilate a patient using this technique; the developers of this cannula themselves recognize this.

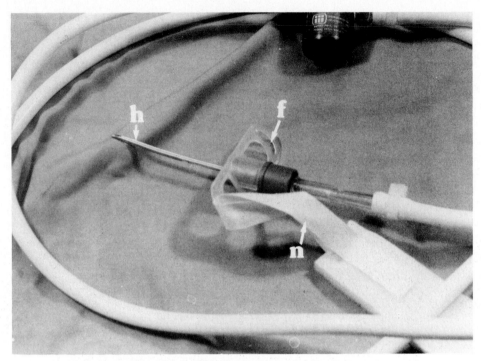

Figure 3-26. A specially-designed 13G cannula for
translaryngeal jet ventilation. Note side-holes (h), flange (f), and
neck strap (n). This is hooked into a 50 psi oxygen source for
adequate ventilation and oxygenation.

Technique: Identification of the cricothyroid membrane is essential to this
technique, although placement between the tracheal rings would probably not
result in major problems.

1.   With continued attempts at ventilation and oxygenation, the crico-
     thyroid membrane is punctured by the cannula firmly attached to a
     5-cc syringe filled with 1 to 2 cc of saline (Figure 3-27). (*Note:* Several
     cubic centimeters of 2% lidocaine can be used instead of saline, to pro-
     duce local anesthesia of the mucosa in the area of the distal port of
     the cannula.)
2.   The cannula is directed downward, with continual aspiration to demon-
     strate entry into the larynx, identified when bubbles of air are readily
     aspirated. At this point, if lidocaine is contained in the syringe, it can
     be injected to provide some anesthesia and prevent the coughing that
     sometimes occurs in those patients who are somewhat responsive.

3.   On entry into the larynx, the cannula is slid off the needle trochar and is held in place while the TLJV is connected to the proximal port of the cannula (Figure 3–28).

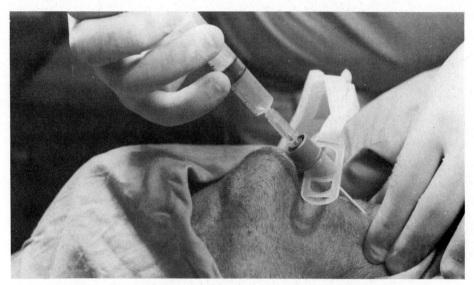

Figure 3–27. Puncture of cricothyroid membrane with jet ventilator cannula. Note syringe in place filled with salinebubbles on aspiration indicate correct intratracheal placement.

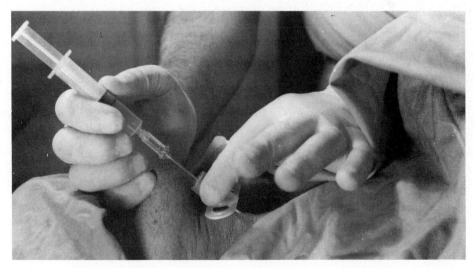

Figure 3–28. Cannula is slid distally off the needle when membrane is punctured.

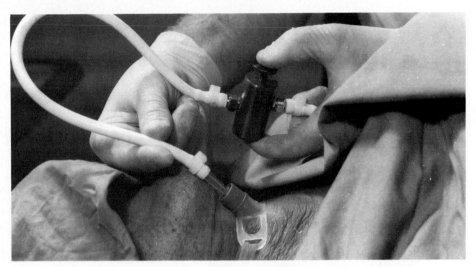

Figure 3–29. Patient is ventilated indefinitely with 1 to 1.5 second bursts of oxygen from a 50 psi source at a rate of 12/20 min.

4. The patient is immediately ventilated using 1-second bursts of oxygen from the 50-psi manual source. The rate used is at least 20 per minute (i.e., an inspiratory/expiratory ratio of 1 : 2; Figure 3–29).

5. If a tie is available, the cannula is fixed in place. Tape can also be used, but it must be fastened firmly to the cannula and then around the patient's neck. Firm pressure at the site of insertion can reduce the small amount of subcutaneous emphysema that usually occurs with this technique.

Although TTJV is usually thought of as a method of last resort, our experience would indicate that it should be considered much sooner in the management of the trauma patient's airway. When properly applied using the appropriate equipment, it can provide adequate ventilation and oxygenation for those in need of airway control.

Summary

The challenge of airway control to the field team is greater in the trauma patient than in almost any other. Prehospital care providers must have options to solve difficulty management problems. They will be called on to assess and manage patients under the most trying conditions. The management of the airway in trauma will require skill, confidence, a planned approach—and a little bit of luck.

Chapter 4

Thoracic Trauma

Andrew B. Peitzman, M.D., and Paul Paris, M.D.

Twenty-five percent of trauma deaths are due entirely to thoracic injuries, and half of trauma victims with multiple injuries have an associated chest injury. Two-thirds of these patients with fatal thoracic trauma are alive to reach the emergency department, and only 15% require surgery. Thus these are salvageable trauma victims. The goal of this chapter is to enable you to recognize signs and symptoms of major thoracic injury and provide appropriate care. Major thoracic injury may result from motor vehicle accidents, falls, gunshot wounds, crush injuries, stab wounds, or other mechanisms.

Anatomy

The thorax is a bony cavity that is formed by 12 pairs of ribs that join posteriorly with the thoracic spine and anteriorly with the sternum. The intercostal neurovascular bundle runs along the inferior surface of each rib.

The inner side of the thoracic cavity and the lung itself are lined with a thin layer of tissue, the pleura. The space between the two pleural layers is normally only a potential space. However, this space may be occupied by air forming a pneumothorax or blood to form a hemothorax. This potential space can hold 3 L of fluid in an adult.

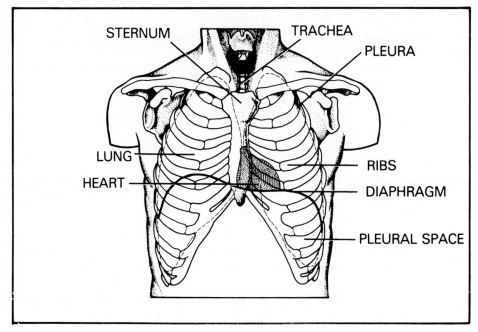

Figure 4–1. Thorax.

As shown in Figure 4–1, one lung occupies each thoracic cavity. Between the two chest cavities is the mediastinum, which contains the heart, aorta, superior and inferior vena cava, trachea, major bronchi, and esophagus. The spinal cord is protected by the vertebral column. The diaphragm separates the thoracic organs from the abdominal cavity. The upper abdominal organs, including the spleen, liver, kidneys, pancreas, and stomach, are protected by

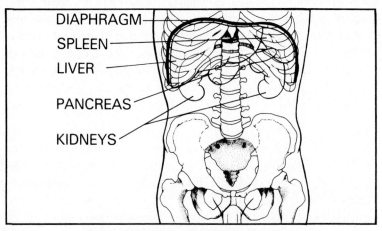

Figure 4–2. Intrathoracic abdomen.

the lower rib cage (Figure 4–2). Any patient with a penetrating thoracic wound at the level of the nipples (fourth intercostal space) or lower should be assumed to have an abdominal injury as well as thoracic injury. Similarly, blunt deceleration injuries such as steering wheel injuries often injure both thoracic and abdominal structures.

Pathophysiology

When evaluating a victim with probable thoracic trauma, always be systematic to avoid missing life-threatening injuries. During the initial survey, search for the most dangerous injuries first to give your patient the best chance for survival. As with any trauma victim, the mechanism of injury is very important in caring for the trauma victim. Thoracic injuries may be the result of blunt trauma or penetrating objects. With blunt trauma, the force is distributed over a large area and visceral injuries occur from deceleration, shearing forces, compression, or bursting. Penetrating injuries, usually gunshot wounds or stab wounds, distribute the forces of injury over a smaller area. However, the trajectory of a bullet is often unpredictable, and all thoracic structures are at risk.

Assessment

The major symptoms of chest injury include shortness of breath, chest pain, and respiratory distress. The signs indicative of chest injury include shock, hemoptysis, cyanosis, chest wall contusion, flail chest, open wounds, distended neck veins, tracheal deviation, or subcutaneous emphysema. An examination of the chest can be completed very quickly. Check the lung fields for presence and equality of breath sounds. Immediately life-threatening thoracic injuries should be identified. Major thoracic injuries may be remembered as the "deadly dozen." The immediately life-threatening injuries include:

1. Airway obstruction
2. Open pneumothorax
3. Tension pneumothorax
4. Massive hemothorax
5. Flail chest
6. Cardiac tamponade

Potentially life-threatening injuries include:

7. Thoracic aortic disruption
8. Bronchial disruption
9. Myocardial contusion
10. Diaphragmatic tear
11. Esophageal injury
12. Pulmonary contusion

Airway management remains a major challenge in the care of the trauma victim. This has been discussed in Chapter 3. Always assume that there is an associated cervical spine injury when securing the airway.

Open Pneumothorax

Open pneumothorax is generally caused by a penetrating thoracic injury and may present as a sucking chest wound. The signs and symptoms are usually proportional to the size of the chest wall defect (Figure 4–3).

Pathophysiology: Normal respiration involves a negative pressure being generated inside the chest by diaphragmatic contraction. As air is drawn through the upper airway, the lungs expand. With a large open wound of the chest, the path of least resistance for airflow is through the chest wall defect. This air will only enter the pleural space. It will not enter the lung and therefore

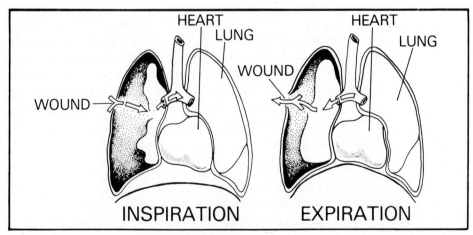

Figure 4–3. Open pneumothorax sucking chest wound.

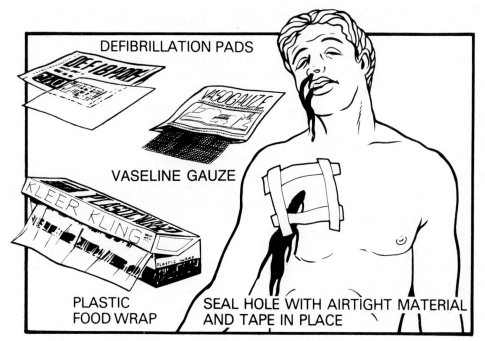

Figure 4–4. Treatment of sucking chest wound.

will not contribute to oxygenation of the blood. Ventilation is impaired and hypoxia results.

Management

1. Ensure an airway.
2. Promptly close the chest wall defect by any available means. This may be accomplished with a defibrillation pad, Vaseline gauze, rubber glove, or plastic dressing. The risk of placing an occlusive dressing is that the patient may then develop a tension pneumothorax. To circumvent this problem, tape the occlusive dressing on three sides, which will produce a flutter valve; air can escape from the chest but not enter it. A chest tube will be needed ultimately, followed by operative closure of the chest wall defect.
3. Administer oxygen.
4. Insert a large-bore IV.
5. Monitor cardiac function.
6. Rapidly transport the patient to the appropriate hospital.
7. Notify medical control.

Tension Pneumothorax

Tension pneumothorax occurs from either blunt or penetrating trauma when a one-way valve occurs, so air can enter but not leave the pleural space (Figure 4–5). This causes collapse of the affected lung and will then push the mediastinum in the opposite direction, with resultant kinking of the superior and inferior vena cavae with loss of venous return to the heart. Shift of the trachea and mediastinum away from the side of the tension pneumothorax will also compromise ventilation of the other lung, although this is a late phenomenon.

Clinical signs of a tension pneumothorax include dyspnea, anxiety, tachypnea, diminished breath sounds and hypertympany to percussion on the affected side, hypotension, and distended neck veins. Tracheal deviation is a late finding and its absence does not rule out the presence of a tension pneumothorax. The development of decreased lung compliance (becomes difficult to squeeze the bag–valve device) in the intubated patient should always alert you to the possibility of a tension pneumothorax.

Management

1. Establish an open airway.
2. Administer high-concentration oxygen.

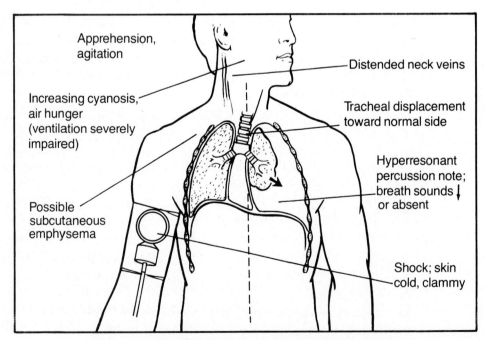

Figure 4–5. Physical findings of tension pneumothorax.

3. Decompress the affected chest by inserting a 14- or 16-gauge plastic catheter over the top of the rib of the fifth or sixth intercostal space in the midaxillary line. This will convert the injury to a simple pneumothorax. A one-way valve may then be made using a Heimlich valve or one of the techniques taught in Advanced Skill Station 9.
    a. Indications to perform emergency decompression of a tension pneumothorax include:
        (1) Loss of the radial pulse
        (2) Loss of consciousness
        (3) Respiratory distress and cyanosis
    b. If the paramedic is not authorized to decompress the chest, the patient must be transported rapidly to the hospital, so this can be performed.
    c. A chest tube will be necessary upon arrival at the hospital. The needle decompression is a temporary, but lifesaving measure.
4. Insert an IV en route.
5. Rapidly transport the patient to the appropriate hospital.
6. Notify medical control.

Massive Hemothorax

Blood in the pleural space is a hemothorax (Figure 4–6). A massive hemothorax occurs as a result of at least a 1500-cc blood loss into the thoracic cavity. Each thoracic cavity may contain up to 3000 cc of blood. Massive hemothorax is more often due to penetrating than blunt trauma, but either injury may disrupt a major pulmonary or systemic vessel.

Pathophysiology: As blood accumulates within the pleural space, the lung on the affected side is compressed. If enough blood accumulates (rare), the mediastinum will be shifted away from the hemothorax. The inferior and superior vena cavae and the contralateral lung are compressed. Thus the on-going blood loss is complicated by hypoxemia.

Signs and symptoms of massive hemothorax are produced by both hypovolemia and respiratory compromise. The patient may be hypotensive from blood loss and compression of the heart or great veins. Anxiety and confusion are produced by hypovolemia and hypoxemia. Clinical signs of hypovolemic shock may be apparent. The neck veins are usually flat secondary to profound hypovolemia, but may *rarely* be distended due to mediastinal compression. Other signs of hemothorax include decreased breath sounds and dullness to percussion on the affected side. See Table 4–1 for a comparison of tension pneumothorax and hemothorax.

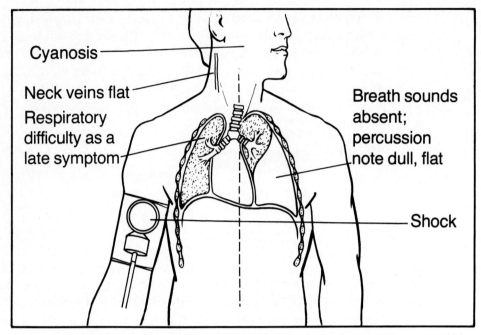

Cyanosis

Neck veins flat

Respiratory difficulty as a late symptom

Breath sounds absent; percussion note dull, flat

Shock

Figure 4-6. Physical findings of massive hemothorax.

Table 4-1 *Comparison of Tension Pneumothorax and Hemothorax*

	Tension pneumothorax	*Hemothorax*
Primary presenting symptom	Difficulty breathing, then shock	Shock, then difficulty breathing
Neck veins	Usually distended	Usually flat
Breath sounds	Decreased or absent on side of injury	Decreased or absent on side of injury
Percussion of chest	Hypertympanic	Dull
Tracheal deviation away from the side of the injury	May be present as a late sign	Usually not present

Management

1. Secure an airway.
2. Supply high-concentration oxygen.
3. Rapidly transport the patient to the appropriate hospital.

4. Provide aggressive volume replacement after IV insertion. Remember that the major problem in massive hemothorax is hemorrhagic shock.
5. Notify medical control.
6. Observe closely for the possible development of a tension hemopneumothorax, which would require acute chest decompression.
7. Although there is some controversy regarding the use of the antishock garment (PASG or MAST) in the treatment of chest injuries, they should probably be utilized.

Flail Chest

Flail chest occurs when three or more adjacent ribs are fractured in at least two places. The result is a segment of the chest wall which is not in continuity with the thorax. A lateral flail chest or anterior flail chest (sternal separation) may result. With posterior rib fractures, the heavy musculature usually prevents the occurrence of a flail segment. The flail segment moves with paradoxical motion relative to the rest of the chest wall (Figures 4–7 and 4–8). The force that is necessary to produce this injury also bruises the underlying lung tissue. This pulmonary contusion will also contribute to the hypoxia.

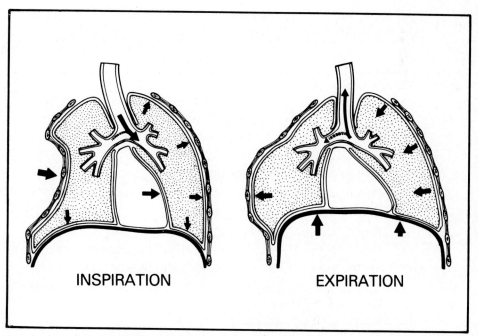

INSPIRATION   EXPIRATION

Figure 4–7. Pathophysiology of flail chest.

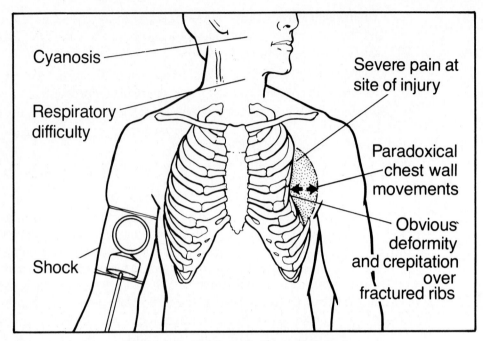

Cyanosis

Respiratory difficulty

Shock

Severe pain at site of injury

Paradoxical chest wall movements

Obvious deformity and crepitation over fractured ribs

Figure 4–8. Physical findings of flail chest.

The patient is at risk for the development of a hemothorax or pneumothorax. With a large flail segment, the patient may be in marked respiratory distress. Palpitation of the chest wall may reveal crepitus in addition to the abnormal respiratory motion.

Management

1. Ensure an airway.
2. Administer oxygen.
3. Assisted ventilation or intubation may be required. Remember that pneumothorax is commonly associated with a flail chest and chest decompression may be needed.
4. Rapid transport to the appropriate hospital.
5. Establish an IV. Attempt to limit fluid administration if appropriate, as volume overload may worsen the hypoxemia.
6. Stabilize the flail segment with manual pressure, then bulky dressings taped to the chest wall (Figure 4–9).
7. Notify medical control.
8. Monitor EKG. Associated myocardial trauma is frequent.

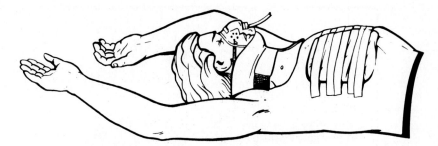

TAPE PAD IN PLACE, EXTENDING TAPE TO BOTH SIDES OF CHEST

Figure 4-9. Thoracic trauma.

Cardiac Tamponade

Cardiac tamponade is usually due to penetrating injury. The pericardial sac is an inelastic membrane that surrounds the heart. If blood collects rapidly between the heart and pericardium from a cardiac injury, the ventricles of the heart will be compressed. A small amount of pericardial blood may compromise cardiac filling. As the compression of the ventricles increases, the heart is less able to refill and cardiac output falls.

Diagnosis of cardiac tamponade classically relies on the triad of hypotension, distended neck veins, and muffled heart sounds. Muffled heart sounds may be very difficult to appreciate in the prehospital setting. The patient may have paradoxical pulse. If the patient loses his peripheral pulse during inspiration, this is suggestive of a paradoxical pulse and the presence of cardiac tamponade. The major differential diagnosis in the field is tension pneumothorax. With cardiac tamponade, the patient will be in shock with a midline trachea and equal breath sounds (Figure 4-10).

Management

1. Maintain airway and oxygen.
2. PASG (MAST).
3. Intravenous infusion of electrolyte solution may increase the filling of the heart and increase cardiac output.
4. This lesion is rapidly fatal and cannot readily be treated in the field. Load the patient and proceed to the appropriate hospital.
5. Notify medical control.

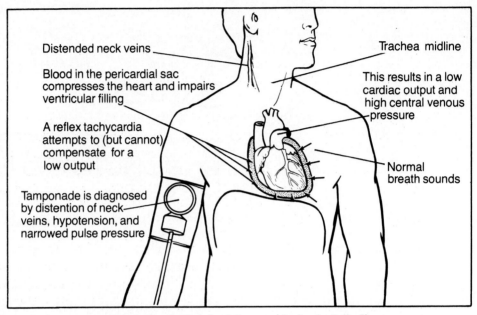

Distended neck veins

Blood in the pericardial sac
compresses the heart and impairs
ventricular filling

A reflex tachycardia
attempts to (but cannot)
compensate for a
low output

Tamponade is diagnosed
by distention of neck
veins, hypotension, and
narrowed pulse pressure

Trachea midline

This results in a low
cardiac output and
high central venous
pressure

Normal
breath sounds

**Figure 4–10. Pathophysiology and physical findings
of cardiac tamponade.**

Traumatic Aortic Rupture

Traumatic aortic rupture is the most common cause of sudden death in motor
vehicle accidents or falls from heights. Ninety percent of these patients die
immediately. For the survivors, salvage is feasible with prompt diagnosis and
surgery. Traumatic thoracic aortic tears are usually due to deceleration injury, with heart and aortic arch moving suddenly anteriorly, which transects
the aorta where it is fixed at the ligamentum arteriosum. Of the 10% who
do not exsanguinate promptly, the aortic tear will be contained temporarily
by surrounding tissues and the adventitia. However, this is temporary and
will usually rupture unless surgically repaired.

The diagnosis of a contained thoracic aortic laceration is impossible in the
field and may be missed even in the hospital. The history from the scene is
critically important since many of these patients have no obvious signs of chest
trauma. Information regarding damage to the car or steering wheel with a
deceleration injury or the height from which the patient fell are vital. Infrequently, the patient may present with upper-extremity hypertension and
diminished lower-extremity pulses.

Management: Management of patients with potential aortic tears includes:

1. Airway
2. Oxygen

3. Rapid transport to the appropriate hospital
4. IV fluids
5. Notify medical control

Tracheal or Bronchial Tree Injury

Tracheal or bronchial tree injury may be the result of penetrating or blunt trauma. Penetrating upper-airway injuries often have associated major vascular injuries and extensive tissue destruction. Blunt trauma may present with subtle findings. Blunt injury usually ruptures the trachea or mainstem bronchus near the carina. Presenting signs of blunt or penetrating injury include subcutaneous emphysema of the chest, face, or neck or an associated pneumothorax or hemothorax.

Management: Management of the airway with tracheal injuries may be quite difficult. Ideally, a cuffed endotracheal tube should be passed beyond the site of the rupture. However, this may not be feasible, and emergency surgical intervention may be needed to obtain an airway. Thus prompt transport to the hospital is important. Observing the patient for signs of a pneumothorax or hemothorax is also necessary.

Myocardial Contusion

Myocardial contusion is a potentially lethal lesion resulting from blunt chest injury. Blunt injury to the anterior chest is transmitted via the sternum to the heart, which lies immediately posterior to it (Figure 4–11). Cardiac injuries from this mechanism may include valvular rupture, pericardial tamponade, and cardiac rupture, but myocardial contusion most commonly occurs. This bruising of the heart is basically the same injury as an acute myocardial infarction and also presents with chest pain, dysrhythmia, or cardiogenic shock. In the field, cardiogenic shock cannot be distinguished from cardiac tamponade. The chest pain may be difficult to differentiate from the associated musculoskeletal discomfort that the patient also suffers as a result of the injury. All patients with blunt anterior chest trauma should be presumed to have a myocardial contusion.

Management

1. Administer oxygen.
2. Establish IV access.
3. Monitor EKG.
4. Treat dysrhythmias as they present.

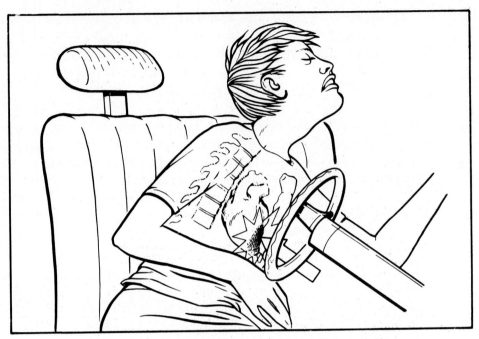

Figure 4-11. Pathophysiology of myocardial contusion.

Diaphragmatic Tears

Traumatic diaphragmatic tears may result from a severe blow to the abdomen. A sudden increase in intraabdominal pressure, such as a seat belt injury or kick to the abdomen, may tear the diaphragm and allow herniation of the abdominal organs into the thoracic cavity. This occurs more commonly on the left than the right, since the liver protects the right hemidiaphragm. Blunt trauma produces large radial tears in the diaphragm. Penetrating trauma may also produce holes in the diaphragm, but these tend to be small.

Traumatic diaphragmatic hernia is difficult to diagnose even in the hospital. The herniation of abdominal contents into the thoracic cavity may cause marked respiratory distress. On examination, the breath sounds may be diminished and infrequently, bowel sounds will be heard when the chest is auscultated. The abdomen may appear scaphoid if a large quantity of abdominal contents are in the chest.

Management

1. Ensure an airway.
2. Administer oxygen.
3. Transport the patient to the hospital.

4. Insert IV. Associated injuries are common and hypovolemia may occur.
5. Use of PASG (MAST) is probably contraindicated with suspected diaphragmatic rupture, as the trousers may increase the herniation of the abdominal organs into the chest and worsen the respiratory distress.
6. Notify medical control.

Esophageal Injury

Esophageal injury is usually produced by penetrating trauma. Management of associated trauma, including airway or vascular injuries, is generally more pressing than the esophageal injury. However, penetrating esophageal injury is lethal if unrecognized in the hospital.

Pulmonary Contusion

Pulmonary contusion is a common chest injury resulting from blunt trauma. This is basically a bruise of the lung which may produce marked hypoxemia. Management consists of intubation, if indicated, oxygen administration, transport, and IV insertion.

Other Chest Injuries

Impalement injuries of the chest may be caused by any penetrating object, usually a knife. As in other areas of the body, the object should not be removed in the field. Stabilize the object, ensure an airway, insert an IV, and transport the patient.

Traumatic asphyxia is an important set of physical findings. The term is a misnomer since the condition is not caused by asphyxia. The syndrome results from a severe compression injury to the chest, such as a steering wheel injury, conveyor belt injury, or compression of the chest under a heavy object. The sudden compression of the heart and mediastinum transmits this force to the capillaries of the neck and head. The victims appear similar to those of strangulation, with cyanosis and swelling of the head and neck. The tongue and lips are swollen, and cyanotic and conjunctival hemorrhage is evident. The skin below the level of the crush injury to the chest will be pink unless there are other problems.

Traumatic asphyxia indicates that the patient has suffered a severe blunt thoracic injury, and major thoracic injuries are likely to be present. Management includes (1) airway maintenance, (2) rapid transport, (3) IV access, and (4) treating other injuries.

Similarly, sternal fractures indicate that the patient has suffered marked blunt trauma to the anterior chest. These patients should be presumed to have a myocardial contusion. Diagnosis can be made by palpation.

A fracture of the scapula or first or second rib requires a large force. The incidence of associated major thoracic vascular injury is high, and these patients should be promptly transported after an airway, and oxygen have been started. Insert IV en route.

Simple pneumothorax may result from blunt or penetrating trauma. Fractured ribs are the usual cause in blunt trauma. This is caused by accumulation of air within the potential space between the visceral and parietal pleura. The lung may be totally or partially collapsed as the air continues to accrue in the thoracic cavity. In a healthy patient this should not acutely compromise ventilation if a tension pneumothorax does not evolve. Patients with less respiratory reserve may not tolerate even a simple pneumothorax well.

Diagnosis of a pneumothorax is based on pleuritic chest pain, dyspnea, decreased breath sounds on the affected side, and hypertympany to percussion. Close observation is required in anticipation of the patient developing a pneumothorax.

Simple rib fracture is the most frequent injury to the chest. If the patient does not have an associated pneumothorax or hemothorax, the major problem is pain. This pain will prohibit the patient from breathing adequately. On palpation, the area of rib fracture will be tender and may be unstable. Give oxygen and monitor for pneumothorax or hemothorax while encouraging the patient to breathe deeply.

Summary

Chest injuries are common and often life-threatening in the patient with multiple injuries. The primary goals in treating the patient with chest trauma are (1) ensuring an airway while protecting the cervical spine, (2) high-concentration oxygen, (3) needle decompression of the chest if needed, (4) stabilization on a backboard, (5) IV access, (6) EKG monitoring, and (7) PASG (MAST) application. These are often "load and go" patients.

The thoracic injuries discussed are life threatening but treatable by prompt intervention and transport to the appropriate hospital. It is mandatory that the injuries presented are recognized in the field and treated appropriately to salvage these patients.

Chapter 5

Shock

Raymond L. Fowler, M.D., F.A.C.E.P.

"Shock" is a condition of inadequate tissue perfusion. Shock may occur for many reasons, such as trauma, fluid loss, and heart problems. The purpose of this chapter is to discuss the shock states caused by trauma, how to diagnose them, and how to intervene in the field.

Normal tissue perfusion requires four intact mechanisms:

1. Functioning pump: the heart
2. Adequate volume of fluid: blood and plasma
3. Adequate air exchange to get oxygen into the blood
4. Intact vascular system to deliver blood throughout the body

The many clinical shock syndromes arise from the failure of one or more of these mechanisms:

1. Failure of the pump
   a. Cardiogenic shock
      (1) Myocardial contusion

(2)   Myocardial infarction (heart attack)
   b.   Pericardial tamponade
2.   Lack of fluid volume
   a.   Blood loss (hemorrhagic shock)
   b.   Fluid loss
      (1)   Burns
      (2)   Vomiting or diarrhea
3.   Lack of adequate air exchange
   a.   Airway obstruction
   b.   Open pneumothorax
   c.   Tension pneumothorax
   d.   Toxic gas inhalation
4.   Lack of adequate vascular system
   a.   Leaking vascular system: results in low volume
   b.   Dilated vascular system: results in high space, thus *relative* lack of volume
      (1)   Spinal shock
      (2)   Anaphylactic shock
      (3)   Septic shock
      (4)   Neurogenic shock (simple fainting)
   c.   Obstructed vascular system
      (1)   Tension pneumothorax
      (2)   Pericardial tamponade
      (3)   Pulmonary embolus

Decreased tissue perfusion results in insufficient oxygen and glucose supply to the cells. The result is that energy is not produced in sufficient quantity to maintain cellular function. The various cells of the body become injured due to the shock state. If this state of inadequate perfusion continues, the cells eventually become injured to the point that they cannot repair themselves even if oxygen and glucose are restored—at this point shock is said to be "irreversible." This state of "irreversible shock" is the main reason that the mortality rate goes up dramatically after the "golden hour."

"Shock" is therefore a condition in which poor tissue perfusion may severely and possibly irreversibly damage the organs of the body.

Types of Shock Commonly Seen in Prehospital Trauma Patients

1.   Mechanical ("obstructive")
2.   Hypovolemic

    a.   Absolute hypovolemia (hemorrhage)
    b.   Relative hypovolemia (spinal)

There are notable differences in the appearances of these conditions. Since interventions depend on the type of shock, it is critical that the paramedic be aware of the signs and symptoms that accompany each condition.

Mechanical Shock

Any shock state caused by the mechanical obstruction of either the airway or the vascular system can be termed "mechanical shock." This is a useful concept because removing the obstruction *immediately* relieves the shock state. The patient will show almost immediate recovery as long as irreversible damage has not occurred.

Airway Obstruction: Rivaling hemorrhagic shock as the most common form of traumatic shock, airway obstruction causes death from hypoxia within a matter of minutes. This is why airway evaluation is the first step in the primary survey. Airway obstruction is one of only two reasons to intervene before finishing the primary survey. Removing the obstruction will immediately relieve the cause of the shock state and the patient should improve immediately.

Common traumatic forms of vascular obstructive shock are tension pneumothorax and pericardial tamponade. In the normal resting state, the heart pumps *out* about 5 L of blood per minute. This means, of course, that the heart takes *in* about 5 L of blood per minute. Any traumatic condition that slows or prevents venous return causes shock by lowering cardiac output and thus tissue perfusion.

The *tension pneumothorax* is so named because of the high air tension (pressure) that develops in the pleural space. This positive pressure on the superior and inferior vena cava and right heart prevents venous filling of the heart and thus causes a decrease in cardiac output. Shifting of the mediastinal structures adds to this effect.

Symptoms of tension pneumothorax include signs of hypoperfusion, respiratory distress, distended neck veins, deviated trachea, diminished breath sounds on the affected side, hypertympany to percussion, cyanosis, and altered sensorium. Cyanosis, altered sensorium, or loss of peripheral pulses (hypotension) may be indications for needle decompression of the pleural space. Needle decompression is done only if permitted by local protocol and state law and with an order by on-line medical control.

Cardiac tamponade occurs when blood, clots, fluid, or restrictive tissue squeeze the heart and prevent the heart from filling. The net result is that the heart cannot fill and cardiac output falls. Distended neck veins, loss of the pulse during inspiration, signs of hypoperfusion, bilateral breath sounds,

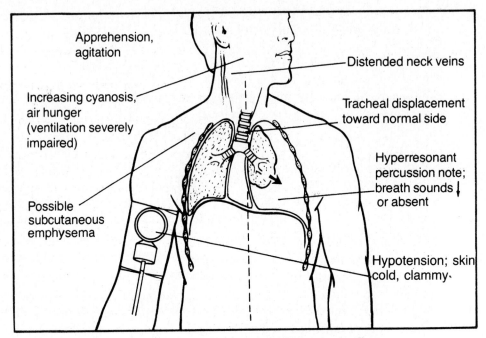

Figure 5–1. Physical findings of tension pneumothorax.

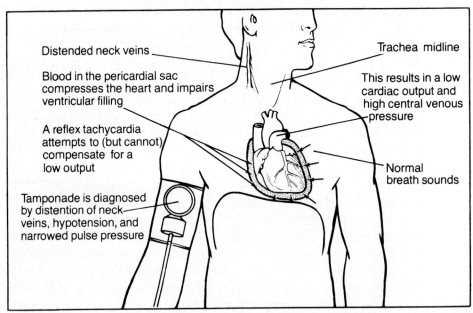

**Figure 5–2. Pathophysiology and physical findings
of cardiac tamponade.**

and evidence of chest trauma are clues to the presence of tamponade. Needle aspiration of the pericardial space may give immediate relief from these symptoms, but this is not a field procedure. Field interventions for pericardial tamponade are MAST (PASG), and IV fluids (to increase filling of the heart), oxygen, and rapid transport to an appropriate hospital where pericardial decompression can be done.

Both forms of vascular obstructive shock give signs of *hypoperfusion*. The brain senses that there is not enough cardiac output, and sends messages down the spinal cord to the adrenal medulla, which releases catecholamines (epinephrine and norepinephrine). The circulating catecholamines cause tachycardia, diaphoresis, and vasoconstriction. The vasoconstriction shunts blood away from the skin to the vital organs, causing an initial rise in the blood pressure and causing the skin to be pale. Decreased perfusion causes weakness, thirst, decreased LOC (confusion, restlessness, or combativeness), worsening of pallor, and hypotension.

Hypovolemic Shock (Hemmorhagic Shock)

Loss of blood volume from injury is called hemorrhage. Major volume loss resulting in shock symptoms is called hemorrhagic shock. Remember, burn shock is also hypovolemic (fluid loss) but is not commonly seen in the prehospital setting because it takes several hours to develop.

The amount of volume that the blood vessels could hold is many liters more than actually flows through the system. It is the action of the sympathetic nervous system in a "steady state" that contracts the vascular space and maintains blood pressure high enough to perfuse vital organs. If blood volume is lost, "sensors" in the aorta and brain signal the adrenal gland to secrete catecholamines, which act through the sympathetic nervous system to cause vasoconstriction and thus further shrink the vascular space and maintain perfusion pressure. If the blood loss is minor, the sympathetics can shrink the space enough to maintain blood pressure. If the loss is critical or continuous, the space cannot be shrunk enough to maintain blood pressure and hypotension occurs. Understanding the effects of catecholamines is important because many of the symptoms of hypovolemic shock are due to the effects of catecholamines. Catecholamines cause the heart to beat fast (tachycardia), stimulate certain sweat glands (diaphoresis), and cause vasoconstriction (skin becomes pale). Therefore, what we commonly call "shock" is in fact a cluster of symptoms due to both poor blood flow and the catecholamines secreted in response to that poor blood flow. The order of development of symptoms in shock is usually:

Weakness: caused by tissue hypoxia and acidosis

Thirst: caused by hypovolemia

Pallor: caused by catecholamine-induced vasoconstriction

Tachycardia: caused by catecholamine's effect on the heart

Tachypnea: (respiratory rate > 24 per minute) caused by acidosis and hypoxia

Diaphoresis: caused by catecholamine's effect on sweat glands

Decreased urinary output: caused by hypovolemia

Hypotension: hypovolemia

Altered sensorium: (confusion, restlessness, combativeness, coma): caused by decreased cerebral perfusion

As shock continues, the prolonged hypoxia causes anaerobic metabolism. This produces metabolic acidosis from large amounts of lactic and pyruvic acids. As acidosis becomes more and more severe, it causes loss of response to catecholamines with precipitous drop in blood pressure. Eventually, the hypoxia and acidosis cause ventricular fibrillation and death.

Classification of Hypovolemic Shock

Early shock: loss of approximately 15 to 25% of the blood volume. This is associated with only slight to moderate tachycardia, pallor, narrowed pulse pressure, thirst, weakness, and delayed capillary refill. *Hypotension is not usually a symptom.*

Late shock: loss of approximately 30 to 45% of the blood volume. This is associated with hypotension and *all* the other symptoms of hypovolemic shock listed above.

Test for Early Shock—Capillary Blanch Test: Low blood volume and catecholamine-induced vasoconstriction cause decreased perfusion of the capillary bed in the skin. Press on the palm of the hand or just proximal to the fingernail. In a child, squeeze the whole foot. The test is suspicious for early shock if the blanched area lasts longer than 2 seconds. This is an example of a test that means something if it is positive but means nothing if it is negative. If capillary refill is delayed, you have strong evidence of early shock. *If capillary refill is normal, you have not ruled out early shock.*

Remember, it is blood that gives the body a pink color. Oxygenated blood is bright red; deoxygenated blood is more purple in color. It is blood that turns "blue" in the setting of hypoxia. If the patient is bleeding severely, there may not be enough blood present within the vascular system to give the patient a cyanotic color in the setting of hypoxia. So, do not depend on cyanosis to tell you a patient is hypoxic: *Give oxygen to all critical trauma patients!*

High Space Shock (Relative Hypovolemia)

As mentioned above, the amount of volume that the blood vessels *could* hold is many liters more than the normal blood volume. Again, it is the action of the sympathetic nervous system in a "steady state" that keeps a portion of the vascular bed constricted in order to maintain perfusion. Anything that disturbs the influence of the sympathetic nervous system on the arterioles may result in loss of this normal vasoconstriction, thus creating a vascular space that is much "too large." In this case the 5 L of blood will be insufficient to maintain blood pressure and tissue perfusion. Such a condition, causing the vascular space to be too large for a normal amount of blood, is called *high space shock*. Although there are several types of high space shock (see the outline on page 105), the only one commonly seen in trauma patients is spinal shock.

Spinal Shock: Control of vasoconstriction of the necessary vessels to maintain blood pressure is through messages sent down the spinal cord from the higher centers. If the spinal cord is injured, no messages are sent to cause vasoconstriction; thus all the vessels remain open and the blood pools in the body and does not return to the heart. When the sensors in the aorta and great vessels detect a drop in blood pressure, there is no way to send messages to the adrenal glands to secrete catecholamines. The pooling of blood continues and blood pressure falls to shock levels. Eventually, acidosis from anaerobic metabolism causes cardiac arrest.

Symptoms of Spinal Shock

1. *Hypotension* (blood pressure <100 mmHg systolic): caused by loss of circulating blood volume (pooled in the body).
2. *Confusion:* caused by decreased perfusion of the brain. This is not as pronounced as would be expected. The victim is usually not restless or combative because he is paralyzed from his spinal injury.
3. *Weakness:* caused by paralysis from spinal injury worsened by hypoxia and acidosis.
4. *Tachypnea* (respiration > 24 breaths per minute): caused by hypoxia and acidosis. This is a late sign. Breathing is usually diaphramatic only, since the intercostal muscles are usually paralyzed.

The clinical presentation of spinal shock differs from hemorrhagic shock in that there is no catecholamine release, thus no pallor, tachycardia, or sweating. The victim will have a decreased blood pressure but the pulse will be normal or slow, the skin warm, dry, and pink. The victim will often be more alert than would be expected for his blood pressure.

Treatment of Shock

Begin with the routine treatment priorities. They were developed to help you pick up critical situations in the correct order of importance.

1. Assess the **airway** while controlling the cervical spine and checking the initial LOC. If there is an airway obstruction, you must interrupt the primary survey long enough to clear the airway. This takes care of airway obstructive shock.
2. Assess **breathing.**
3. Assess **circulation.**
4. Stop major bleeding.
5. Determine transport decision and critical interventions.

At this point you should have enough information to diagnose shock. If shock is present, you must expose the victim and perform the MAST survey. Then transfer to a backboard and begin field interventions. Most field treatment of shock will be done in the ambulance on the way to the hospital. Shock is a "load and go" condition.

The treatment of shock is directed toward the causes of the problem:

1. Oxygen must be administered by a high-flow delivery system. This is begun by a second rescuer during the primary survey. Use a non-rebreather mask with an attached reservoir; nasal cannulas are reserved only for those who will not tolerate a mask. Unconscious patients should have their airways secured with an endotracheal tube or EGTA.
2. The patient must be placed in the horizontal or even Trendelenburg position. Place the victim on a spine board. You may elevate the foot of the board.
3. The size of the vascular space must be decreased; this is accomplished by using the MAST (PASG).
4. The volume in the vascular space must be increased; this is done with the use of intravenous fluids (Ringer's lactate or normal saline) through multiple large-bore catheters.

The "treatment" of shock certainly includes the rapid mobilization of the patient to an appropriate hospital to manage the problem. This transport is rapid, but with careful monitoring of the patient, including frequent repeat surveys. Do not delay to start IVs at the scene. Get the MAST on and move!

Keep the patient warm. It takes energy to maintain a normal temperature, and it takes oxygen for energy; the patient in shock has no oxygen to spare.

Monitor vital signs and level of consciousness at least every 5 minutes. The best way to do this is to repeat the entire primary survey—*all the steps*—every 5 minutes.

Antishock Garment*

Principle

No one has proven how the antishock garment works, but the most likely mechanism is an increase in peripheral resistance by way of circumferential compression. The important thing is that they do work. They improve blood pressure and cerebral circulation in the hemorrhagic and spinal shock victim. They may also be used to tamponade bleeding and immobilize fractures of the pelvis and lower extremities.

Indications for Use in Trauma

1. Systolic blood pressure less than 80 mmHg
2. Shocklike symptoms and systolic blood pressure of 100 mmHg or less
3. Pelvic fracture
4. Fracture of lower extremity
5. Spinal shock
6. Massive abdominal bleeding

Contraindications

1. Pulmonary edema
2. Abdominal injury with protruding viscera (may use leg compartments)
3. Pregnancy (may use leg compartments)
4. Diaphragmatic hernia (may use leg compartments)

Head injuries do not produce shock except in a very late state of deterioration. If a patient with a head injury develops symptoms of shock, he prob-

*Also known as military antishock trousers (MAST) or pneumatic antishock garment (PASG).

ably has hypovolemic shock from internal or external blood loss, or he may have spinal shock. This is not a contraindication of the use of the antishock garment. The use of the antishock garment improves cerebral circulation, decreases cerebral ischemia, and inhibits the development of cerebral edema.

Thoracic injuries also are not a contraindication to the use of MAST, although certain preliminary and nonconclusive data suggest that patient outcome *may* not be improved by the use of MAST in the setting of penetrating thoracic trauma. These data are new and untested, so until further studies are done, you may use the MAST in the setting of thoracic trauma. It would be prudent to inflate only until the systolic blood pressure is raised to the range 100 to 110 mmHg.

Use of the Antishock Garment

The technique of applying and removing the garment is covered in Basic Skill Station 7. Three variations of the garment are available:

1. Plain garment with no pressure gauges
2. Garment with one gauge that can be rotated among the three compartments
3. Garment with three gauges, one for each compartment.

For trauma use the plain garment. It is superior since the only gauge you need is a blood pressure cuff on the patient's arm. The danger with having extra gauges is that one tends to become more concerned with the pressure in the suit than the pressure in the patient.

Important Points in Use of the Antishock Garment

1. Application of the garment takes 1 to 2 minutes and immediately improves the patient's condition. Note the time of inflation on the run report.
2. Transportation of a patient with the garment inflated will minimize displacement of pelvic and other fractures. If a traction splint is required, apply it after the garment is in place and then inflate the garment.
3. Once the garment has been placed on a patient, it should not be deflated until there has been adequate fluid resuscitation and the patient is in the hospital under a physician's care. The only exception to this is the development of pulmonary edema. If the patient develops pulmonary edema the garment should be completely deflated immediately. The

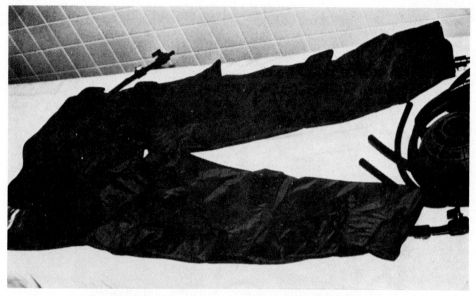

**Figure 5–3(a). Military anti-shock trousers (MAST)—
no pressure gauges.**

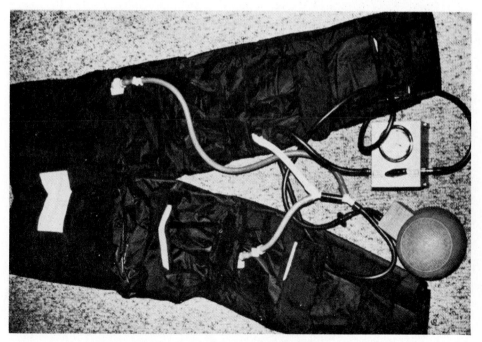

**Figure 5–3(b). Military anti-shock trousers (MAST)—
one pressure gauge.**

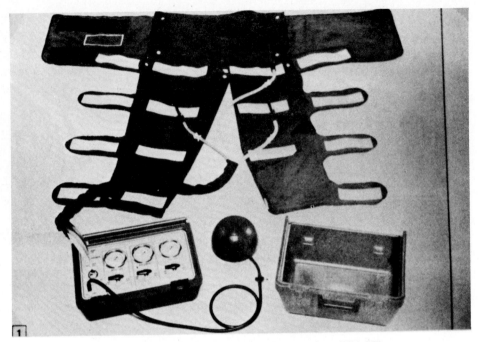

Figure 5–3(c). Military anti-shock trousers (MAST)—three pressure gauges.

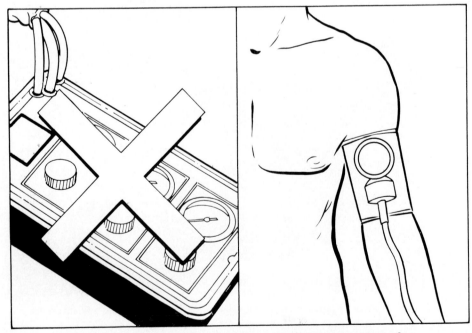

Figure 5–4. Blood pressure gauge and air pressure gauge for MAST. The pressure in the victim is what is important!

correct procedure for deflation is to deflate each compartment separately (beginning with the abdomen) while monitoring the blood pressure constantly. A blood pressure drop of 5 mmHg signals a halt to deflation until more fluid can be replaced. The greatest danger associated with utilization of the suit is rapid removal by persons unaccustomed to its use.

Summary

Shock is a critical condition that occurs just before death. In the past, treatment has tended to be "too little and too late." However, successful resuscitation is almost always possible if careful, alert evaluation is teamed with aggressive fluid replacement and vascular space control early in the shock syndrome.

Chapter 6

Spinal Trauma

James J. Augustine, M.D.

We have all immobilized C-spines enough to do it in our sleep, right? We know that it takes about $1.5 million to support a spinal-cord-injury victim for a lifetime. The question is: Which one of the victims that you as an EMT treat, who have fallen, wrecked, been beaten, shot, or stabbed, will you need to be supporting for the rest of their life? The answer is: You don't know! Even after years of research, no formula has been devised to predict who has the unstable fracture or cord injury that will be aggravated by improper packaging. The only safe course of action is constant suspicion of spinal injury combined with proper patient handling and packaging. In this chapter we review this process.

Normal Anatomy and Physiology

Spinal Column

It is important to begin by differentiating the spinal column from the spinal cord. The spinal column is a flexible girder that supports the body in an upright position, allowing us to use our extremities in a more worthwhile fashion. It also serves as a rigid tube around the delicate spinal cord. The column is composed of 33 bony vertebrae: 7 cervical, 12 thoracic, 5 lumbar, and the remainder fused together as the posterior portion of the pelvis (sacrum and coccyx). The bones, each separated by a fibrous disc, are aligned in an S-shaped curve. This curve has inflection points in the C5-6 and T12-L1 areas, making these areas the most susceptible to injury.

Spinal Cord

The spinal cord is an electrical conduit. It is an extension of the brainstem which continues down to the level of the first lumbar vertebra. The cord is 10 to 13 mm in diameter and is suspended in the vertebral foramen. The cord is composed of specific bundles of nerve tracts which are arranged in a predictable manner. These arrangements cause the various clinical presentations of spinal cord injuries. Input to and output from the spinal cord occurs along

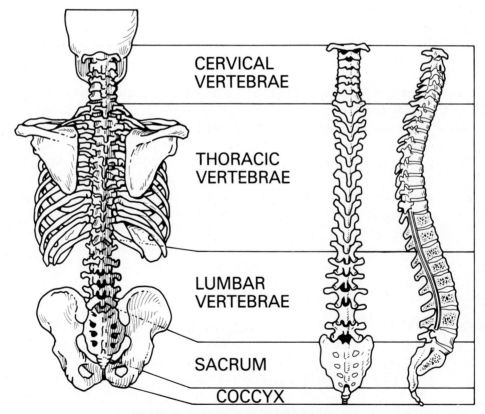

Figure 6–1. Anatomy of spinal column.

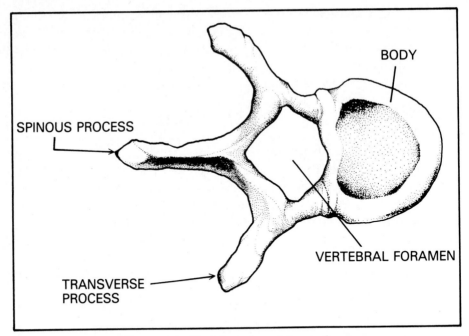

SPINOUS PROCESS

BODY

VERTEBRAL FORAMEN

TRANSVERSE PROCESS

Figure 6–2. Vertebra viewed from above.

the nerve roots that exit at each vertebral level. The roots lie adjacent to the intervertebral discs and the lateral portions of the vertebrae, making the nerve roots themselves prone to injury with trauma to these areas of the spinal column.

The spinal cord is assessed by testing its motor, sensory, and reflex functions. Motor levels are more predictable anatomically than sensory levels, but sensory levels are easier to determine in the conscious patient in the prehospital setting. Reflexes are helpful for distinguishing complete from partial spinal cord injuries, but are best left for emergency department management. The spinal cord is also an integrating center for the autonomic nervous system, which assists in controlling heart rate, vascular tone, and blood flow to the skin. Injury to this component of the spinal cord results in "spinal shock."

Spinal Injuries

Spinal Column

Sudden deceleration, producing flexion, extension, or lateral stresses of the head or trunk may damage the bony or connective tissue components of the spinal column. Although most common in motor vehicle accidents, column damage occurs from falls, recreational activities, electrical shock, and falling

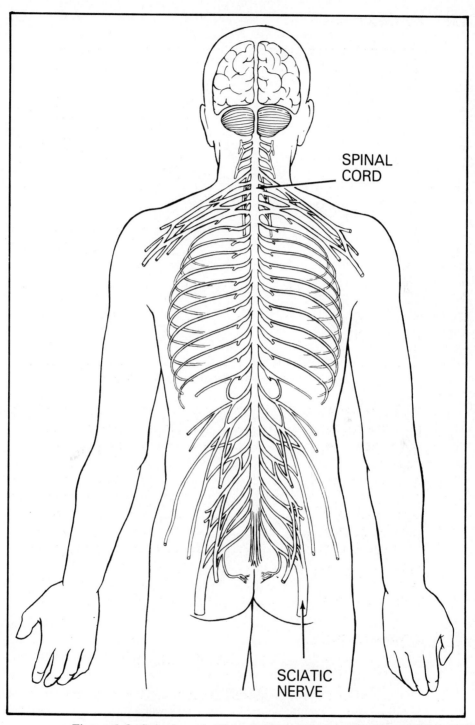

SPINAL
CORD

SCIATIC
NERVE

Figure 6–3. Spinal cord. The spinal cord is a continuation
of the central nervous system outside of the skull.

123

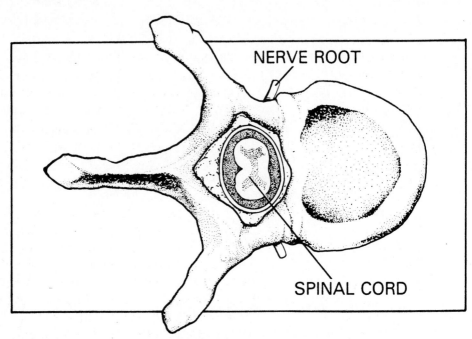

Figure 6–4. Relationship of spinal cord to vertebra.

objects. Any of these mechanisms of injury merit spinal column immobilization. Motor vehicle accidents most commonly cause rapid flexion/extension injuries, with the cervical spine being at highest risk. Falls or recreational activities mainly place the cervical and lumbar areas at risk. Electrical shock produces violent muscle spasm and then a fall, with unpredictable risks to all areas. Elderly persons with wear-and-tear changes to the bony column and supporting connective tissue are at greater risk for injury and merit immobilization for lesser degrees of trauma.

Injury to the spinal column manifests in several ways. Pain is the most common symptom, but it may be completely absent or unnoticed by the patient. Local muscle spasm may occur. Injury to individual nerve roots occur and results in localized pain, paralysis, or sensory dysfunction. Spinal cord injury is of greatest concern, but it is important to remember that only 14% of all *column* injuries have evidence of spinal *cord* damage. In the cervical spine it is much more prevalent, with almost 40% of column injuries having cord damage. Conversely, only 63% of spinal cord injuries have evidence of spinal column damage. The unconscious trauma victim carries a higher risk (15 to 20%) of spinal column and cord damage, and thus should be immediately and consistently immobilized.

Spinal Cord

Cord injury results in a defect in the signal conducting function, manifesting as a loss of motor function and reflexes, loss or change in sensation, and/or spinal shock. The delicate structure of the nerve tracts in the cord make it very sensitive to any form of trauma. Primary damage occurs with the direct injury itself. Secondary damage occurs from damage to blood vessels, swelling, compression of the cord from surrounding hemorrhage, hypotension, or generalized hypoxia. Since primary injury cannot be prevented by the EMT, all efforts are directed at preventing secondary damage through meticulous packaging of the victim and attention to the ABCs.

Spinal shock is the malfunction of the autonomic nervous system in regulating vascular tone and cardiac output. Classically, this means that a victim is hypotensive, with normal skin color and temperature and an inappropriately low heart rate. Normally, blood pressure is maintained by the controlled release of catecholamines from the adrenal glands. Catecholamines cause constriction of the vascular bed and increase heart rate and strength of contraction (they also stimulate sweat glands). Sensors in the aortic arch and cartoid arteries monitor the blood pressure and, through the brain and spinal cord, signal the adrenal glands to release catecholamines to keep the blood pressure in a normal range. In *hemorrhagic shock,* these sensors detect the hypovolemic state and compensate by constricting the vascular bed and speeding the heart rate. This is accomplished by release of high levels of catecholamines, resulting in pallor, tachycardia, and sweating. The mechanism of shock from spinal cord injury is just the opposite. There is no blood loss, but there is also *no* signal going to the adrenals (the cable is out), so *no* catecholamines are released. The vascular bed dilates, blood pools, and the blood pressure cannot be maintained. The brain cannot correct this because it cannot get the message to the adrenal glands. The patient is not vasoconstricted and does not have tachycardia or sweating because he has no catecholamines to cause those signs. Since spinal shock is caused by vasodilation it responds to antishock trousers (which work by circumferential compression) or by infusion of vasopressors (dopamine or norepineprine). The danger of using vasopressors is that the victim may have both spinal shock and hemorrhagic shock. Due to the loss of sensation and muscle tone in the abdomen, it is very easy to miss abdominal bleeding in a patient with a cord injury. The patient with spinal shock cannot show the signs of pallor, tachycardia, and sweating because the cord injury prevents release of catecholamines. Spinal shock is a diagnosis of exclusion, after all other potential causes of shock have been ruled out. In the prehospital setting this is difficult, since these are often victims of multiple trauma and have inconclusive abdominal examinations due to sensory loss and flaccid abdominal muscles. In the field it is wiser to treat spinal shock the same as hemorrhagic shock, with MAST and IV fluids.

Spinal cord injury is usually devastating, with approximately 50% dying, 25% having permanent neurologic dysfunction, and 25% having little or no permanent sequelae. Of the average 12,000 cord injuries per year, 56% involve motor vehicle accidents (including pedestrians), 19% falls, 12% penetrating wounds, 7% recreational activities, and the remaining 6% from all other causes. Injury to the cord occurs in about 10% of all multiple-trauma victims, and in 15 to 20% of those with serious head injury.

Patient Management

Preparation for managing spinal column or cord injury can begin en route to the emergency. On dispatch to the scene of a motor vehicle accident, fall, explosion, head injury, or neck injury, the initial immobilizing device should be prepared and taken to the victim. This device (rigid extrication collar) can be placed on the victim as airway assessment is being made. These one- or two-piece collars are not definitive devices for cervical spine control, but should be used only as a reminder that cervical immobilization is necessary, and to prevent gross neck movement. In general, any patient with an injury above the clavicles should be treated for potential cervical spine injury. Suspect thoracic and lumbar spine injuries from sudden deceleration accidents or direct torso injuries. Victims who have had seizures or who are "found unconscious" should also be managed as if they had spinal injury.

In all cases, the most easily applied and readily available method of cervical immobilization is with your hands or knees. They should be placed to stabilize the neck in relation to the long axis of the spinal column. "Pulling traction" is *not* a prehospital option, as it will result in further instability of any spinal column injury. The hands may be supplemented by the use of an immobilization collar as described above. The hands are removed only when the head and spinal column has been definitely immobilized on a spinal board with an attached immobilization device.

Patient management then proceeds with initial assessment and interventions. In the critically unstable victim, rapid extrication may be necessary before spinal column immobilization can be performed. This form of extrication is used in victims whose risk/benefit ratio favors rapid removal from the vehicle or structure. This occurs when the vehicle or structure is in danger of fire, explosion, or collapse or when the victim's vital signs or clinical condi-

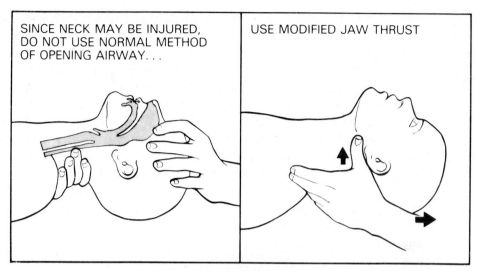

SINCE NECK MAY BE INJURED, DO NOT USE NORMAL METHOD OF OPENING AIRWAY...

USE MODIFIED JAW THRUST

Figure 6–5. Modified jaw thrust.

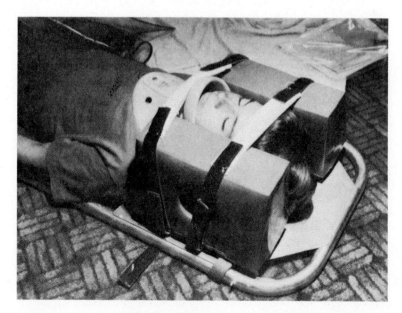

Figure 6–6. Spine board with rigid extrication collar and padded immobilization device. Collars do not give adequate lateral support—use padded immobilization device also.

tion is unstable and will be worsened during routine immobilization and removal. Rapid extrication requires multiple rescuers, who remove the victim along the long axis of the body, using the hands to maintain cervical immobilization (see Basic Skill Station 4).

Routine removal involves the use of spinal boards for total spinal column immobilization. Short boards or their adaptations (KED or XP-1) are used in sitting patients to provide the initial immobilization of the thoracic and cervical spinal column and to facilitate the movement of the patient onto a long backboard. Definitive immobilization occurs when the body is strapped securely to the board, with cushions (Bashaw device or similar secured cushion device), blanket, or towel rolls maintaining the head and cervical spine in line with the rest of the spinal cord. Sandbags have been used for head immobilization and perform well when the victim is supine. However, if the board is tilted or the victim and board are rotated (as to prevent aspiration when victim vomits), the weight of the sandbags may cause a large degree of head movement. Lighter-weight bulky objects, such as towel rolls, blanket rolls, or head cushions, are a better tool for this job. When applied properly, these devices allow removal of the collar and observation of the neck. Cervical spine immobilization is achieved only when the *body* is also securely strapped to the backboard. Failure to strap the head *or* the body adequately will allow movement of the neck. Total body immobilization is probably best

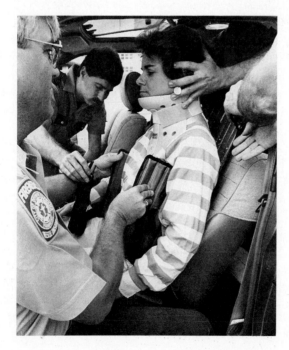

Figure 6–7. "KED® BEING APPLIED TO A SITTING VICTIM."

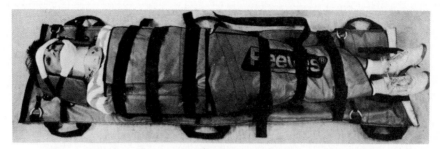

Figure 6-8. A victim immobilized on a Reeve's Sleeve. The arms can be positioned inside the vinyl panels, between the panels and the straps, or outside the panels and the straps.

accomplished by use of a long backboard and a Reeve's Sleeve or Miller Body Splint.

Immobilization must occasionally be performed in less conventional circumstances. These include: closed space or water rescue, victims in a prone or standing position, pediatric patients, and patients with disfiguring or penetrating neck wounds. Closed-space rescues are performed in a manner appropriate for the clinical condition of the patient. The only general rules that can be applied to these rescues are to prevent gross cervical spine movement and to move victims in line with the long axis of the body. Water rescues are again performed, moving the patient in line, preventing gross cervical movement. When the rescuers are in a stable position for immobilizing the victim, the backboard is floated under the victim and the victim is then secured and removed from the water.

Prone and standing victims are immobilized in a manner that minimizes spinal column movement, ending with the victim in the conventional supine position. Prone victims are log-rolled onto a long board with careful coordination of head and chest rescuers. Prone victims can also be immobilized using adaptations of the long board, such as the Miller Body Splint. Standing victims may be strapped to the long board while upright and then lowered to the supine position, or may be carefully lowered to the sitting position on a long board and then even more carefully supported as they are extended back to the supine position.

Pediatric patients are difficult to manage using the conventional collars, which, in addition, may frighten the child and compromise the airway. It is therefore best to assume that initial immobilization will be with the rescuer's hands, and that the use of cushions or towel rolls is the most consistent and flexible approach on an appropriate board or device. The Clark Pediatric Unit is an excellent device for immobilizing small children.

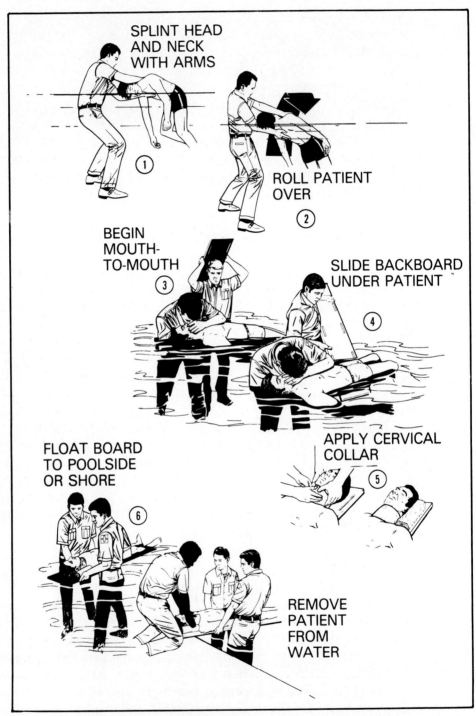

Figure 6–9. Extricating suspected diving accident victim.

Victims with penetrating or disfiguring wounds of the neck or lower face also require more flexibility in their immobilization. Cervical collars will prevent continued examination of the wound site and they may compromise the airway in wounds with expanding hematomas or subcutaneous air. If the mandible is fractured, the collar may again cause airway compromise. Therefore, in this class of victims it may be wise to avoid collars, using manual stabilization and then head cushion devices or blanket rolls for cervical immobilization.

Trauma victims with paralysis or spinal shock have lost vascular control and thus cannot control blood flow to the skin. They may lose heat rapidly. Unless the weather is very warm, they should be covered to prevent hypothermia.

Field Evaluation of Spinal Cord Function

All trauma victims are evaluated in the same manner by way of the priority plan. Evaluation of spinal cord function is part of the neurological exam. The neurological exam (except for level of consciousness) is performed in the secondary survey. This often means that it is done after the victim is loaded into the ambulance. For this reason all victims of multiple trauma are treated as if they had a spinal injury until such an injury can be ruled out. The neurological exam has already been covered in Chapter 2. To review: The exam of peripheral neurological function is kept brief and simple. If the conscious patient can move his fingers and toes, the motor nerves are intact. If the conscious patient has normal sensation in his fingers and toes, the sensory nerves are intact. Anything less than normal sensation (tingling or decreased sensation) is suspicious for cord injury. The unconscious victim may withdraw if you pinch his fingers and toes. If so, you have demonstrated intact motor and sensory nerves and thus an intact cord. Flaccid paralysis, even in the unconscious head injury victim, usually means cord injury. These are important findings; document them.

Airway Control and Spinal Immobilization

When the rescuer performs spinal immobilization in any manner, the patient loses some of his ability to maintain his own airway. The rescuer must then assume this responsibility until the patient has a controlled airway or has the spinal column cleared and is released from the immobilizing equipment. This is particularly critical in children, who have a greater potential for vomiting and aspiration following a traumatic injury.

Airway manipulations in the trauma victim require careful consideration. Current research indicates that any airway intervention will cause some movement of the spinal column. In line, manual stabilization is the most effective manner for minimizing this movement. Cervical collars do *little* to prevent movement. Nasotracheal, orotracheal, or cricothyroid intubation all induce bony movement. The priority plan should include airway control with *manual* immobilization, using the method which the individual provider is most skilled at performing. In weighing the risks and benefits of each airway procedure, recall that the risk of dying with an uncontrolled airway is greater than the risk of inducing spinal cord damage using a careful approach to intubation.

Summary

Spinal cord injury is a devastating sequelae of modern-day trauma. Unstable or incomplete damage to the spinal column or cord is not predictable, and therefore trauma victims who are unconscious or have any mechanism of injury affecting the head, neck, or trunk should have spinal immobilization performed. Once immobilized, the rescuer is responsible for controlling the victim's airway and must be prepared at all times to intervene should the victim vomit or have evidence of airway compromise.

Chapter 7

Head Trauma

Paul S. Auerbach, M.D.

Approximately 40% of serious trauma victims have central nervous system (CNS) injuries. This group has a death rate twice as high (35% versus 17%) as that of victims without CNS injuries. It has been estimated that head injuries account for 25% of all trauma deaths and up to one-half of all motor vehicle fatalities. As with other injuries, prompt and organized evaluation and treatment give the patient the greatest chance of complete recovery. To manage the head-injured victim most effectively, the rescuer should have a working knowledge of the basic anatomy and physiology of the head and brain. Head injuries may represent bruising of the brain tissue with severe swelling, injured blood vessels with bleeding and increased intracranial pressure, or penetrating injuries of the skull which directly damage brain tissue. *The rescuer must always assume that a serious head injury is accompanied by an injury to the cervical spine and spinal cord.*

Anatomy of the Head

The head (excluding the face and facial structures) includes the following:

1. Scalp

133

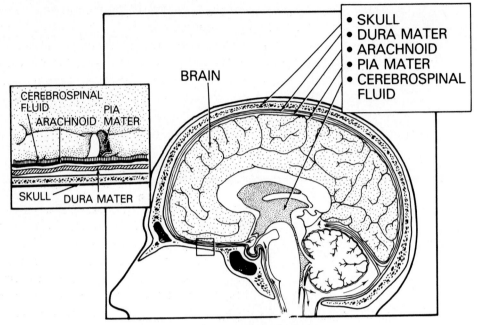

Figure 7–1. The head.

2. Skull
3. Fibrous coverings of the brain (meninges)
4. Brain tissue
5. Cerebrospinal fluid
6. Vascular compartments

The scalp is very vascular and bleeds freely when lacerated. Because many of the small blood vessels are suspended in an inelastic matrix of supporting tissue, the normal protective vasospasm that would limit bleeding is inhibited, which may lead to prolonged bleeding and significant blood loss.

The skull is like a closed box, the only significant opening through which pressure can be released is the foramen magnum at the base where the brain stem ends and the spinal cord originates. The rigid and unyielding bony skull contributes to several injury mechanisms in head trauma. Because of the way the brain is situated in the skull, there is greater movement at the top of the brain than at the base. This is a factor on impact. The temporal bone (temple) is quite thin and easily fractured.

The fibrous coverings of the brain include the dura mater ("tough mother"), which covers the entire brain; the thinner pia arachnoid (called simply the arachnoid), which lies underneath the dura and in which are suspended both arteries and veins; and the very thin pia mater ("soft mother"), which lies underneath the arachnoid and is adherent to the surface of the brain. The cerebrospinal fluid is found beneath the arachnoid and pia mater.

The brain fills the volume of the skull, which virtually excludes any adaptation to swelling. This is of great importance in the pathophysiology of head tissue.

Cerebrospinal fluid ("spinal fluid") is created within the brain at a rate of $\frac{1}{3}$ mL/min. This nutrient fluid bathes the brain and spinal cord.

Pathophysiology of Head Trauma

Most brain injuries are not from direct injury to brain tissue, but occur as a result of external forces applied against the exterior of the skull or from movement of the brain inside the skull. In deceleration injuries, the head usually strikes an object such as the windshield of an automobile, which causes a sudden deceleration of the skull. The brain continues to move forward, impacting first against the skull in the original direction of motion, and then rebounding to hit the opposite side of the inner surface of the skull. Thus injuries may occur to the brain in the area of original impact ("coup") or on the opposite side ("contrecoup").

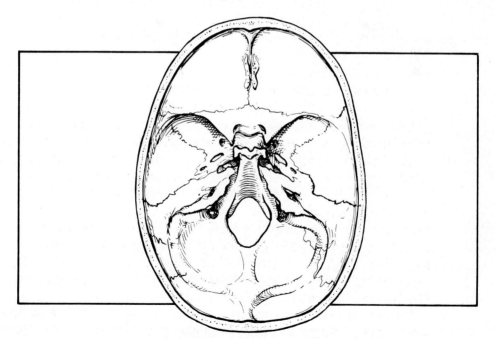

Figure 7–2. Base of skull.

The interior base of the skull is rough. Movement of the brain over this area may cause various degrees of injury to the brain tissue or to blood vessels supporting the brain.

The initial response of the bruised brain is swelling. This is from increased blood volume because of vasodilatation and increased cerebral blood flow to the injured areas. The increase in blood volume exerts pressure upon the brain, eventually causing decreased blood flow to the uninjured parts of the brain. The increase in cerebral water (edema) does not occur immediately but develops over the next 24 to 48 hours. Early efforts to decrease the initial vasodilatation in the injured area can have a profound effect on the patient's immediate and long-term outcome.

The blood level of carbon dioxide (CO_2) has a critical effect on cerebral blood vessels. The normal measurement is 40 mmHg. An *increase* in the partial pressure of CO_2 ($PaCO_2$) promotes *vasodilatation* (of the small veins), while *decreasing* the $PaCO_2$ causes *vasoconstriction*. If a head-injured patient is poorly ventilated, the rise in $PaCO_2$ causes vasodilatation and contributes to the increase in intracerebral pressure. Conversely, hyperventilation (>24 breaths per minute) can decrease the $PaCO_2$ to levels about 25 mmHg, causing rapid cerebral vasoconstriction. Therefore, prompt definitive airway management which incorporates hyperventilation will help to minimize the development of cerebral edema and allow better perfusion of the entire brain. Early in the course of the injury, hyperventilation is more important than the administration of mannitol or furosemide (Lasix). Because mannitol and furosemide are diuretics, they require more time for full effect and should not be relied on to replace vigorous oxygenation and ventilation. There are rare instances where early administration of mannitol to a head-injured victim may briefly worsen the situation by causing vasodilatation and thus increasing intravascular volume. Any victim who shows signs of increasing intracranial pressure or decreasing level of consciousness should have *immediate hyperventilation*.

Intracranial Pressure

Within the skull and fibrous coverings of the brain are the brain tissue, cerebrospinal fluid, and blood. An increase in the volumes of one of these components must be at the expense of the other two because the adult skull (a "rigid box") cannot expand. Although there is some "give" to the volume of cerebrospinal fluid, it accounts for little space and cannot offset rapid brain swelling. Blood supply cannot be compromised, for the brain requires a constant supply of blood (oxygen and glucose) in order to survive. Thus, since none of the supporting components of the brain can be compromised, an increase in brain swelling can be rapidly catastrophic.

The pressure of the brain contents within the skull is termed *intracranial pressure*. The pressure of the blood flowing through the brain is termed the *cerebral perfusion pressure*. Its value is obtained by subtracting the intracranial (intracerebral) pressure from the mean arterial blood pressure. If the brain swells or if there is bleeding inside the skull, intracranial pressure increases and the perfusion pressure decreases. The body has protective reflex (Cushing response or reflex) that attempts to maintain a constant perfusion pressure: As the intracerebral pressure increases, the systemic blood pressure increases to try to preserve blood flow to the brain. As the situation becomes more critical, the pulse rate drops (bradycardia) and eventually the respiratory rate declines. The pressure within the skull continues in an upward spiral until a critical point, at which time the head injury becomes overwhelming and all vital signs deteriorate, culminating in the patient's death.

Herniation Syndrome

When the brain swells, particularly after a blow to the head, a sudden rise in intracranial pressure may occur. This may force portions of the brain downward, obstructing the flow of cerebrospinal fluid and applying great pressure to the brainstem. This is a life-threatening situation characterized by deteriorating level of consciousness which rapidly progresses to coma, dilation of the pupil, and outward/downward deviation of the eye on the side of the injury,

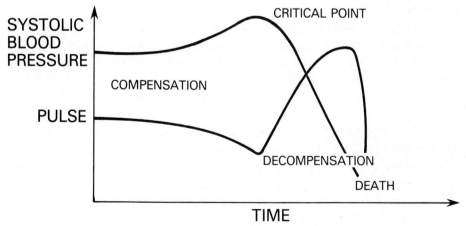

Figure 7-3. Cushing response.

paralysis of the arm and leg on the side opposite the injury, and decerebrate posturing (described below). The victim may soon cease all movement, stop breathing and die. The syndrome often follows an acute subdural hemorrhage.

Anoxic Brain Injury

Injuries to the brain from lack of oxygen (e.g., cardiac arrest, choking, near-drowning) affect the brain in a serious fashion. If the brain is without oxygen for a period greater than 4 to 6 minutes, irreversible damage almost always occurs. Following a nontraumatic anoxic episode, spasm develops in the small cerebral arteries, so that if the brain is reperfused, blood will not flow to the cortex and the patient will ultimately die from brain failure. One theory is that this arterial spasm is related to the flow of calcium into arterial muscle cells; complete spasm does not occur for approximately 90 minutes. Although it is currently accepted that the brain cannot be effectively resuscitated after 4 to 6 minutes of anoxia, there are exceptions to the rule, notably the condition of hypothermia. Current research is directed toward the use of drug therapy in concert with vigorous resuscitation. With the recent development of calcium channel blocking drugs, there may be hope of brain recovery if resuscitation is accompanied by drug therapy within 90 minutes of anoxic injury.

Head Injuries

Scalp Wounds

The scalp is very vascular and often bleeds briskly when lacerated, rapidly resulting in significant blood loss. This can be very important in children, who bleed as freely as adults but do not have the same blood volume. A child may develop shock from a briskly bleeding scalp wound, whereas it is a very uncommon cause of shock in an adult. As a general rule, adults with scalp injuries who are in shock usually have another site of bleeding (often internal), but one should not underestimate the blood loss from a scalp wound. Most bleeding from the scalp can be easily controlled in the field with direct pressure.

Skull Injuries

Skull injuries can be linear nondisplaced fractures, depressed fractures, and compound fractures. There is very little that can be done for these injuries

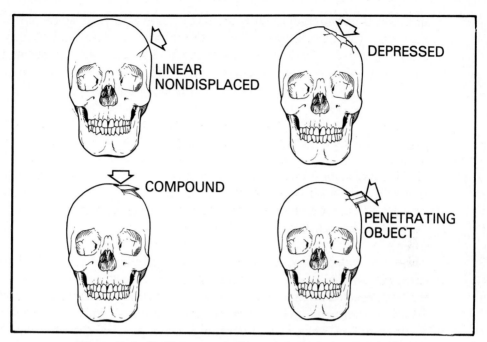

Figure 7–4. Skull fracture—linear nondisplaced, depressed, compound, and penetrating object.

in the field except to avoid placing direct pressure on an obvious depressed or compound skull fracture. Penetrating objects in the skull should be left in place (*not removed*) and the victim transported immediately to the emergency department. In a gunshot wound to the head, unless there are clear entrance and exit wounds in a perfectly linear path, assume that the bullet has ricocheted and may be lodged in the neck near the spinal cord.

Any head injury in a child without a clear explanation should arouse suspicion for child abuse. Pay particular attention to the setting from which the child was rescued and request police or social service assistance if the circumstances suggest child abuse. In an adult, if there is a large contusion or darkened swelling in the scalp, suspect an underlying skull fracture.

Brain Injuries

There are several types of brain injuries. In the following outline we briefly discuss some of these.

1. Concussion: A concussion implies no significant injury to the brain. There is usually a history of trauma to the head with a variable period of unconsciousness or confusion and then a return to normal consciousness. There may be amnesia from the injury. This amnesia usually extends to some point before the injury (retrograde short-term amnesia) so that often the patient will not remember the events leading to the injury. Until the patient becomes fully oriented to his surroundings and situation, he may repeat questions over and over as if he has not been paying attention to your answers. There may be dizziness, headache, ringing in the ears, and/or nausea. If unconsciousness exceeds 3 to 5 minutes, the emergency physician or neurosurgeon will usually admit the patient to the hospital for observation.

2. Cerebral Contusion: A patient with cerebral contusion (bruised brain tissue) will have a history of prolonged unconsciousness or serious alteration in state of consciousness (e.g., profound confusion, persistent amnesia, abnormal behavior). Brain swelling may be rapid and severe. The victim may have focal neurological signs or appear to have suffered a cerebrovascular accident (stroke). Depending on the location of the contusion, the victim may have personality changes, such as inappropriately rude behavior. A patient with a suspected cerebral contusion should be transported rapidly to the emergency department, where he will be evaluated [often with computed tomography (CT scan)] and admitted to the hospital for observation.

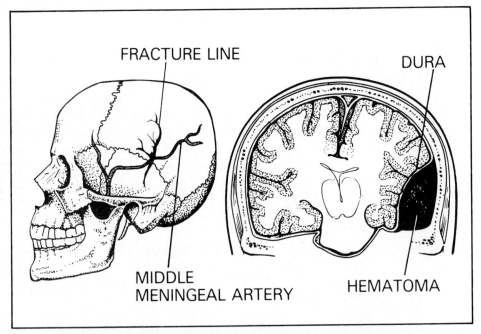

Figure 7–5. Acute epidermal hematoma. This hemorrhage may follow injury to the extradural arteries. The blood collects between the fibrous dura and the periosteum.

3. Intracranial Hemorrhage: Hemorrhage can occur between the skull and dura (the fibrous covering of the brain), between the dura and the arachnoid, between the arachnoid and the brain, or directly into the brain tissue.

a. *Acute epidural hematoma.* This injury is most often caused by a tear in the middle meningeal artery, which is often associated with a linear skull fracture in the temporal or parietal region. Because the bleeding is arterial (although it may be venous from one of the dural sinuses), the collection of blood and pressure can increase rapidly, so death may occur quickly. Surgical removal of the blood and ligation of the ruptured blood vessel often allows full recovery if the underlying brain tissue is not injured. Symptoms of an acute epidural hematoma include a history of head trauma with initial loss of consciousness, followed by a period during which the patient is conscious and coherent (the "lucid interval"). After a period of 30 minutes to 2 hours, the patient will develop signs of increasing intracranial pressure (vomiting, headache, altered mental status), lapse into unconsciousness, and develop body paralysis on the side opposite from the head injury. There is often a dilated and fixed (no response to bright light) pupil on the side of the head injury. Usually, this is followed rapidly by death. The classic example is the boxer who is knocked unconscious, wakes up, and is allowed to go home, only to

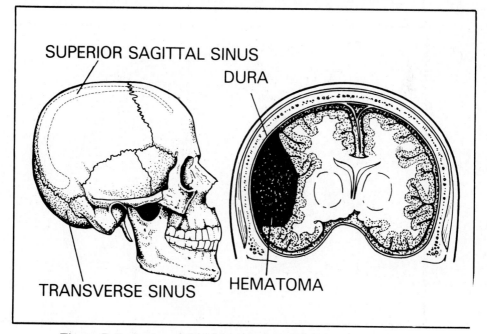

Figure 7–6. Acute subdural hematoma. This usually occurs following the rupture of dural vessels (veins). Blood collects and often severely compresses and distorts the brain.

be found dead in bed the next morning. Any victim who awakens from unconsciousness and complains of a severe headache should be observed for a minimum of 6 hours for the development of an epidural hematoma. The mortality rate from an acute epidural hemorrhage is approximately 20%.

b. *Acute subdural hematoma.* This is caused by bleeding between the dura and the arachnoid and is associated with injury to the underlying brain tissue. Because the bleeding is venous, pressure increases more slowly, and often the diagnosis is not apparent until hours or days after the injury. The signs and symptoms include headache, fluctuations in the level of consciousness, and focal neurological signs (e.g., specific weakness, hemiparesis, altered deep tendon reflexes, slurred speech). Because of underlying brain tissue injury, prognosis is often poor. Mortality is very high (60 to 90%) in victims who are comatose when found. Early surgery may favorably influence outcome, with a reduction in mortality rate from 80 to 90% (surgery performed more than 4 hours after the injury) to 30 to 40% (surgery performed less than 4 hours after the injury). Always suspect a subdural in an alcoholic with any degree of altered mental status following a fall.

c. *Intracerebral hemorrhage.* This is bleeding within the brain tissue. With regard to trauma, it is always associated with penetrating injuries and often associated with blunt injuries. Unfortunately, surgery is usually not helpful.

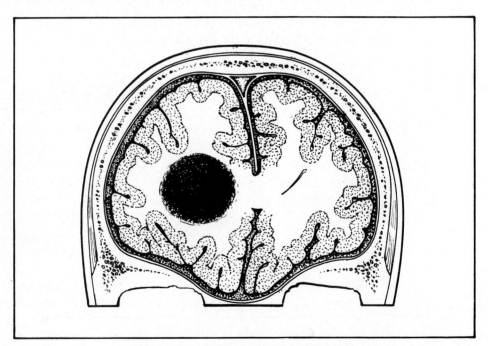

Figure 7–7. Intracerebral hemorrhage.

The signs and symptoms depend on the regions involved and the degree of injury, in patterns similar to those that accompany a stroke.

Evaluation of the Head Trauma Victim

The head-injured victim will rarely be cooperative and is often under the influence of alcohol. As a rescuer, you must pay extraordinary attention to detail and never lose your patience with a combative patient. Remember that every trauma victim is initially evaluated in the same sequence:

1. Secure the **airway** as you control the cervical spine and check initial level of consciousness.
2. Assess **breathing.**
3. Assess **circulation.**
4. Control major **bleeding.**
5. Determine transport decision and critical interventions.
6. Perform secondary survey:
    a. Vital signs
    b. History of patient and trauma event
    c. Head-to-toes exam (including *neurological*)
    d. Further bandaging and splinting
    e. Continuous monitoring

Control of the airway cannot be overemphasized. The supine, restrained, and unconscious victim is prone to having the tongue fall backward into the pharynx or to choking on blood, vomit, or other secretions. Vomiting is very common within the first hour following a head injury. The airway should be protected by endotracheal intubation, placement of an oral or nasal airway, positioning the victim on his side (in the absence of suspicion for a cervical fracture), and constant suctioning. Endotracheal intubation of the head-injured patient should be performed as rapidly and smoothly as possible, to avoid patient agitation, straining, and breath holding that may contribute to elevated intracranial pressure. Before beginning intubation, hyperventilate with high-flow oxygen.

In general, evaluation for head injury is begun as you obtain your initial level of consciousness by speaking to the patient. A much more detailed neurological exam is done during the secondary survey. Obviously, a patient with a history and physical examination that indicates an epidural hematoma should be transported in greater haste than would be an alert post-concussion victim. It is very important that all observations be recorded because the treatment is often dictated by detection of the deterioration of clinical stability. The goals of the evaluation are to determine quickly if the victim is brain injured, and if so, is he deteriorating? Level of consciousness is your most sensitive indicator of brain function.

It is essential to obtain as thorough a history about the event as possible. The circumstances of the head injury may be extremely important for management of the victim, and may be of prognostic importance with regard to the ultimate outcome. Pay particular attention to reports of near-drowning, electrocution, lightning strike, drug abuse, smoke inhalation, hypothermia, and seizures. Be absolutely certain to inquire about the victim's behavior from the time of the head injury until the time of your arrival.

Primary Assessment

1. Level of Consciousness: A change in the level of consciousness is the first indicator of a brain injury or increase in intracranial pressure. Keep your evaluation and report simple so that everyone can understand you. The AVPU method is quite adequate.

A   Patient is alert
V   Patient responds to vocal (voice) stimuli
P   Patient responds to painful stimuli
U   Patient is unresponsive

To be consistent with the Champion Trauma Score and other field triage scoring systems, you should be familiar with the Glasgow Coma Scale, which is simple, easy to use, and has good prognostic value as to eventual outcome.

Glasgow Coma Scale: The victim should be scored by the best response. This is a dynamic score and can be calculated multiple times during resuscitation and transport of a victim.

Eye opening	
Spontaneous	4
To voice	3
To pain	2
None	1
Motor response	
Obeys	6
Localizes	5

Withdraws	4
Flexion (decorticate)	3
Extension (decerebrate)	2
None	1
Verbal response	
Oriented	5
Confused	4
Inappropriate	3
Incomprehensible	2
None	1
Total	3 to 15

2. Vital Signs: These are extremely important in following the course of a patient with head trauma. Most important, they can indicate changes in intracranial pressure. You should observe and record vital signs at least every 5 minutes.

a. *Blood pressure:* Increasing intracranial pressure causes increased blood pressure. Other causes of hypertension include fear and pain. Hypotension associated with a severe head injury should always be treated as hemorrhagic shock, because if the low blood pressure is caused by the head injury, the prognosis is grim. If possible, the systolic blood pressure should be maintained in the range 100 to 140 mmHg to avoid hypotension that might compromise cerebral perfusion and hypertension that might contribute to raised intracranial pressure.

b. *Pulse.* Increasing intracranial pressure causes the pulse rate to decrease.

c. *Respirations.* Increasing intracranial pressure causes the respiratory rate to increase, decrease, and/or to become irregular. Unusual respiratory patterns may reflect the level of brain/brainstem injury. Preterminally, the patient may demonstrate central neurogenic hyperventilation, which is a rapid, noisy respiratory pattern. Because respiration is affected by so many factors

Comparison of Vital Signs in Shock and Head Injury

	Shock	Head Injury with Increasing Intracranial Pressure
Blood pressure	↓	↑
Pulse	↑	↓
Respiration	↑	↓
Level of consciousness	↓	↓

Figure 7–8.

(e.g., fear, hysteria, chest injuries, spinal cord injuries, diabetes), it is not as useful an indicator as are the other vital signs in monitoring the course of head injury.

Secondary Assessment

All patients with head or facial trauma have a cervical spine injury until proven otherwise. Stabilization of the cervical spine should accompany airway and breathing management.

Once the primary survey is completed and recorded, begin with the scalp and quickly, but carefully, examine for obvious injuries such as lacerations or depressed or open skull fractures. The size of a laceration is often misjudged because of the difficulty in assessment through hair matted with blood. Feel the scalp gently for obvious unstable areas of the skull. If none are present, you may safely apply a pressure dressing or hold direct pressure on a bandage to stop the bleeding.

A basilar skull fracture may be indicated by bleeding from the ear or from the nose, clear fluid running from the nose, swelling and/or discoloration behind the ear (Battle's sign), and/or swelling and discoloration around both eyes (raccoon eyes).

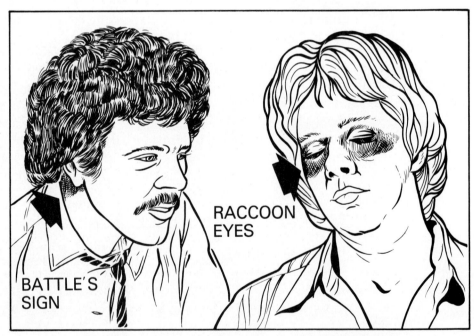

RACCOON
EYES

BATTLE'S
SIGN

Figure 7-9. Signs of basilar skull fracture—Battle's sign and raccoon eyes.

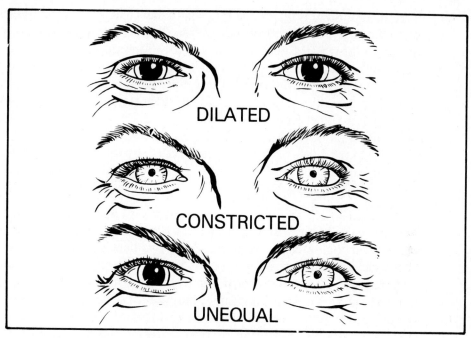

Figure 7–10. Pupils of the eyes.

Pupils: The pupils are controlled in part by the third cranial nerve. This nerve takes a long course through the skull and is easily compressed by brain swelling, so it may be affected by increasing intracranial pressure. Following a head injury, if both pupils are dilated and do not react to light, the patient probably has a brainstem injury and the prognois is grim. If the pupils are dilated but still react to light, the injury is often still reversible, so every effort should be made to get the patient quickly to a facility capable of treating a head injury. A unilaterally dilated pupil that remains reactive to light may be the earliest sign of increasing intracranial pressure, which affects the third cranial nerve that regulates constriction of the pupil. The development of a unilaterally dilated pupil ("blown pupil") while you are observing the patient is an extreme emergency and mandates rapid transport. Other causes of dilated pupils that may or may not react to light include hypothermia, lightning strike, anoxia, optic nerve injury, drug effect (e.g., atropine), or direct ocular trauma. Fixed and dilated pupils signify head injury only in patients with decreased level of consciousness. If the patient is alert, the fully dilated pupil is not from head injury.

Fluttering eyelids are often seen with hysteria. Slow lid closure (like a curtain falling) is rarely seen with hysteria.

If the brainstem is intact, the eyes will remain synchronized (conjugate gaze) when the head is turned from side to side. The eyes turn in the opposite direction from the way the head is turned. Since this resembles the way a toy doll's eyes move, this test is called the doll's eye reflex (oculocephalic reflex). *This test is never done in the field* on a trauma victim who may have a neck injury, since turning the head from side to side may cause a serious spinal cord injury. (In the emergency department, it should be performed only after cervical spine films have been obtained, to rule out a cervical spine fracture.)

Testing for a blink response (corneal reflex) by touching the cornea, testing for a gag reflex, or applying overly noxious stimuli to a victim to test for response to pain are primitive field techniques that are unreliable and *do not* contribute to prehospital care.

Extremities: Note sensation and motor function in the extremities. Can the patient feel you touch his hands and feet? Can he wiggle his fingers and toes? If the victim is unconscious, note his response to pain. If he withdraws or localizes to the pinching of his fingers and toes, he has grossly intact sensation and motor function. This usually indicates that there is normal or minimally impaired cortical function.

Both decorticate posturing or rigidity (arms flexed, legs extended) and

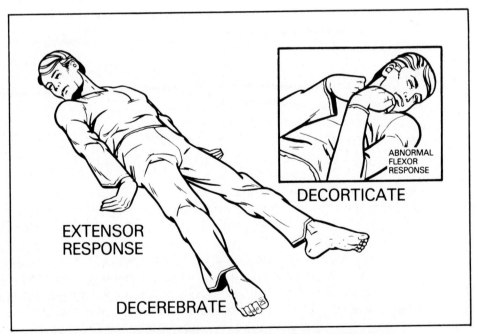

Figure 7–11. Decorticate and decerebrate posturing.

decerebrate posturing or rigidity (arms and legs extended) are ominous signs of deep cerebral hemispheric or upper brainstem injury. *Flaccid paralysis usually denotes spinal cord injury.*

Decisions on the management of the head trauma patient are made on the basis of changes in all parameters of the physical and neurological examination. You are establishing the baseline from which later judgments must be made; record your observations.

Management of the Head Trauma Victim

There is not a great deal that you can do for the head trauma patient in the field. It is extremely important to make a rapid assessment and then transport the victim to a facility capable of managing head trauma. The important points of management in the field are:

1. *Secure the airway and provide good oxygenation.* The brain does not tolerate hypoxia, so good oxygenation is mandatory. *The head trauma patient should be hyperventilated* (>24 breaths per minute). This decreases intracranial pressure. The neck should be immobilized in a rigid collar and a padded head-immobilization device. If the patient is comatose, he should undergo endotracheal intubation. This prevents aspiration and allows better oxygenation and ventilation. Because head-injured victims are prone to vomiting, be prepared to log-roll the immobilized victim and to suction the oropharynx, particularly if an endotracheal tube has not been placed.

2. Record baseline observations. This includes recording the Glasgow Coma Scale, which includes measures of eye opening, motor response, and verbal response. Also record the blood pressure, respirations (rate and pattern) pupils (size and reaction to light), sensation, and voluntary motor activity. If the victim develops hypotension, suspect hemorrhage or spinal injury.

3. Frequently monitor and record the observations listed above. If it is important enough to examine a victim the first time, the examination should be repeated.

4. You may be ordered to insert an intravenous catheter and administer fluids. Unless the victim is hypotensive, the purpose of this maneuver is to administer medications. Fluids are generally restricted in victims with isolated head trauma. A paramedic or physician may administer an osmotic diuretic such as mannitol, which draws excess fluid from the brain and promotes urination.

Potential Problems

Always anticipate a cervical spine injury in the head-injured patient.

1. *Seizures.* Head trauma, particularly intracranial hemorrhage, may cause seizures. The seizing patient becomes hypoxic and hyperthermic, so persistent seizure activity may worsen his condition. You may be ordered to administer diazepam (Valium) intravenously to control the seizures. It is not uncommon for seizures to be related to poor airway control, so remember that oxygenation and ventilation are of extreme importance.

2. *Vomiting.* A patient with head trauma almost always vomits. You must remain alert to prevent pulmonary aspiration. If the victim is unconscious, he should be intubated. Otherwise, keep mechanical suction available and be prepared to log-roll the victim onto his side (maintaining immobilization of the cervical spine).

3. *Rapid deteriorating condition.* A patient who shows rapid deterioration of vital signs or rapid progression of his brain injury (e.g., dilated pupil, decorticate or decerebrate posturing) should be transported rapidly to a trauma center. There is nothing definitive that you can do in the field. You may be ordered to administer mannitol or furosemide intravenously to decrease intracranial pressure. Radio ahead so that a neurosurgeon can be available and the operating room prepared by the time you arrive at the hospital. A rapid field response and transport will not compensate for the time lost in the emergency department or a delay to the operating room.

4. *Shock.* Think "spinal cord injury or bleeding."

5. *Metabolic abnormalities.* Remember to administer naloxone (Narcan) to any victim with altered mental status when narcotic abuse is a possibility. Remember to administer thiamine and dextrose to any victim with altered mental status who is diabetic, alcoholic, or who might otherwise be suffering from hypoglycemia.

Summary of Management

1. Stabilize the cervical spine.
2. Secure and maintain the airway.
3. Hyperventilate.
4. Record baseline vital signs, observations of pupils, neurological examination, Glasgow Coma Scale.
5. Continuously monitor and record all observations.
6. Transport rapidly.

Chapter 8

Extremity Trauma

Daniel G. Sayers, M.D.

The prehospital professional must never let distorted or wounded extremities occupy his attention when there may be more-life-threatening injuries present. Extremity injuries are easy to identify upon first encountering the victim and may be disabling, but are rarely immediately life threatening. It is quite important to remember that the movement of air through the airway, the mechanics of breathing, the maintenance of circulating blood volume, and the appropriate treatment of shock always come before the splinting of any fracture.

Hemorrhagic shock is a potential danger of very few musculoskeletal injuries. Only direct lacerations of arteries or fractures of the pelvis or femur are commonly associated with enough bleeding to cause shock. Injuries to the nerves or vessels that serve the hands and feet are the most common complications of fractures and dislocations. Such injuries cause the loss of function that we lump under the term "neurovascular compromise." Thus evaluation of sensation and circulation (pulses, color, and movement) distal to fractures is very important.

Injuries to the Extremities

Fractures

Fractures may be open (compound), with the broken end of the bone still protruding or having once protruded through the skin, or they may be closed (simple), and no communication to the outside. Fractured bone ends are extremely sharp and are quite dangerous to all the tissues that surround the bone. Since nerves and arteries frequently travel near the bone, across the flexor

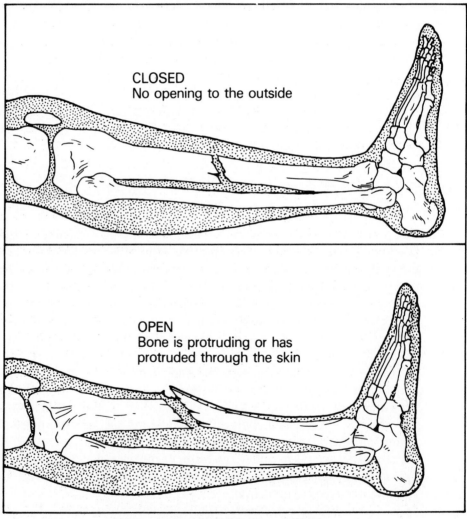

CLOSED
No opening to the outside

OPEN
Bone is protruding or has
protruded through the skin

Figure 8–1. Classification of fractures.

side of joints, or very near the skin (hands and feet), they are frequently injured. Such neurovascular injuries may be due to lacerations from bone fragments or from pressure due to swelling or hematomas. Closed fractures can be just as dangerous as open fractures because injured soft tissues often bleed profusely. It is important to remember that any break in the skin near a fractured bone may be considered to be an opening for contamination.

A closed fracture of one femur can cause the loss of up to two units of blood, and two fractured femurs can cause life-threatening hemorrhage. A fractured pelvis can cause extensive bleeding into the abdomen or behind the peritoneum. The pelvis usually fractures in several places and may have a unit of blood loss for each fracture. Pelvic fractures may lacerate the bladder or the large pelvic blood vessels. Either of these structures can cause exsanguinating hemorrhage into the abdomen. Remember, multiple fractures can cause life-threatening hemorrhage without any *external* blood loss.

Open fractures add the dangers of contamination as well as loss of blood outside the body. If protruding bone ends are pulled back into the skin when the limb is aligned, bacteria-contaminated debris will be pulled into the wound. Infection from such debris may prevent healing of the bone and may even cause death from septic complications.

Dislocations

Joint dislocations are extremely painful injuries. They are almost always easy to identify because of distortion of the normal anatomy. Major joint dislocations, although not life-threatening, are often true emergencies because of the neurovascular compromise, which can, if not treated quickly, lead to amputation. It is impossible to know whether or not a fracture exists in combination with a dislocation. It is very important to check for sensation, pallor, and pulses distal to major joint dislocations. Ordinarily, you splint injuries in the position in which you find them. There are certain exceptions to this rule. It is universally true, however, that one can apply only gentle traction to any distorted extremity in an effort to straighten it. In the few instances that you would use traction to straighten, use no more than 10 pounds of force. Most often the best treatment for the patient is padding and splinting the extremity in the most comfortable position and rapidly transporting to a facility that has orthopedic care available.

Amputations

These are disabling and sometimes life-threatening injuries. They have the potential for massive hemorrhage, but most often, the bleeding will control

ESTIMATING BLOOD LOSS BY SITE
AND NUMBER OF FRACTURES

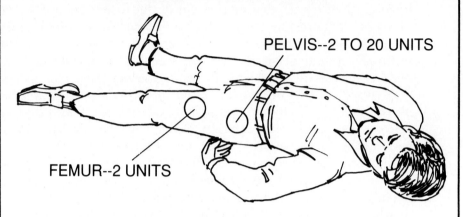

PELVIS--2 TO 20 UNITS

FEMUR--2 UNITS

FRACTURE BLEEDING WILL USUALLY BE
50% COMPLETE IN THE FIRST 4 TO 6 HOURS.

THE MOST SEVERE BLOOD LOSS OCCURS IN
FRACTURE OF THE PELVIS

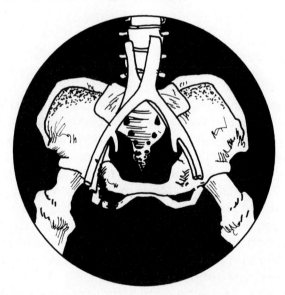

PELVIC FRACTURE. ANYWHERE FROM 2 TO 20 UNITS OF
BLOOD MAY BE LOST IN A SEVERE PELVIC FRACTURE.

Figure 8–2. Internal blood loss from fractures.

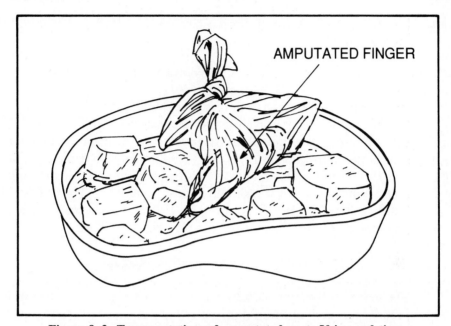

AMPUTATED FINGER

Figure 8–3. Transportation of amputated part. If ice and time are available, seal part in small container and place this in large container of ice and water. Do not use dry ice. Do not place amputated part directly on ice. If no ice is available, place part in plastic bag and seal so that the part will not lose moisture. Do not wrap part in moistened dressing.

itself quite readily with ordinary pressure applied to the stump. The stump should be covered with a damp sterile dressing and an elastic wrap that will apply uniform, reasonable pressure across the entire stump. If bleeding absolutely cannot be controlled with pressure, a tourniquet may be used. In general, a tourniquet is to be avoided whenever possible.

You should make an effort to find the amputated part and bring it with you. This sometimes neglected detail can have serious implications for the patient in the future, since parts can frequently be used for graft material. Reimplantation is usually not done in patients over a certain age, in avulsion or crush injuries, or in injuries to the very distal portions of the extremity. For this reason, it is very important for the EMT not to discuss reimplantation with the patient during the prehospital phase of treatment.

Small amputated parts should be placed in a plastic bag. If ice is available, place the bag in a larger bag or container containing ice and water. Do not use ice alone and *never* use dry ice. Cooling the part slows the chemical processes and will increase the viability from 4 hours to several times that length of time. It is important to bring amputated parts even if reimplantation appears to you to be impossible.

Wounds

Cover wounds with a sterile dressing and bandage carefully. Gross contamination such as leaves or gravel should be removed from the wound and smaller pieces of contamination can be irrigated from the wound with a normal saline drip in the same manner that you would irrigate a chemically contaminated eye. Bleeding can almost always be stopped with pressure dressings or pneumatic splints. Tourniquets should almost never be used to stop bleeding from a wound if amputation is not present. If necessary, a blood pressure cuff or pressure on a larger artery proximal to the injury may be appropriate.

Neurovascular Injuries

The nerves and major blood vessels generally run beside each other, usually in the flexor area of the major joints. They may be injured together, and loss of circulation and/or sensation can be due to disruption, swelling, or by compression by bone fragments or hematomas. Foreign bodies or broken bone ends may well impinge on delicate structures and cause them to malfunction. Pulses and sensations are always checked before and after any extremity manipulation, application of splint, or traction.

Sprains and Strains

These injuries cannot be differentiated from fractures in the field. Treat them as though they are fractures.

Impaled Objects

Do not remove them. Apply a very bulky type of padding to hold the object in place and transport the patient with the object in place. The skin is a pivot point in these cases, and any motion outside the body is translated or magnified within the tissues where the end of the object may lacerate or harm sensitive structures. The cheek of the face is the only exception to this rule.

Compartment Syndrome

When bleeding occurs in a closed space surrounded by membranes that will not stretch, pressure is transmitted to the blood vessels and nerves. This pressure may compress the blood vessels in such a manner that circulation is impossible. The nerve may also be compromised. Sometimes the only way to identify these injuries is to note the absence of the distal pulse or function in the hand or foot. This particular condition may be found in either the forearm or the lower leg.

Assessment and Management

History

This is especially important in extremity trauma because the apparent mechanism of injury and the condition of the extremity when you arrive may give you important information about how severe the injury actually is. This process should be almost instantaneous, and no time should be wasted in trying to elicit a verbal history until airway, breathing and circulatory status is clearly established. In the conscious patient, you should obtain the history during the secondary survey. Ordinarily, the history follows examination of the trauma patient. The history becomes especially important in extremity trauma because certain mechanisms of injury predispose to extremity injuries that may not be immediately obvious.

Foot injuries from long jumps (falls landing on the feet) often have associated lumbar spine injuries. Any injury to the knee when the patient is in the sitting position may have severe injuries to the hip. In a like manner, hip injuries may refer pain to the knee, so the knee and the hip are intimately connected and must be evaluated together rather than separately. Falls onto the wrist frequently injure the elbow, so wrist and elbow must be evaluated together. The same is true of the ankle and the proximal fibula of the outside of the lower leg.

Any injury that appears to be in the shoulder must be examined carefully because it may easily involve either the neck, chest, or shoulder. Fractures of the pelvis are usually associated with very large amounts of blood loss. Whenever a fracture in the pelvis is identified, shock must be suspected and proper treatment begun.

Assessment

During the secondary survey, you should quickly palpate the full length of each extremity, checking for deformity and areas of spasm, swelling, or tenderness. Check the joints for pain and movement. Check and record distal pulses and sensation. Pulses may be marked with ball-point pen to identify the area

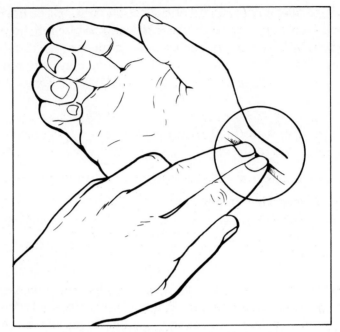

Figure 8–4(a). Palpation of radial pulse.

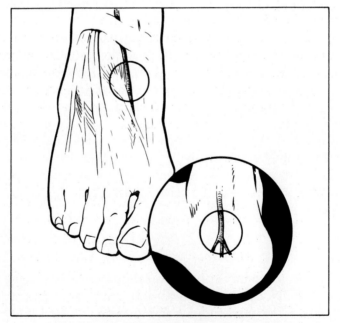

Figure 8–4(b). Location of posterior tibial and dorsalis pedis pulses.

in which the pulse is best felt. Crepitation or grating of bone ends is a definite sign of fracture, and once identified, the bone ends should be immediately immobilized to prevent further soft tissue injury.

General Management of Extremity Injuries

Proper management of fractures and dislocations will decrease the incidence of pain, disability, and serious complications. Treatment in the field is directed at proper immobilization of the injured part by the use of an appropriate splint.

Purpose of Splinting: The objective is to prevent motion in the broken bone ends. The nerves that cause the most pain in a fractured extremity lie in the membrane surrounding the bone. The broken bone ends irritate these nerves, causing a very deep and distressing type of pain. Splinting not only decreases pain, but also eliminates further damage to muscles, nerves, and blood vessels by preventing further motion of the broken bone ends.

When to Use Splinting: There is no simple rule that will determine the precise sequence to follow in every trauma patient. In general, the seriously injured patient will be better off if only minimal (spinal) immobilization is done before transport. The multiply traumatized patient with severe injuries to the trunk may have the lower extremities briefly examined (MAST survey) and splinted with a MAST suit almost immediately after the primary survey. This rapidly and effectively saves very critical time. The patient who requires a "load and go" type of approach can be adequately immobilized by careful packaging on the long spine board. This does not mean that the EMT has no responsibility to identify and protect extremity fractures, but rather implies that some splinting can be done in the vehicle en route to the hospital. It is never appropriate to sacrifice time immobilizing a limb to prevent *disability* when that time may be needed to save the patient's *life.*

General rules of splinting

1. You must adequately visualize the injured part. Clothes should be cut off, not pulled off unless there is only an isolated injury that presents no problem with maintaining immobilization.
2. Check and record distal sensation and circulation before and after splinting. Check movement distal to the fracture if possible (e.g., ask the conscious patient to wiggle his fingers or observe the motion of the unconscious patient with the application of painful stimulus). Pulses may be marked with a pen to identify where they were last discovered.
3. If the extremity is severely angulated, you should apply gentle traction in an attempt to straighten it. This traction should never exceed

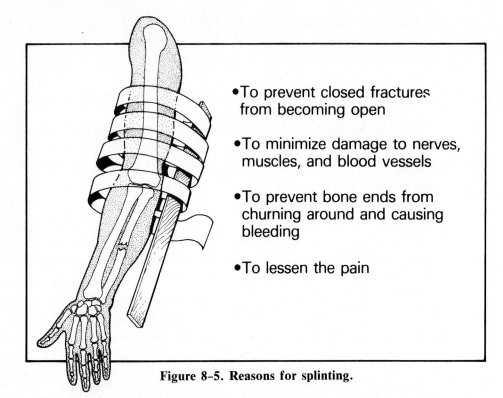

• To prevent closed fractures from becoming open

• To minimize damage to nerves, muscles, and blood vessels

• To prevent bone ends from churning around and causing bleeding

• To lessen the pain

Figure 8–5. Reasons for splinting.

10 pounds of pressure. If resistance is encountered, splint it in the angulated position. It is very important for the EMTs who are attempting to straighten an extremity to be honest with themselves with regard to resistance in that it takes very little force to lacerate the wall of a vessel or to interrupt the blood supply to a large nerve. If in doubt and the transport time is reasonable, always splint in the position found.

4. Open wounds should be covered with a sterile dressing and occasionally moistened before you apply the splint. Splints should always be applied on the side of the extremity away from open wounds in order to prevent pressure necrosis.

5. Use the splint that will immobilize one joint above and below the injury.

6. Pad the splint well. This is particularly true if there is any skin defect or if bony prominences may press against a hard splint.

7. Do not attempt to push bone ends back under the skin. If you apply traction and the bone end retracts back into the wound, do not increase the amount of traction. You should not use your hands or any tools to try to pull the bone ends back out, but be sure to notify the receiving physician. Bone ends should be carefully padded by bandages

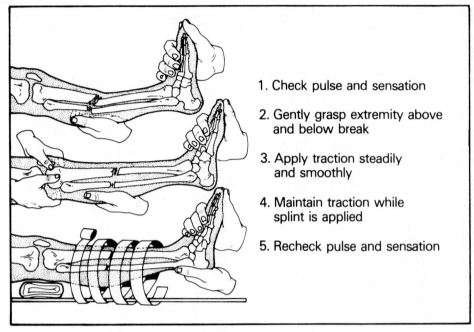

1. Check pulse and sensation

2. Gently grasp extremity above and below break

3. Apply traction steadily and smoothly

4. Maintain traction while splint is applied

5. Recheck pulse and sensation

Figure 8-6. Straightening angulated fractures.

prior to the application of the MAST suit to the lower extremities. The healing of bone is improved if the bone ends are kept moist when transport time is prolonged.

8. When there is a life-threatening situation, injuries may be splinted as the patient is being moved. In cases where the injury is less severe, splint all injuries before moving the patient.

9. If in doubt, splint a possible injury.

Types of splints

1. *Rigid splint.* This type of splint can be made from many different materials and includes all of the cardboard, hard plastic, metal, and wooden types of splints. The type of splint that is made rigid by evacuating air from a moldable splint is also classified as a rigid splint. Rigid splints should be padded well and always extend one joint above and below the fracture.

2. *Soft splint.* This type includes air splints, pillows, and sling and swathe splints.

Air splints are good for fractures of the lower arm and lower leg. The MAST suit is an excellent air splint. Air splints have the advantage of compression, which helps to slow bleeding, but they have the disadvantage of increasing pressure as the temperature rises or the altitude increases. They *should not*

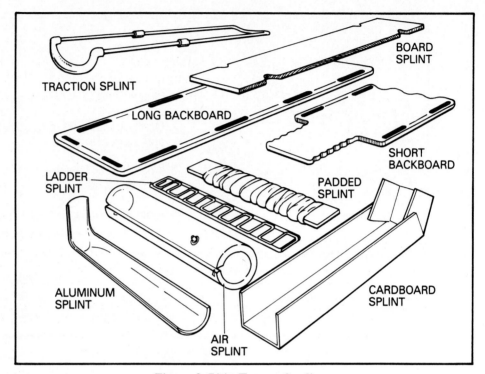

Figure 8–7(a). Types of splints.

be put on angulated fractures since they will automatically apply straightening pressure.

Other major disadvantages of air splints include the fact that the extremity pulses cannot be monitored while the splint is in place; also, the splints often stick to the skin and are painful to remove.

Inflating the splints requires the EMT to blow them up by mouth or by hand or foot pump (never by compressed air) until they give good support and yet can easily be dented with slight pressure from a fingertip. When using air splints, you must constantly check the pressure to be sure that the splint is not getting too tight or too loose (they often leak).

Remember that if air splints are applied in a cold environment and the patient is moved into the warm environment of the ambulance, the pressure will increase as the splints warm up. Where air ambulances are available, it must be remembered that the pressure in air splints increases if they are applied on the ground and then subsequently the patient is air lifted to the hospital. Also remember that if pressure is released while in flight, the pressure will be too low when the patient is returned to the ground.

Pillows make good splints for injuries to the ankle or foot. They are also helpful along with a sling and swathe to stabilize a dislocated shoulder.

Slings and swathes are excellent for injuries to the clavicle, shoulder, upper arm, elbow, and sometimes the forearm. They utilize the chest wall as a solid foundation and literally hold the arm against the chest wall. It should be borne in mind that some shoulder injuries cannot be brought close to the chest wall without significant force being applied. In these instances, pillows are used to bridge the gap between the chest wall and the upper arm.

3. *Traction splint.* This device is designed for fractures of the lower extremities. It holds the fracture immobile by the application of a steady pull on the extremity by applying countertraction to the ischium and the groin. This steady traction overcomes the tendency of the very strong thigh muscles to spasm. If traction is not applied, there is worse pain because the bone ends tend to impact or override. Traction also prevents free motion of the ends of the femur, which may lacerate the femoral nerve, artery or vein. There are many designs and types of splints available to apply traction to the lower extremity, but each must be carefully padded and applied with care to prevent excessive pressure on the soft tissues around the pelvis. It is also necessary to use a great deal of care in applying the ankle hitch so as not to interfere with the circulation of the foot. Many of these devices can be used with a Buck's Boot as an alternative to the ankle hitch.

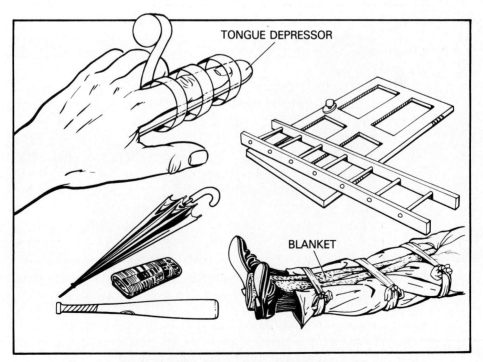

Figure 8–7(b). Improvised splinting materials.

Management of Specific Injuries

Spine: This is covered elsewhere in the book but included here to remind you that if there is any chance of spinal injury, proper immobilization must be done to prevent life-long paralysis or even death from a spinal cord injury. In the most urgent cases, careful packaging of the patient on the long spine board may be adequate splinting for a number of different extremity injuries. Remember that certain mechanisms of injury such as a fall from a height in which a victim lands on both feet may cause lumbar spine fracture because forces are transmitted all the way up the body.

Pelvis: It is practical to include injuries to the pelvis with extremities because they are frequently associated. These injuries are usually caused by motor vehicle accidents or by severe trauma such as falls from heights. They must be identified by pressure being placed on the iliac crests, hips, and pubis during patient survey.

There is always the potential for serious hemorrhage in pelvic fractures, so shock should be expected and measures should be taken to prevent the development of shock. The patient with a pelvic injury should always be transported on a spine board. Pelvic fractures can be associated with very

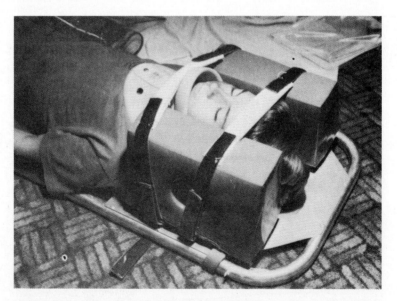

Figure 8–8. Spine board with rigid extrication collar and padded immobilization device. Collars do not give adequate lateral support—use padded immobilization device also.

severe abdominal bleeding; therefore, antishock trousers may be used to splint and simultaneously to tamponade bleeding.

Femur: The femur usually fractures at the midshaft, although hip fractures are quite common. Very often these fractures have open wounds in association with them and they must be presumed to be open fractures. The soft tissues surrounding the femur are heavy and will allow a great deal of bleeding into the tissue of the thigh. Bilateral femur fractures can be associated with a loss of up to 50% of the circulating blood volume. This implies that one should whenever possible have the MAST suit in place and an intravenous line established. Use a traction splint or the inflated MAST suit on femur fractures to prevent movement and to reduce pain.

Hip: Hip fractures are most often in the narrow "neck" of the femur, where strong ligaments may occasionally allow this type of fracture to bear weight. The ligaments are very strong and there is very little movement of the bone ends in the most frequent type of hip fracture.

The EMT must consider hip fractures in any elderly person who has fallen and has pain in the knee, hip, or pelvic region. This type of presentation and pain should be considered a fracture until x-ray proves otherwise. In this age group, pain is frequently well tolerated and sometimes even ignored or denied.

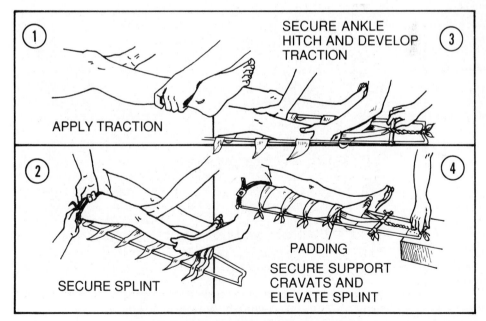

Figure 8–9(a). Applying a traction splint.

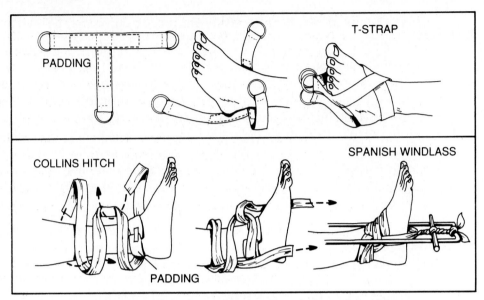

PADDING

T-STRAP

COLLINS HITCH

SPANISH WINDLASS

PADDING

Figure 8–9(b). Applying a traction hitch to the ankle.

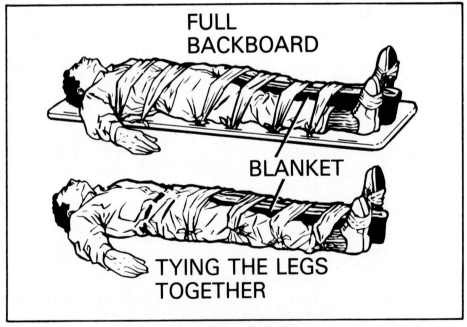

FULL
BACKBOARD

BLANKET

TYING THE LEGS
TOGETHER

Figure 8–10. Hip fracture.

In general, the tissues in the elderly patient are more delicate and less force is required to disrupt a given structure. Always remember that isolated knee pain may well be coming from damage to the hip in the child and in the elderly patient.

Hip dislocation is a different story. Most hip dislocations are a result of the knees being struck by the dashboard, forcing the relatively loose, relaxed hip out of the posterior side of its cup in the pelvis. Thus any patient in a severe automobile accident with a knee injury must have the hip examined very carefully. Hip dislocation is an orthopedic emergency and requires reduction as soon as possible to prevent sciatic nerve injury or necrosis of the femoral head due to interrupted blood supply. This is a very difficult reduction to perform because the amount of force required is very great and the movement must be quite precise.

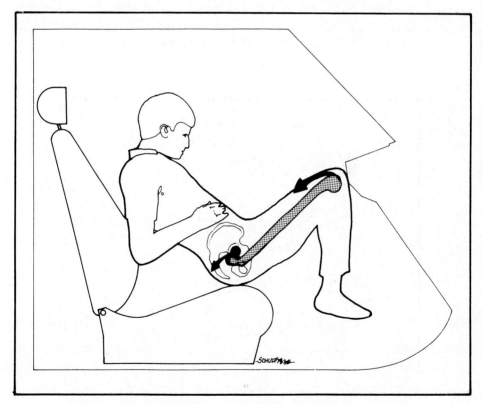

Figure 8–11. Mechanism of posterior dislocation of the hip. "Down and Under."

The dislocated hip will usually be flexed and the victim will not be able to tolerate having the leg straightened. The leg will almost invariably be rotated toward the midline. A hip dislocation should be supported in the most comfortable position by the use of pillows and by splinting to the uninjured leg. This patient requires rapid transport.

Knee: Fractures or dislocation here are quite serious because the arteries are bound down above and below the knee joint and are often bruised or lacerated if the joint is in an abnormal position. There is no way to know whether or not a fracture exists in an abnormally positioned knee, and in either case, the decision must be based on the circulation and neurological function below the knee in the foot. Some authorities state that about 50% of knee dislocations have associated injuries to the vessels and many knee injuries later require amputation. It is important to restore the circulation below the knee whenever possible.

Prompt reduction of knee dislocation is very important. If there is a loss of pulse or sensation, you should apply gentle traction, which may be by hand or with a traction splint. You must be careful to apply *no more than 10 pounds*

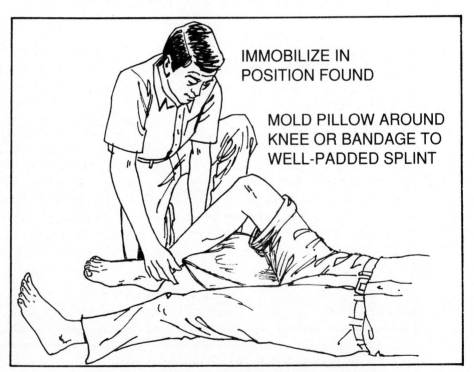

IMMOBILIZE IN POSITION FOUND

MOLD PILLOW AROUND KNEE OR BANDAGE TO WELL-PADDED SPLINT

Figure 8–12. Splinting posterior dislocation of the hip.

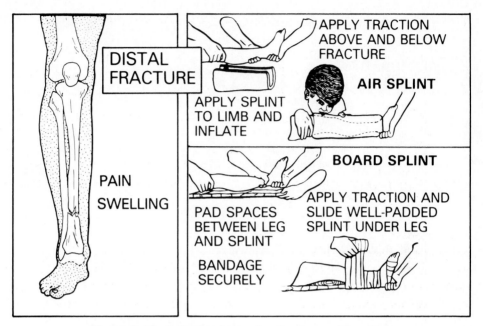

Figure 8–13. Splinting lower leg fractures. Air splint or board splint.

of force and this force must be applied along the long axis of the leg. If there is resistance to straightening the knee, splint it in the most comfortable position and transport the patient rapidly. This may be considered to be a true orthopedic emergency.

Tibia/Fibula: Fractures of the lower leg are frequently the results of accidents. They are often open due to thin skin over the front of the tibia and often have significant internal and/or external blood loss. Internal blood loss can interrupt the circulation to the foot if a compartment syndrome develops. It is rarely possible for patients to bear weight on fractures of the tibia. Fractures of the lower tibia/fibula may be splinted with a rigid splint, air splint, or pillow. The MAST suit will adequately splint upper tibia fractures. Here again it is important to dress any wound and pad any bone ends that may be put under an air splint or MAST suit.

Clavicle: This is the most frequently fractured bone in the body but rarely causes problems. It is best immobilized in the field with a sling and swathe. Rarely there may be injuries to the subclavian vein and artery or to the nerves of the arm when this area is injured. It is also very important that the ribs and chest be very carefully evaluated whenever an injury to the shoulder or clavicle is discovered.

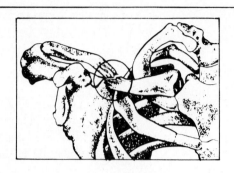
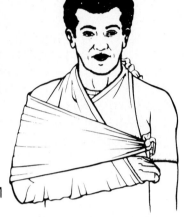

- SHOULDER BENT FORWARD
- ELBOW FLEXED AND FOREARM HELD ACROSS CHEST
- PAIN IN SHOULDER AREA
- SWELLING OR LUMP

FOLD ARM OF INJURED SIDE ACROSS CHEST

PLACE ARM IN SLING AND SECURE IT TO BODY WITH SWATHE

Figure 8–14. Fractured clavicle.

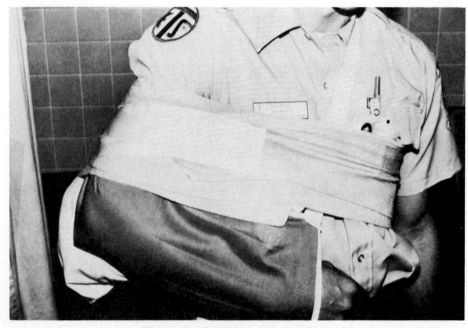

Figure 8–15. Dislocated shoulder.

Shoulder: Most shoulder injuries are not life threatening, but they may be associated with severe injuries of the chest or of the neck. Many shoulder injuries are dislocations or separations of joint spaces and may show as a defect at the upper outer portion of the shoulder. The upper humerus is fractured with some degree of frequency, however. The radial nerve travels quite close around the humerus and may be injured in humeral fractures. Injury to the radial nerve results in an inability of the patient to lift the hand (wrist drop). Dislocated shoulders are very painful and quite often require a pillow between the arm and body to hold the upper arm in the most comfortable position. Shoulders that are held in abnormal positions should never be forced into a more anatomic alignment.

Elbow: It is often difficult to tell whether there is a fracture or dislocation; both can be serious because of the danger of damage to the vessels and nerves which run across the flexor surface of the elbow. Elbow injuries should always be splinted in the most comfortable position and the distal function clearly evaluated. Never attempt to straighten or apply traction to an elbow injury because the tissues are quite delicate and the structure is very complicated.

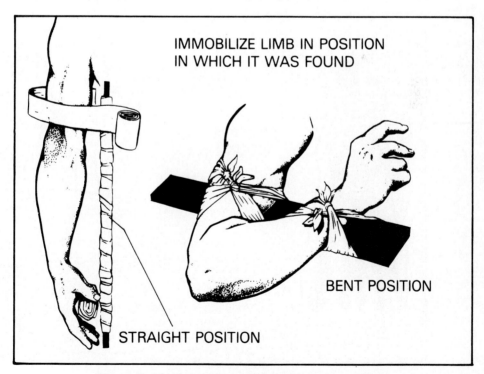

Figure 8–16. Fractures or dislocations of the elbow.

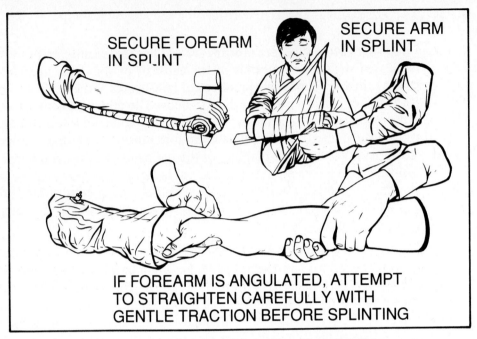

Figure 8–17. Fractures of the forearm and wrist.

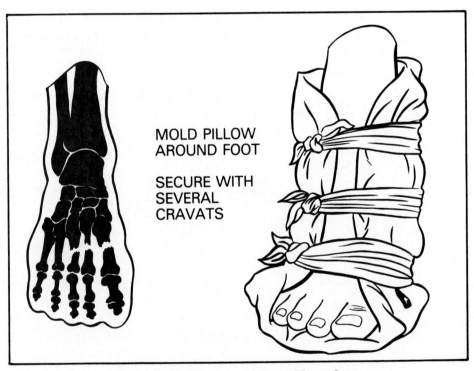

Figure 8–18. Fracture of the ankle or foot.

Forearm and Wrist: This is a very common fracture, usually as a result of a fall on the outstretched arm. Usually, it is best immobilized with a rigid splint or an air splint. If a rigid splint is used, a roll of gauze in the hand will hold the arm in the most comfortable position of function. The forearm is also subject to internal bleeding, which can interrupt the blood supply to the fingers and the hand (compartment syndrome).

Hand or Foot: Many industrial accidents involving the hand or the foot produce multiple open fractures and avulsions. These injuries are often gruesome in appearance but are seldom associated with life-threatening bleeding. A pillow may be used to support these injuries very effectively. An alternative method of dressing the hand is to insert a role of gauze in the palm, then arrange the fingers and thumb in their normal position. The entire hand is then wrapped as though it were a ball inside a very large and bulky dressing. Elevating the isolated hand or foot injury above the level of the heart will almost always reduce bleeding dramatically during transport.

Review of Important Points

1. Be very alert to the mechanism of injury so that you know what fractures to suspect and so that you can predict possible complications.
2. Remember the ABCs.
3. Visualize the injured part.
4. Be prepared for hemorrhagic shock when major bones are fractured.
5. Always record sensation and circulation initially and after any manipulation, particularly splinting.
6. Pad joints and hard spots very carefully. Make sure that all splints are well padded.
7. Examine and immobilize one joint above and below any suspected fracture.
8. Splint the patient at an appropriate time. The axial skeleton is splinted after the primary survey, but extremities should be splinted en route if a critical situation exists.
9. If in doubt, splint a potential fracture. In major trauma, the axial skeleton is always splinted on a long spine board.
10. Do not waste the "golden hour." Be cautious but be rapid.

Chapter 9

Abdominal Trauma

Gail V. Anderson, Jr., M.D., F.A.C.E.P.

Injury to the abdomen can be a difficult condition to evaluate even in the hospital. In the field it is usually more so. An abdominal gunshot wound obviously needs immediate medical attention. Blunt injuries may be more subtle, but just as deadly. The role of prehospital management of abdominal trauma has been the subject of some controversy. However, there are studies which demonstrate that appropriate and timely intervention by well-trained paramedics can improve the hemodynamic status of critically injured patients with wounds to the abdomen.

In the field, you only need to remember a few things in order to manage the abdominal trauma patient. These concepts are important, however, because blood loss from an abdominal injury can be fatal if appropriate care is not rendered in a rapid and efficient fashion.

Anatomy

The abdomen is traditionally divided into three regions: the thoracic abdomen, the true abdomen, and the retroperitoneal abdomen. The thoracic abdomen is located underneath the diaphragm and the lower ribs and contains the liver,

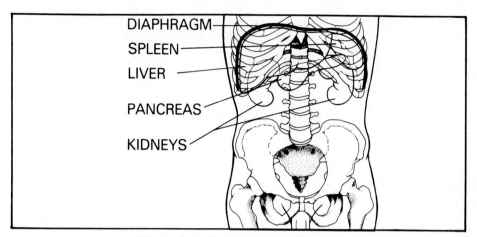

Figure 9–1. Intrathoracic abdomen.

gallbladder, spleen, and stomach. Injury to the liver and spleen can result in considerable hemorrhage.

The true abdomen contains the large and small intestines and the bladder. Damage to the intestines can result in infection, peritonitis, and shock. In the female, the uterus, fallopian tubes, and ovaries are considered to be part of the pelvic portion of the true abdomen.

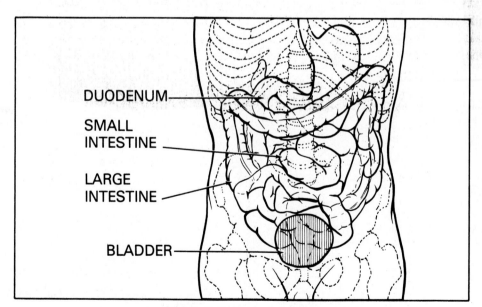

Figure 9–2. True abdomen.

The retroperitoneal region lies behind the thoracic and true portions of the abdomen. This area includes the kidneys, ureters, pancreas, part of the duodenum, abdominal aorta, and inferior vena cava. Because of location, injuries here are difficult to evaluate. While hemorrhage in the true abdomen may cause the anterior abdominal wall to become distended, extensive bleeding in the retroperitoneal space may go undetected unless a high index of suspicion is maintained.

Types of Injury

Injuries to the abdomen are usually described as being blunt or penetrating. The penetrating group is subdivided into gunshot and stab wound categories. Blunt abdominal injuries have relatively high mortality rates of 10 to 30%, usually because of the frequency of accompanying injuries to other parts of the body. As mentioned previously, the blunt trauma patient may have little external evidence of injury, which may create a false sense of security in the examiner.

Gunshot wounds to the abdomen, as a rule, will be explored in the operating room. These patients have mortality rates of between 5 and 15%. These rates are much higher than those of stab wounds because of greater tendency of injury to abdominal viscera from the gunshot(s).

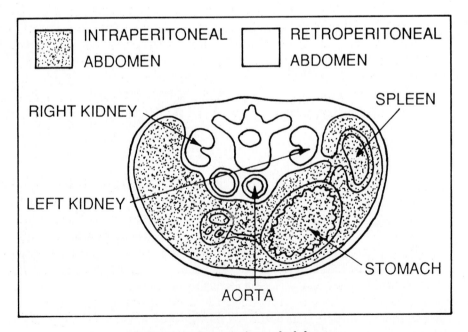

Figure 9-3. Retroperitoneal abdomen.

The mortality rate from abdominal stab wounds is relatively low (1 to 2%). Unless the knife penetrates a major vessel or organ, such as the liver or spleen, the patient may not initially appear to be in shock at the scene. However, some of these patients can develop life-threatening peritonitis over the next few hours. These wounds need to be carefully evaluated in the hospital.

It should be remembered that the path of the penetrating object may not be readily apparent from the wound location. A stab to the chest may penetrate the abdomen, and vice versa. The course of a bullet may pass through numerous structures in different body locations. In the prehospital phase, the abdominal injury you must be most concerned about is intraabdominal bleeding with hemorrhagic shock.

Evaluation and Stabilization

History

Much important information can be gleaned from the scene by noting the circumstances surrounding the patient's injury. If the patient was involved in a motor vehicle accident, quickly observe the damage to the vehicle (passenger compartment intrusion, broken windows, bent steering wheel, etc.) as you approach the vehicle. If the patient needs to be extricated, note the location of the safety belts. (Although they certainly save lives, incorrectly worn safety belts can cause blunt abdominal injuries.) The person who is stabbed or shot may be able to give you some idea of the size of the instrument or trajectory of the bullet. Often, a bystander may be able to provide such information. However, it is important not to spend a great deal of time in attempting to obtain a history. Be sure to report to the receiving physician any mechanism that would suggest abdominal injury. The major cause of delayed mortality in abdominal injury is *delayed diagnosis and treatment.*

Examination

As in any other traumatic condition, the patient with abdominal injury first needs to have the ABCs secured. The essence of the prehospital physical examination is rapid visual evaluation and palpation. Observe for wounds, bruises, evisceration, and distension. Note any tenderness or tenseness. A painful or expanding abdomen is an indication for immediate transportation to the hospital. Little is gained and critical time is lost by auscultation or percussion in the field.

Signs of intraabdominal injury usually do not appear early, so if present in the prehospital phase, there is usually significant injury and shock is probably imminent.

Stabilization

Two large-bore intravenous (IV) lines should be started and an infusion of Ringer's lactate begun. If the patient is in shock, this should be done en route to the hospital.

Any organ or viscera protruding from a wound should be gently covered with gauze moistened with saline or water (if the intestines are allowed to dry, they may be irreversibly damaged). Do not try to push the intestines back into the abdomen.

If a foreign body (e.g., knife, glass shard, etc.) is impaled in the abdomen, do not attempt removal. Carefully secure the object to the patient without moving it.

The patient should be placed in MAST (noninflated) and readied for transport. If the patient becomes shocky, the IV fluids should be administered

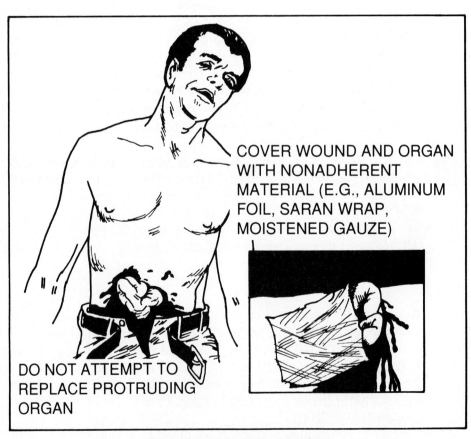

Figure 9–4. Protruding intestines.

at a wide-open rate and the MAST inflated following the guidance of medical control. The inflated abdominal compartment may help to tamponade intra-abdominal hemorrhage. Do not inflate the abdominal portion of the MAST if:

1. Any viscera is protruding
2. A foreign object is impaled
3. The patient is pregnant
4. The patient is a small child
5. You suspect a diaphragmatic hernia

Only the leg sections should be inflated in such circumstances.

Summary

Effective prehospital management of the patient with abdominal trauma entails:

1. Pertinent history
2. Rapid visual inspection and palpation
3. IVs, MAST (en route if patient in shock)
4. Rapid transport to hospital

The enemies of the patient are bleeding and time. If you can minimize on-scene delays, you will help to maximize the patient's chance for survival.

Chapter 10

Trauma in Pregnancy

Ron W. Lee, M.D.

The traumatic injured pregnant patient represents a unique challenge for the prehospital provider. The pregnant patient is often at risk for a higher incidence of accidental trauma. The increase in fainting spells, hyperventilation, and excess fatigue that are common in early pregnancy, as well as the changes in the physiological parameters of the pregnant patient, such as the loosening of pelvic joints, add to the risk of minor accidental trauma. It is estimated that accidental injury may complicate 6 to 7% of all pregnancies. The pregnant patient with minor injuries rarely represents a problem for the prehospital provider and therefore our discussion will be centered around moderate to severe traumatic injuries. It is important to remember that the pregnant patient represents two patients with separate requirements, those of the mother and those of the fetus. Therefore, any intervention must have the twin goals of supporting the mother and identifying the needs of the fetus.

To understand the unique aspects associated with trauma in pregnancy, it is important to recall certain physiological processes that are peculiar to pregnancy. The pregnant patient is known to have an extraordinary unique response to stress and trauma.

The cardiopulmonary changes that occur during pregnancy are significant. The cardiac output will increase by 20 to 30% during the first 10 weeks of gestation. This increase in cardiac output peaks at term and approximates

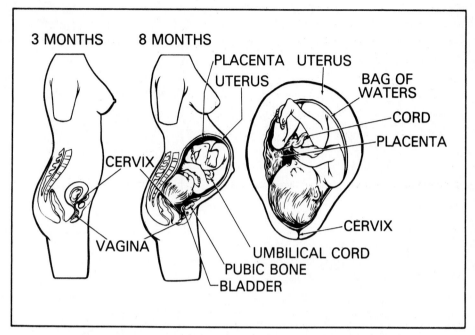

Figure 10–1. Anatomy of pregnancy. Uterus at 3 months and 8 months.

6 to 7 L/min. The average maternal heart beat will increase by 10 to 15 beats per minute, while the systolic and diastolic blood pressure will often lessen by 10 to 15 mmHg when compared to the nonpregnant patient.

The respiratory status of the patient is submitted to significant changes because of the enlarging uterus that will elevate the diaphragm and decrease the overall volume of the thoracic cavity. There tends to be some flaring out of the rib margins in order to compensate for this decrease in capacity. There is also an increase in the amount of gas exchange occurring over each minute that leads to a relative alkalosis.

The pregnant patient also undergoes a change that is described as the "hypervolemia" of pregnancy. This represents an increase of both red blood cells and plasma, yielding an increase in the total blood volume of approximately 45 to 50%. However, since there is a greater increase in plasma over blood cells, the patient tends to manifest a relative anemia.

This enlargement in plasma volume is particularly important since the patient may lose 30 to 35% of the circulating blood volume before vital signs changes occur where one would identify hypotension. This expansion in circulating blood volume also mandates that any significant maternal hypovolemia must be replaced with large amounts of fluids.

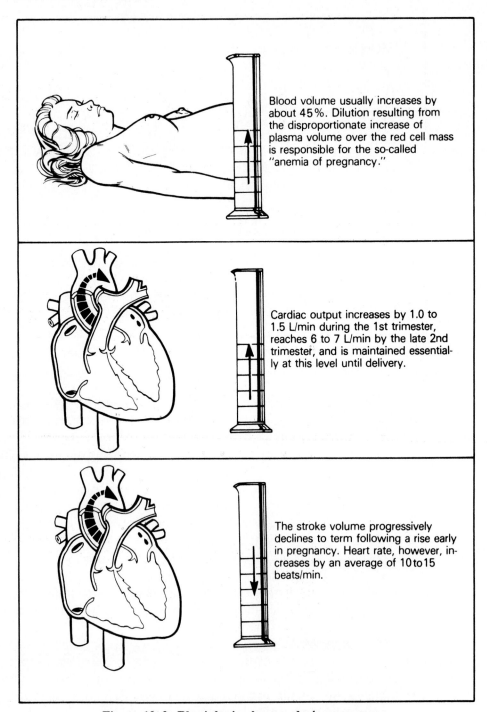

Blood volume usually increases by about 45%. Dilution resulting from the disproportionate increase of plasma volume over the red cell mass is responsible for the so-called "anemia of pregnancy."

Cardiac output increases by 1.0 to 1.5 L/min during the 1st trimester, reaches 6 to 7 L/min by the late 2nd trimester, and is maintained essentially at this level until delivery.

The stroke volume progressively declines to term following a rise early in pregnancy. Heart rate, however, increases by an average of 10 to 15 beats/min.

Figure 10–2. Physiologic changes during pregnancy.

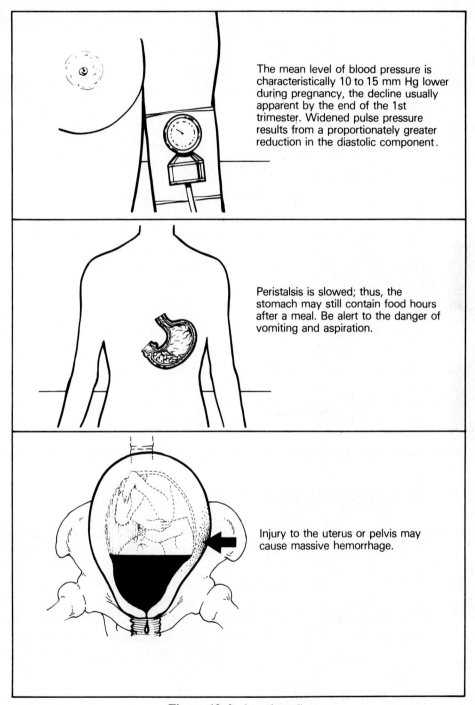

The mean level of blood pressure is characteristically 10 to 15 mm Hg lower during pregnancy, the decline usually apparent by the end of the 1st trimester. Widened pulse pressure results from a proportionately greater reduction in the diastolic component.

Peristalsis is slowed; thus, the stomach may still contain food hours after a meal. Be alert to the danger of vomiting and aspiration.

Injury to the uterus or pelvis may cause massive hemorrhage.

Figure 10-2. (continued).

The major physiological changes in the gastrointestinal system are secondary to the enlarging uterus that leads to several considerations.

1. It causes a compartmentalization of the organs within the abdomen. This compartmentalization now displaces most of the small bowel upward, while the uterus becomes the largest organ within the abdominal cavity. This has major consideration when trying to identify organ systems that are injured from either penetrating or blunt trauma.

2. There is a general decrease in GI motility, with a resulting delay in gastric emptying. This often places the traumatically injured pregnant patient in great risk for regurgitation and aspiration.

The changes in the urinary system are many; however, the most significant is the displacement of the bladder anteriorly and superiorly, placing it in a position where penetrating or blunt trauma is more likely to do greater harm.

The multiple changes in the reproductive system are significant in that the uterine blood flow, which is normally approximately 2% of the cardiac output, now increases to approximately 20%. It is important to realize that the vessels supplying the uterus are low-resistant vessels and that there is very little autoregulation available to the uterus as there is within the brain, heart, kidneys, and muscles. The α-adrenegic response predominates over the β-adrenegic response in the uterus. Therefore, under periods of stress there may be significant vasoconstriction with a reduction of blood flow to the uterus. Furthermore, the uterus is not as responsive to vasodilation and cannot increase the blood flow to the uterus in times of placenta hypoperfusion.

Responses to Hypovolemia

The response to acute blood loss results from a decrease in circulating blood volume. The cardiac output decreases as the venous return falls. This hypovolemia causes the arterial blood pressure to fall, resulting in an inhibition of vagal tone, thereby causing tachycardia, and the rest of the autonomic system comes into play by causing a vasoconstriction of the vascular bed. The vasoconstriction profoundly affects the uterus. This leads to a reduction of uterine blood flow by 20 to 30%. This reduction in uterine blood flow may occur prior to any detectable change in the blood pressure of the maternal system. The fetus reacts to this hypoperfusion by a drop in arterial blood pressure and a decrease in heart rate. The fetus now begins to suffer from a reduction in oxygen concentration in the maternal circulation. It is important to remember that some methods for oxygenation of the hemorrhagic maternal patient in shock may not always provide adequate oxygenation of the fetus. Therefore, it is important to give large amounts of supplemental oxygen in order to provide sufficient oxygen to the fetus, who suffers from both oxygen starvation and inadequate nutrient supply.

Another cause of hypotension in the pregnant patient results from the decrease in venous return when the patient is in the supine position. The enlarging uterus can cause significant compression of the vena cava, which reduces venous return. This effect is particularly evident after the twentieth week of gestation. The reduced venous return has been shown to lead to maternal hypotension, syncope, and fetal bradycardia. Therefore, all pregnant patients should be transported in the left lateral decubitus or decubent position. This should be done only if this can be done without risk to the patient. If the type of patient trauma prevents this type of maneuver, the vena cava obstruction can be prevented or can be alleviated by one of the following methods.

1. Tilt or rotate the backboard 20 to 30° to the left.
2. Manually displace the uterus to the left side during transport.

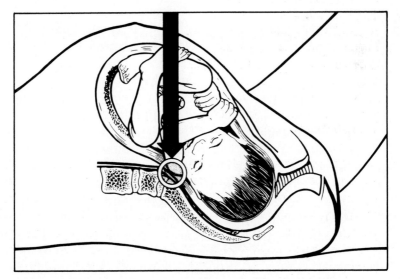

Figure 10–3. Venous return to the heart may be greatly compromised by uterine compression. Transport victim on her left side or tilt spine board to the left.

Types of Injuries

A pregnant patient is subject to all manners of accidental injury, including falls, automobile accidents, gunshot wounds, and electrical and thermal injuries.

Vehicular Accidents

The most common cause of maternal mobility is the blunt injury resulting from vehicular accidents. A review of this type of injury indicates that where there is only minor damage to the vehicle, fewer than 1% of pregnant patients will sustain injury. The liklihood of a major life-threatening injury is directly related to the damage inflicted on the vehicle. The factors important in predicting the severity of injury are related to the following questions:

1. How fast was the vehicle traveling at impact?
2. What was the position of the patient in the vehicle at the time of impact?
3. Were any restraints utilized?
4. Which body parts sustained the impact?
5. On what side of the automobile did the impact occur in relationship to the patient?

The most common cause of death in these patients was due to head injury. The internal injuries that occurred in those pregnant patients that died tended to be multiple, and death resulted from uncontrolled hemorrhage. The old concern that an injury to the fetus is likely to occur with the seat belt on was based on early data, which revealed that with the use of the lap belt alone, there was an increased incidence of injury to the uterus and fetus. However, the overall vehicular mortality for pregnant patients declined with the use of seat restraints. The use of lap restraints, however, did change the types of presenting injuries. It is clear that the mortality was reduced because more patients were restrained from being thrown from the car. This reduction in mortality was a direct result of putting the restraining device over the abdomen. The acceleration/deceleration injuries associated with use of only the lap belt probably contributed to more cases of uterine rupture and placental separation. However, the use of a lap belt with shoulder restraint has not shown any increase in uterine injuries.

The most common cause of fetal death is maternal death. Fetal death with maternal survival occurs most often in abdominal trauma with placental separation or placental abruption. Here the patient presents with vaginal bleeding, abdominal pain, an irritable uterus, and often some degree of hypotension.

Vehicular accidents have associated injuries, such as pelvic injuries, that often result in placental separation and concealed hemorrhage within the retroperitoneal area. The retroperitoneal area, because of its low-pressure venous system, can show a loss of 4 or more liters of blood into that area with few clinical signs. It should be noted that fetal skull fractures are much more common when maternal pelvic fractures occur.

Penetrating Injuries of the Abdomen

The most common type of penetrating injury to the pregnant patient is the gunshot wound. The likelihood of any abdominal organ being struck by a bullet is directly related to the size of the organ and the space it occupies within

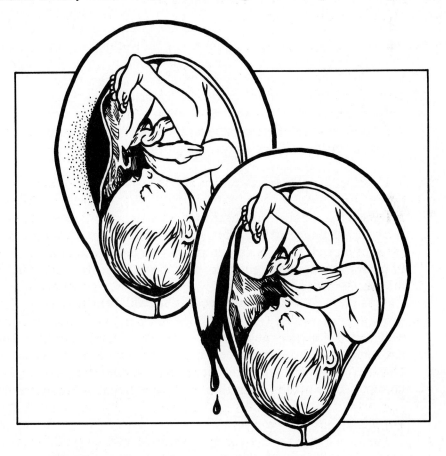

Figure 10–4. Blunt trauma to uterus. Blunt trauma may cause separation of the placenta or rupture of the uterus. Massive bleeding may occur.

the peritoneal cavity. Therefore, in early pregnancy the likelihood of uterine injury or fetal injury is low. However, as the pregnancy progresses toward term, the chance for injury increases proportionately. The most common organs injured from gunshot wounds to the nonpregnant patient are the small bowel, liver, colon, and stomach, in decreasing order. The mortality and complication rates are related to the number of organs injured. It should be noted that there has been no recorded maternal mortality secondary to gunshot wounds to the uterus since 1912. Note that 19% of women who do sustain gunshot wounds to the uterus will have associated visceral injuries. Fetal injuries from gunshot wounds to the uterus vary from 60 to 90%, with a mortality of 40 to 70%. Fetal death is secondary to direct injury to the fetus or injuries to the membranes, cord, or placenta.

The second most common cause of penetrating abdominal wounds is the stab wound. Stab wounds to the abdomen have an associated mortality of approximately 1.4% in the nonpregnant individual. The enlarged uterus protects the pregnant patient from serious organ injury when lower abdominal stab injuries occur. However, due to the compartmentalization, stab wounds to the upper abdomen often carry a higher incidence of visceral injury especially to the small bowel. Fetal mortality in these injuries is related directly to maternal mortality, and when isolated fetal death occurs it is usually secondary to either direct fetal injury or to prematurity.

Falls

The incidence of significant injury to the pregnant patient resulting from a fall is proportional to the force of impact and the specific body part that sustains the impact. Injuries associated with pelvic fractures manifest an increase in placental separation and fetal fractures of the skull and long bones.

Trauma from Thermal Injuries

.The overall mortality and morbidity resulting from thermal injuries to the pregnant patient is not markedly different from the nonpregnant individual. However, it is important to remember that the fluid requirements for the pregnant patient is greater than that in the nonpregnant individual.

Evaluation

The evaluation of the traumatized pregnant patient does not differ from that of the nonpregnant patient. The priorities remain the same.

1. Secure the **airway** and stabilize the cervical spine.
2. Assess **breathing.**
3. Assess **circulation.**
4. Stop the bleeding.
5. Determine transport decision and critical interventions.
6. Perform a secondary survey.
7. Transport with continuous monitoring.

Things to Remember: The pregnant patient has a resting pulse that is 10 to 15 beats faster than normal and the blood pressure is 10 to 15 mmHg lower than normal. Therefore, it is important not to mistake normal vital signs in pregnant individuals as signs of shock. However, it is also important to realize that a blood loss of 30 to 35% can occur in these patients before there is a significant change in the blood pressure. Therefore, these patients must be managed expectantly. Remember, more volume replacement will be needed for fluid resuscitation of the pregnant individual in shock. It is important to realize that trauma to the abdominal compartment can cause occult bleeding in either the intrauterine or retroperitoneal area. Keep in mind that gradual stretching of the abdominal wall during pregnancy, along with hormonal changes within the body, make the peritoneal surface less sensitive to irritable stimuli. Therefore, bleeding can occur intraperitoneally, and the signs of rebound, guarding, and rigidity may not be present.

Management of the Pregnant Patient

The management of most injuries are the same as discussed in other chapters. However, severe hemorrhagic shock can occur from injuries to the uterus because this very vascular organ can bleed profusely. Fluid resuscitation should include one to two intravenous lines of lactated ringers. The MAST suit can be utilized, but generally only the leg compartments should be inflated. Inflation of the abdominal compartment may impair blood flow to the fetus.

Oxygen Administration

Oxygen requirements for women in late pregnancy has been reported to be 10 to 20% greater than normal. Maternal shock of *any degree* will cause vasoconstriction of the uterus with a marked decrease in oxygenation of the fetus. *Any injured pregnant patient should receive high-flow oxygen immediately.*

Transport

The transport of any pregnant patient whose pregnancy is greater than 20 weeks should occur with the patient on her back, with the uterus displaced to the left to prevent inferior vena cava obstruction. If there is no danger of spinal injury, you can transport the patient on her left side. If there is a possibility of spinal injury, secure the patient appropriately to the long spine board but prop up the board slightly on the right side so that the uterus is tilting to the left. An alternative method is to manually hold the uterus to the left side.

Important Points to Remember

1. It is imperative to recall that you are treating two patients; however, the mortality of the fetus is related to the treatment provided to the mother. The goal of prehospital intervention is to maximize the chances of maternal survival, which will provide the fetus with the best chance for survival.

2. Treat shock expectantly; do not wait for definitive signs or symptoms of classic shock. Treat the patient early and remember that replacement volume will be greater than usual.

3. Hypoxemia of the fetus may go unnoticed in the traumatized pregnant patient. Treatment may include high-flow oxygen.

4. Transport must include appropriate spinal immobilization, extremity splints, and prevention of vena cava obstruction.

5. Reassessment and constant monitoring are paramount during transport.

6. If the mother dies, continue CPR and notify the hospital to be prepared for immediate cesarean section.

7. Cardiac arrest in the pregnant patient is treated the same as for other victims. Defibrillation settings and drug dosages are exactly the same.

Chapter 11

Pediatric Trauma

Carden Johnston, M.D., F.A.A.P.

Everyone in the health care profession has had an episode of "freezing" when approaching an injured or seriously ill child. This occurs less often and less severely if the provider has had practice drills involving children's mannequins and is secure with his pediatric knowledge, equipment, and skills.

Predictable Pediatric Problems

There are conditions that you anticipate when you hear that a man is down. There should be conditions that you anticipate when you hear that a child is down. One of the most frequent is Waddell's triad—a combination of injuries occurring to the child crossing the street and getting hit by a car. In countries where automobiles are driven on the right side of the road, generally the bumper of the car hits the child's left femur while the fender hits the spleen area. The child flies through the air and lands on the opposite side of his head. So anticipate children hit by a car to have femur, spleen, and opposite side-of-the-head injuries.

Statistically, when you hear that a child is down, you should anticipate head injury, as this is the leading cause of death in children. Head injuries occur most frequently in motor vehicular accidents, although in some areas of the country, falls are the primary cause of death. If a call from home does not involve a fall, anticipate an airway foreign body, a seizure, or SIDS (sudden infant death syndrome).

Children come with parents, which means that you have two patients even if the adult is not injured. You have to have the confidence of the parents to help and even allow you to treat the child. This is no easy task in itself. The parents are anxious, upset, and probably feel guilty. They will transfer these emotions to you, so they may put unreasonable blame on you as well as unreasonable expectations.

The best way to get the parent's confidence is to show your competency in managing the child, using appropriately sized equipment. Involve the parent in the care of the child and try not to separate family members. The parents can do simple tasks such as hold a pressure dressing (or just hold the child's hand) and can explain to the child what you are doing. Show your concern for the child—but don't freeze. One technique is to pretend that the parent is one of your examiners and you are talking your way through the examination of a multiply injured patient.

You can gain confidence from the parent and child if you talk to the child in a language appropriate for age and examine the child like you are playing games. At the same time you are performing an overall assessment and obtaining information about mental status. A child who can be consoled or distracted by you, a friend, or a toy reflects an assessment that the brain is being perfused with oxygen and nutrients with an adequate blood pressure. On the other hand, a child who cannot be consoled or distracted may be in shock, experiencing hypoxia, or severe pain. Changes in distractibility and consolability are important observations that should be recorded and reported just as you would report changes in level of consciousness for the adult.

A child less than 9 months old likes to hear "cooing" sounds, the tinkle and sight of keys, and usually enjoys the flashlight. For the child less than 2, the flashlight is a good distracter. As the child knows a lot of "ah" sounds, like "mama" and "papa," try to use those. The 2-year-old is typically negative, and little you do will distract or comfort the child. Unfortunately, that behavior is normal. Try making faces, word sounds, and smile a lot. All questions you ask the child will probably be answered "no." The preschool child can benefit from a toy or doll. If the child had one in the car or nearby, ask the parent to get it, as it will make the trip to and through the hospital easier. Or you can make a doll out of a rubber glove or a balloon (from your pediatric box), or an airplane out of two tongue blades.

Don't get caught in the trap of asking the child if he wants to take a trip in the ambulance or to be placed in a cervical collar. The child will answer "no" most of the time. Tell the child what you are doing with a smile on your face. If you can put a collar on the mother or a sibling to show that it does not hurt, it will help your compliance with the patient. Size is intimidating. Paramedics spend a lot of field time on their knees, and in the care of the child, it is very appropriate. When approaching a child, try to make yourself small by getting on the child's level.

Try not to use the word "hurt," even in a negative sense, until you are ready to do something painful. Tell the child when it will hurt and when the pain will be over. This will establish some trust with the child.

Parents and children do not understand packaging. Explain to the parent why you are doing it, and although the chances are low that anything serious is wrong with the spine, the stakes are high if there is. Make a game of packaging with the child. If the parent refuses to let you package, write it down on your run sheet and get the parent to sign it.

Frightened children, especially around the ages of 2 to 4, will try to defend themselves by biting, spitting, or hitting. They are acting out of fear. Stay calm, recognize that the behavior is normal, reassure the child, and use firm, not painful, physical control of the patient as needed.

Many states do not allow transport or treatment of the pediatric patient without the consent of the parent. Paramedics have to make a decision whether or not it will take too long to find a parent to obtain consent. In a situation of a child needing emergency care (e.g., an asphyxiated infant where the mother is unconscious), you must treat that child appropriately. Transport before permission is received, document why you are transporting without permission, and notify medical control of this action.

The parent or legal guardian is responsible for approving therapy and transport. If they do not want you to transport or treat and you cannot persuade them, document your actions on the run sheet and try to get them to sign it. If abuse is suspected, notify the authorities.

Before you leave the scene with the child, be sure to ask the parent about other children. Sometimes they are so concerned about one that they forget about other small children who may be in a high-risk situation, such as alone in the house.

Equipment

Table 11-1 contains a list of suggested equipment for the prehospital provider. You would not want to approach a 170-pound man having a heart attack with a 3.5-mm endotracheal tube, so a child should not be approached with adult equipment. The equipment is listed for different ages and could be kept in different trauma boxes so that everything for that age child would

Table 11-1 *Prehospital Pediatric Equipment and Supplies*

Pediatric femur traction splint
Pediatric backboard
Pediatric and child antishock trousers
Pediatric cervical collars
Pediatric bag–valve–mask resuscitator with newborn and child-size masks
Blood pressure cuffs, infant and child
Sandbags
Endotracheal tubes, sizes 2.5 to 9 m
Infant and child laryngoscope blades, straight and/or curved, sizes 0 to 3

Nasogastric tubes, sizes 8, 10, 12, 14
Bone marrow needles, sizes 16 to 18
Epinephrine, 1 mg/10 mL (1:10,000); 10-cc syringe
Atropine sulfate, 0.1 mg/mL
Dextrose, 0.5 g/mL (50%); 50-cc syringes
Sodium bicarbonate, 1 mEq/mL; 10-mL syringes
Oral airways, 0 to 5
Butterfly cannulas, 23 and 25 gauge
Twenty-two and 24 gauge over the needle catheters

be at your fingertips. That is, you could have a box for the 0- to 1-year-old child, another for the preschool child, and one for the preadolescent. Having needed equipment readily available can be timesaving and would be very reassuring to the parent.

Approach

The approach to the injured child is the same as for the adult:

1. Airway with C-spine stabilization
2. Breathing assessment
3. Circulatory assessment
4. Control major bleeding
5. Decision
    a. Critical situation present:
        Backboard

        Immediate transport
        Lifesaving interventions en route
        Secondary survey en route
  b. Critical situation not present:
        Backboard
        Secondary survey
        Transport
 6. Medical control notification

Children are different not only in size but also in anatomy and physiology. Fortunately, most often children are easier to manage than adults. Children are portable and they can (and should) be transported rapidly. *There are very few procedures that should be done in the field.* Pediatric procedures are difficult, even in a warm, dry, well-lighted emergency department.

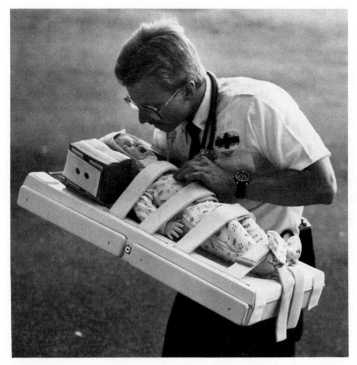

Figure 11–1. Example of an infant immobilized on a Clark Pediatric Unit®.

Airway with C-Spine Stabilization and Initial LOC

This is the same as for the adult, but for the child is easier. It is true that the child's tongue is large, the tissue is soft, and the airway is easier to obstruct, but other anatomical characteristics, such as the short distance from the mouth to the larynx, make it easier. For example, neonates are obligatory nose breathers, so just opening the mouth or clearing the nose with a bulb syringe can be lifesaving. To use the bulb syringe, collapse the bulb end of the syringe, put the pointed end in the nose of the child, and release the bulb. Remove the syringe from the nose, empty the mucus, and repeat. The bulb syringe can be used to remove secretions from the posterior pharynx of infants as well.

So that the neck does not have to be moved, jaw thrust should be tried first in the unconscious child who has sustained trauma. Be sure that the neck is stabilized in a neutral position. The occiput is so big in a child that if he is lying flat, the neck automatically will be flexed and may occlude the airway.

Nasopharyngeal airways are too small to work predictably in children; do not depend on them. Nasopharyngeal airways are quite narrow for their length; it takes very little mucus to obstruct them, and the child produces copious secretions.

For the unconscious child, oral airways are very helpful to get the tongue out of the way and keep the airway open. Choose an oral airway that goes from the corner of the mouth to the ear, and place it in after opening the mouth with a tongue blade. Placing oral airways in upside down and then rotating them may dislodge already loose teeth and cause them to fall into the airway. If a tooth is knocked loose, be sure to remove it from the mouth so that the child does not choke on it. The oral airway can stimulate a gag reflex, which is very sensitive in the child.

Cervical collars are useful and they can help remind the patient and the providers not to move the head. However, in small children they do not fit well and allow some motion. Do not depend on the cervical collar; immobilize the head with tape and head immobilizer.

Check the neck for signs of injury, carotid pulse, distended neck veins, and deviated trachea. Comparing carotid and radial pulses is not useful in a child.

Assessment of Breathing

Look at the chest rise, listen for air going in and out, and feel the air coming out of the nose. If there is no movement or ventilation is inadequate, you *must* breathe for the child. On a small child you may use mouth-to-mask and include the nose. If the face mask you have does not fit well, try turning it upside down for a better seal. Give the breaths slowly at low pressure, to keep

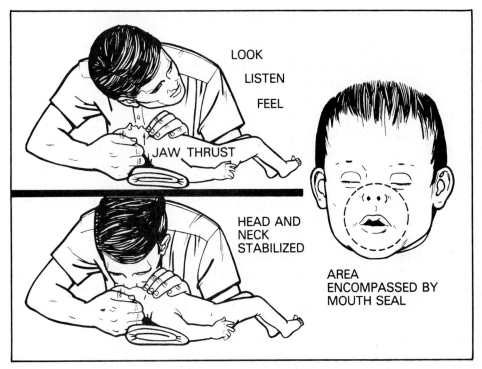

Figure 11–2. Mouth-to-mouth ventilation in a child.

from inflating the stomach. The rates are 40 per minute for neonates, 20 per minute for infants, 15 per minute for a child, and 12 per minute for an adolescent. The amount of pressure to be used is less than 20 cmH$_2$O pressure. The esophageal valve will open at about this pressure and allow air into the stomach. Most important, watch for chest rise. If the chest is rising, air is getting into the lungs. Check air entry on both sides of the chest with your stethoscope.

Some self-inflatable bags may have a pop-off valve at about 40 cmH$_2$O pressure. This is more than adequate most of the time. However, sometimes lungs are stiff either from a near-drowning, hypercarbia, or aspiration, and more pressure is needed. Make sure that your bag does *not* have a pop-off valve at 40 cmH$_2$O pressure.

You would rather not intubate the child in the field. It is extremely difficult to do even in a dry, well-lighted emergency department. If you have to intubate at the scene, choose a tube about the size that slips through the child's nose—about the size of the little fingernail. Another guide is:

$$\frac{16 + \text{age in years}}{4} = \text{size of tube (mm)}$$

Do not use a cuffed endotracheal tube until the tube size is at least 6 mm.

If intubation must be performed, the oral route should be used. Blind nasotracheal intubation is difficult if not impossible in the child less than 8 years old, as the larynx is too far anterior. There is a significant risk of neck movement with oral tracheal intubation, so have someone immobilize the neck while intubation is performed. Endotracheal intubation is easier in the small child than in the adult because the larynx is closer to the mouth. Use a straight blade, gently move the tongue to the left by entering on the right side of the mouth, place the blade in the vallecula, and lift. As opposed to the adult, this technique is often effective in the small child. If you cannot see the cords, advance the laryngoscope blade to the epiglottis and lift again. The cords should be easily seen. Remember to hold your breath during the period of time you are not breathing for the child. As soon as you get an urge to breathe, but not more than 15 seconds, stop trying to intubate, bag the child to re-oxygenate him, and try again in a few minutes. Another effective method to remind you when to ventilate is to have the team member who is stabilizing the neck count aloud to 15 slowly. Check to see if the tube is in place by following the confirmation protocol (see Chapter 3). Be sure to make the tube stay in. A simple flexion of the neck can push the tube in the right mainstem bronchus, and an extension can pull the tube out of the trachea completely. Firmly tape the tube to the corner of the mouth and immobilize the head.

Assessment of Circulation

Capillary refill is the easiest, quickest, and most reproducible mechanism to access circulation. Either compress the nailbed or entire foot and release to see how quickly the blood returns. It should return to the precompressed state within 1 to 2 seconds. To the inexperienced, blood pressure can be time consuming in a frightened pediatric patient. To make it easier and more reliable to obtain in an emergency situation, practice taking it at every opportunity. The rule of thumb for blood pressure cuff size is to use one that is the largest that will fit snugly on the patient's arm. If there is too much noise, you can perform a blood pressure by palpation. Find the radial pulse, pump up the blood pressure cuff to above the point you feel the pulse, and allow air to leak slowly while observing the dial on the BP cuff. Record the blood pressure at which you first feel the pulse and label it "p" for palpation. This will be a systolic blood pressure only and will be slightly lower than a blood pressure that can be auscultated. As a general rule, a blood pressure less than 80 is a sign of shock.

Children's skin can become mottled and is a normal finding in a child less than 6 months of age, but it may also be a sign of poor circulation, so document it. Extremities can be cold because of nervousness, cold weather, or poor circulation.

Heart rate increases for many reasons in children, but a weak, rapid pulse is still a sign of shock. As pulses feel different in a child than they do in an adult, practice feeling them on most of your prediatric runs as well as on your own children. A dorsalis pedis pulse is sometimes easier to feel than a femoral and causes a lot less anxiety in a child. The brachial is a pulse that is usually easy to feel. A weak rapid pulse with a rate over 130 is usually an early sign of shock.

The circulation can be poor even though the child appears awake. But if the child is consolable by the parent, there is enough circulation to allow the child's brain to be working. Another sign is if the child is distractable. If the child responds to your flashlight, peek-a-boo games, keys, drawings on tongue blades, or use of the stethoscope as a telephone, circulation is felt to be intact. Yawning is also a good sign that shock is not imminent. When you contact medical control, they would like to know whether the child is consolable and/or distractable. This is a helpful finding in the pediatric patient.

Initial therapy for shock is the antishock garment (MAST or PASG). They are available in child and infant sizes. If the child is too small, try placing both of the child's legs into one of the legs of the antishock garment to see if that will help increase the child's blood pressure. While you are getting the antishock garment out, place the backboard in Trendelenburg position. This in itself may raise the blood pressure, so the garment may not have to be inflated. Wrapping the legs with an Ace bandage or using an air splint can be tried.

The abdominal portion of the antishock garment is not inflated as a routine, as it compresses abdominal contents and makes breathing more difficult. Remember, older children wearing popular, tight-fitting pants are wearing a form of antishock garment. As a drop in blood pressure may occur when the pants are cut off, try to start your IV first. When it *must* be given in the field, intravenous fluid replacement is a bolus of 20 cc per kilogram of Ringer's lactate or normal saline. If there is no response, another 20 cc/kg can be given. Look around for the best vein. Time spent finding a vein and getting it dilated so that it can be stuck on the first try is time well spent. Scalp vein needles are easier to start and can be used. They do not stay in as long, but in an emergency situation can get your initial bolus of fluids in before a plastic catheter can be inserted. If you cannot see or feel a vein, you may need to perform intraosseous infusion.

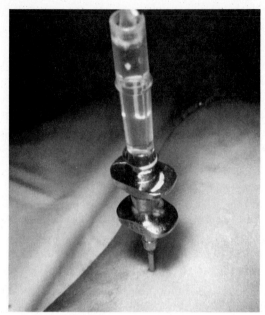

Figure 11-3. An intraosseous needle in a child's proximal tibia being used for intravenous access.

Control of Bleeding

Obvious bleeding sources must be controlled to maintain circulation. Remember, the child's blood volume is about 80 to 90 cc per kilogram, so a 10-kg child has less than 1 L of blood. Three or four lacerations can cause enough blood loss to lose 200 cc, which is about 20% of the child's total blood volume! Pay closer attention to blood loss in a child than you do in an adult as the loss volume—although in cubic centimeters—represents a larger percentage of the total volume in the child.

Use pressure firm enough to control arterial bleeding and then ask the parent or a bystander to help. Use a bandage tight enough to control venous bleeding, not one that will just soak up the blood so that you do not see it.

Decision: Critical

If you have found a critical trauma situation, the child needs rapid transport. Log-roll the child onto a pediatric spine board and go. Minutes count—especially in children—so your field time hopefully is less than 5 minutes. Administer 100% oxygen to all critical pediatric patients.

If the child is unconscious, has a dilated pupil, or has a decreasing level of consciousness, he needs rapid transport to a trauma center equipped to manage a child with head trauma.

Not all emergency departments are equipped with equipment or personnel to handle pediatric emergencies. See Table 11–2 for a partial list of severe mechanisms of injury. Discuss in advance with your medical control these as well as pediatric burns, near-drowning, and head injuries with loss of consciousness, so that you know where seriously injured children of different age groups should go. Transfer arrangements should be worked out in advance so that when the injury occurs, confusion will be minimized and time will be saved.

A child with a Glasgow Coma Scale (Table 11–3) below 10, or a Pediatric Trauma Score (Table 11–4) below 8, or a severe mechanism of injury should be transported to an emergency department approved for pediatrics or a pediatric trauma center.

If the child needs a procedure, a decision is made about how long it will take to do that procedure or procedures versus how long it will take to get better lights and temperature with more equipment and personnel. If you have a 3-minute procedure (an IV) and a 30-minute transport, the IV should be started. If you are awaiting the arrival of a helicopter, you may also attempt the procedure, but be sure to have the child packaged and ready when transportation arrives. Even physicians flying on a helicopter to the scene of trauma perform very few procedures on the critical patient. They prefer to perform lifesaving procedures en route and rapidly transport to a predesignated emergency department. Your lifesaving procedures can also be performed in the ambulance while en route to the hospital. Call ahead so that the emergency department can have cut-down trays open, endotracheal tubes at bedside, and chest tube drainage sets ready. They may need to have IV fluids or O-negative blood primed in a warmer.

Table 11–2 *Severe Mechanisms of Injury*

1. Fall from a height of 20 feet or more
2. An accident with fatalities
3. Ejected from an automobile in a motor vehicular accident
4. In a motor vehicular accident, the engine entered the passenger compartment
5. Hit by a car as a pedestrian or bicyclist
6. Fractures in more than one extremity
7. Significant injury to more than one system

Table 11-3 *Glasgow Coma Scale*

		>1 year	*<1 year*
Eyes opening	4	Spontaneously	Spontaneously
	3	To verbal command	To shout
	2	To pain	To pain
	1	No response	No response

		>1 year	*<1 year*
Best motor response	6	Obeys	
	5	Localizes pain	Localizes pain
	4	Flexion-withdrawal	Flexion-normal
	3	Flexion-abnormal (decorticate rigidity)	Flexion-abnormal (decorticate rigidity)
	2	Extension (decerebrate rigidity)	Extension (decerebrate rigidity)
	1	No response	No response

		>5 years	*<2-5 years*	*0-23 months*
Best verbal response	5	Oriented and converses	Appropriate words and phrases	Smiles, coos, cries appropriately
	4	Disoriented and converses	Inappropriate words	Cries
	3	Inappropriate words	Cried and/or screams	Inappropriate crying and/or screaming
	2	Incomprehensible sounds	Grunts	Grunts
	1	No response	No response	No response

Decision: Not Critical

If after assessing airway, breathing, circulation, and control of bleeding no critical trauma situation is found, transfer to a backboard and proceed methodically to a secondary survey in a timely fashion.

Secondary Survey

As in adults, record accurate vital signs, take an *ample* history, and perform a complete head-to-toes exam, including a more detailed neurological exam. A brief neurological check such as AVPU is useful. A preschool child does

Table 11-4 *Pediatric Trauma Score*

PTS	+2	+1	−1
Weight	>44 lb (>20 kg)	22–44 lb (10–20 kg)	<22 lb (<10 kg)
Airway	Normal	Oral or nasal airway	Intubated tracheostomy invasive
Blood pressure	Pulse at wrist >90 mmHg	Carotid or femoral pulse palpable 50–90 mmHg	No palpable pulse <50 mmHg
Level of consciousness	Completely awake	Obtunded or any ↓ LOC	Comatose
Open wound	None	Minor	Major or penetrating
Fractures	None	Closed fracture	Open or multiple fracture

not respond to stimuli like an adult, but like the circulation check, you can note if the child can be consoled or distracted. A sleeping preschool child can look unconscious; they can even sleep through a gentle pupillary check with a flashlight. However, they will awake with pain. A child who does not respond to a pinch has very little cerebral function, which in the trauma situation indicates shock, head trauma, or seizure. Finish bandaging and splinting and transport the child with continuous monitoring. Notify medical control.

Injuries

Head Injury

Because the child's head is larger in proportion to his body than the adult's, the head is the primary focus of injury in the child.

1. Give oxygen! With head injury brain cell metabolic rate is increased, blood flow is decreased in at least part of the brain, and oxygen may be very helpful.
2. Keep blood pressure up! Blood has got to get to the brain to carry oxygen, so systolic pressure should be at least 80 mmHg in the preschool child and 90 mmHg in older children.

3. Lower intracranial pressure! If the child is not in shock, elevation of the head to 30° will help lower intracranial pressure and allow blood into the intracranial vault. Do not flex the neck. Increase the rate and depth of ventilation by about 50%, so an infant's respiration rate would go to 45 per minute, a child's to 30 per minute, and an adolescent's to 25 per minute. This contracts blood vessels in the brain and lowers the pressure. Let the blood out of the brain. Do not compress jugular veins by pressure, rotation of the neck, or tight-fitting collars.

Changing level of consciousness is the best indicator for head trauma. A child entering the emergency department with a Glasgow Coma Scale of 10, who has come down from 13, will receive a very different approach from the child who has a Glasgow Coma Scale of 10, who has come up from 7. A pediatric Glasgow Coma Scale is helpful (Table 11-3). Assessments using words like "semiconscious" are not helpful. Note whether the child is distractible, consolable, or reacts to pain or voice instead of using words such as "lethargic" or "semiresponsive."

Pupil assessment is as important in the child as in the adult. Note also whether the eyes are moving both left and right or whether they are set in one position. Do not move the head to determine this! Children with head injury often fare much better than adults with the same degree of injury. If you see a child with tire tracks across his face, do not freeze. Although only minimally responsive to painful stimuli on reaching the hospital, one child with tire tracks on his face went home in 2 days, having obtained his normal level of activity (Figure 11-4).

On the other hand, children with head injury may need immediate surgical intervention to give the brain a maximal chance of complete healing. Children with serious head injury should be quickly transported to a trauma center that is appropriately equipped to provide definitive care and should arrive at that source of care well oxygenated with an adequate blood pressure.

Although it is taught that it is impossible to go into shock from intracranial blood loss, the exception to that rule is the young infant. It is not uncommon for a neonate to bleed intracranially enough to decrease blood volume, enough to enter shock. Fortunately, these children are not often involved in trauma. However, if you see an infant in shock and no obvious source of bleeding, intracranial blood loss should be considered.

Chest Injury

Because the chest is small, difference in breath sounds from side to side will be subtle, so listen carefully. Neck vein distention is not a consistent sign in children as it is in adults. However, children are easier to assess, as they will

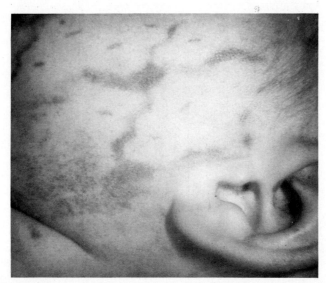

Figure 11-4. A child who had been playing behind a car and got rolled over leaving tire tread marks on his face.

give you visible signs of respiratory distress. Tachypnea, grunting, flaring, and retraction are signs that mean there is something wrong with the pulmonary system in the child. Tachypnea is a rapid respiratory rate, so count the respiratory rate. A rate over 40 usually indicates distress. Grunting indicates that the child has a need for ventilatory assistance. A few grunts are not significant, but persistent grunting is. Flaring relates to dilatation of the nares on inspiration. A child in respiratory distress will breathe with his nose like a rabbit.

Table 11-5 *Normal Vital Signs, By Age*

Age	Respiration	Blood pressure	Pulse
Newborn	50	70–75 sys.	120
12 wk	40	85 sys.	120
6 mo	35	90/60	110
1 yr	30	95/65	110
2–4 yr	24	95/65	100
5–7 yr	21	95/65	100
8–10 yr	20	95/65	90
12 yr	16	105/70	85
14 yr	16	110/75	80
16 yr	16	120/75	75

Table 11-6 *Pediatric Drugs and Dosages*

Weight [kg (lb)]	Sodium bicarbonate (1 mEq/mL)		Epinephrine (1:10,000)		Atropine (0.1 mg/mL)		Dextrose 50% (dilute 1:1 with sterile water for injection)	
	Dose (mEq)	Volume (mL)	Dose (mg)	Volume (mL)	Dose (mg)	Volume (mL)	Dose (G)	Volume (mL)
1 (2.2)	1	1	0.01	0.1	0.1	1.0	0.5	1.0
5 (11)	5	5	0.05	0.5	0.1	1.0	2.5	5.0
7.5 (16.5)	7.5	7.5	0.075	0.75	0.1	1.0	3.75	7.5
10 (22)	10	10	0.1	1.0	0.1	1.0	5.0	10.0
12.5 (27)	12.5	12.5	0.125	1.25	0.125	1.25	6.25	12.5
15 (33)	15	15	0.15	1.5	0.15	1.5	7.5	15.0
20 (44)	20	20	0.2	2.0	0.2	2.0	10.0	20.0
25 (55)	25	25	0.25	2.5	0.25	2.5	12.5	25.0
30 (66)	30	30	0.3	3.0	0.3	3.0	15.0	30.0
35 (77)	35	35	0.35	3.5	0.35	3.5	17.5	35.0
40 (88)	40	40	0.4	4.0	0.4	4.0	20.0	40.0
50 (110)	50	50	0.5	5.0	0.5	5.0	25.0	50.0

Retraction relates to either diaphragm, suprasternal area, or the intercostal area caving in on inspiration. These are signs to indicate that the lungs are stiff or the child is having to work harder to breathe. If any of these signs are persistent, they should be noted and alert you that something is wrong with the pulmonary system.

In children with blunt injury to the chest, place an "X" over the point of maximum impulse (PMI) of the heart. If a pneumothorax develops, the heart should shift away from the side of the pneumothorax. This will help confirm the stethoscope findings, which are difficult in the field. Also, the trachea will shift away from the side of the pneumothorax. A child arriving at the emergency department in respiratory distress whose PMI has shifted since the last time you marked it will make much easier your decision as to the side in which to put the chest tube.

Pneumothorax is not uncommon in pediatric trauma, and the chest tube can be lifesaving. In a small child, a 14-gauge angiocath can be placed either anterior in the second intercostal space in the midclavicular line or preferably in the anterior axillary line at nipple level, the fourth intercostal space. Place it just over the top of a rib and insert until you can aspirate air. Attach it to a one-way flutter valve.

Pericardial tamponade, flail chest, and aortic rupture are seldom seen in the preadolescent age group because of the elasticity of their chest wall.

Abdominal Injury

The second leading cause of death in most pediatric trauma centers is rupture of the liver. The liver and spleen both protrude below the ribs in children, exposing them to blunt trauma. The liver and spleen tear easily because they are relatively large and poorly protected in children. As a child goes into shock, blood flow decreases, as does the rate of blood loss. A delicate clot may form. As the child is moved and blood pressure increases, bleeding may restart. If a child has blunt injury to the chest or abdomen, be prepared to treat for shock. If a child with blunt trauma is in shock with no obvious source of bleeding, the decision should be made to "load and go." Lifesaving interventions should be made en route to the hospital. If the child has not responded to a total of 40 cc per kilogram of fluid, many centers will take the child with blunt trauma directly to the operating room. Children who respond to fluid are frequently conservatively treated with close observation and fluid replacement. Children with abdominal or head injuries are likely to vomit; be prepared.

Spinal Injury

The neck is short, the head is big, and the ligaments are loose, but fortunately C-spine injuries are uncommon in children before adolescence. However, it does occur, and children must have their spines stabilized. Immobilize the cervical spine using a padded immobilization device. A C-collar is not necessary if the head is properly immobilized in a padded device. Again, try to make a game of packaging the child, stating that you will give him a ride in the ambulance as a reward after you get him all wrapped up and ready. Utilize a parent or familiar person if possible.

Car Seats

A child in a wreck while in a car seat may be transported to the emergency department in that car seat. If the child is not in shock, the head can be taped directly to the car seat. If the child is showing early signs of shock, the car seat can be laid on its back, elevating the child's legs. Check to make sure

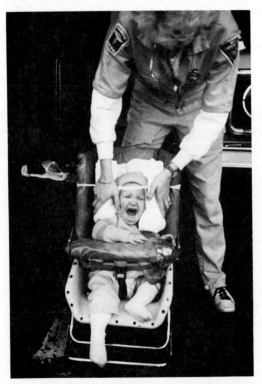

Figure 11–5. Infant immobilized in infant car seat.

that there are no hidden sources of bleeding. If the child was properly restrained in the car seat and the car seat properly attached, external bleeding should be on exposed areas only.

Prevention

All of us involved in the care of the seriously injured child should also be concerned about prevention. Car seats, seat belts, water safety, and fire drills are within our area of concern. Currently, there is an alarming increase in the number of injuries with all-terrain vehicles (ATVs). Children are not equipped with the coordination, judgment, or experience to control these vehicles and should not be allowed on one as a passenger or as a driver. We should donate our time to teach safety and we should speak out for laws (infant seat restraints, seat belts, drunk driving) that save lives.

Chapter 12

Burns

Richard C. Treat, M.D.

There are about 2 million burn injuries per year in the United States with more than 12,000 deaths as a result of these injuries. Multiple agents (Table 12-1) can cause burn injuries, but in general, the skin pathologic damage is similar. Differences between the types of burns are discussed in later sections.

Anatomy and Pathology

The skin is actually the largest organ of the body. Anatomically, the skin is made up of two layers. The outer layer that we can see on the surface is called the *epidermis*. It serves as a barrier between the environment and our body. Underneath the thin epidermis is a thick layer of collagen connective tissue called the *dermis*. This layer contains the important sensory nerves and also the support structures such as hair follicles, sweat glands, and oil glands (Figure 12-1). The skin has many important functions, including a mechanical barrier between the body and the outside world, and a protective barrier to seal fluids inside and prevent bacteria and other microorganisms from readily entering the body. The skin is also a vital sensory organ that provides input to the brain on general and specific environmental data and serves a primary role in temperature regulation.

Table 12-1 *Types of Burn Injuries*

A. Flame
B. Electrical
C. Chemical
D. Steam
E. Radiation
F. Scald

Burn damage to the skin occurs when heat or caustic chemicals come in contact with the skin and damage the chemical and cellular components that make up the skin. In addition to actual tissue injury, there is body inflammatory response to the skin damage. Burns are characterized as first, second, or third degree, based on the depth of tissue damage and skin response. First-degree burns result in actual minor tissue damage to the outer epidermal layer only, but result in an intense and painful inflammatory response. Although no medical treatment is usually required, various medications can be prescribed, which significantly speed healing and reduce the painful in-

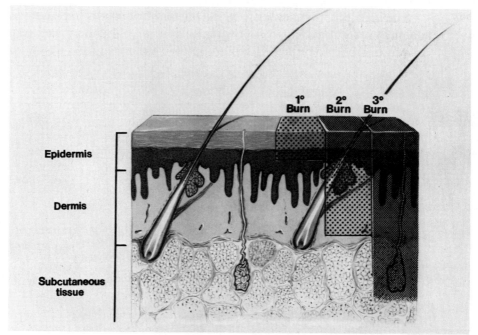

Figure 12-1. Anatomy of the skin.

flammatory response. Second-degree burns cause damage through the epidermis and into a variable depth of the dermis. These injuries will heal (usually without scarring) because the cell lining at the deep level of the epidermis (which also lines the deeper hair follicles) will multiply and result in the growth of new skin for healing. Antibotic creams or various specialized types of dressings are standardly used to treat these burns, and therefore, appropriate medical evaluation and care should be provided for patients with these injuries.

Flash burns are virtually always first- or second-degree burns. A flash burn occurs when there is some type of explosion but no actual fire. The single heat wave traveling out from these explosions results in such short patient-heat contact that only more superficial burns occur. Only areas directly exposed to the true heat wave will be injured. *In situations of possible flash explosion risk, proper protective clothing should always be worn by the paramedic or EMT.* Other injuries (fractures, internal injuries, blast chest injuries, etc.) may well occur as a result of explosion. Third-degree burns cause damage to all layer of the epidermis and dermis. No more skin cell layers are left, so healing is impossible except in small third-degree burns, which usually scar in from the sides. All third-degree burns leave scars. Deeper third-degree burns usually result in skin protein becoming denatured and hard, leaving a firm leatherlike covering that is referred to as *eschar*. Characteristics of these burns are listed in Table 12–2, and the depth levels are shown in Figure 12–1.

The inflammatory response to the burn injury results in progressive tissue damage for a day or two following burn injury; this may well result in an increase in burn depth. Any condition that either reduces circulation to this

Table 12–2 *Characteristics of Various Depths of Burns*

	First degree	*Second degree*	*Third degree*
Cause:	Sun or minor flash	Hot liquids, flashes, or flame	Chemicals, electricity, flame, hot metals
Skin color	Red	Mottled red	Pearly white and/or charred translucent and parchment-like
Skin surface	Dry with no blisters	Blisters with weeping	Dry with thrombosed blood vessels
Sensation	Painful	Painful	Anesthetic
Healing	3–6 days	2–4 weeks, depending on depth	Requires skin grafting

damaged tissue or itself causes further tissue damage will lead to burn progression with increasing burn depth. Because of the process of burn progression, it is not essential to be able to determine the burn depth exactly in the field. The EMT should be able to discern clearly between superficial and deep burns.

First-degree and second-degree burns are commonly referred to as partial thickness burns because there are still some layers of skin cells left that can multiply with resultant healing. Third-degree burns may also be referred to as full-thickness burns because all layers of the skin have been destroyed and no skin cells are left to allow healing. The magnitude of burn injury depends on the extent and depth of the burn. Initial care, which is directed specifically toward the burn, concentrates on limiting any progression of these two factors.

Initial Field Care

1. Remove the burn source. The most important concept in removing the burn source is the maintenance of safety. This involves both maintaining patient safety and maintaining EMT safety. There are specific and significant dangers to removing the burn source in all types of burn injuries. In the progression of a building fire, there is a point at which "flashover" occurs. Flashover is the *sudden* explosion into flame of everything in the room, with the temperature rising instantaneously to over 3000°F. There is no warning before this happens; thus *removal of victims from burning buildings takes priority over all other treatment*. Chemicals are usually easy to detect either on patients or on other objects in the environment. Severe chemical burns to rescuers have occurred because of the inability to note sources of toxic and caustic chemicals. Electricity is exceptionally dangerous, and handling high-voltage wires is extremely hazardous. Specialized training and knowledge are required to deal appropriately with these situations, and the EMT should not attempt to remove wires unless specifically trained to do so. Even objects commonly felt to be safe, such as wooden sticks, manila rope, and even firefighters gloves, may not be protective and may result in EMT electrocution. If at all possible, the source of electricity should be turned off before any attempt at rescue.

2. Provide patient care. People do not actually die rapidly from burn injuries. Even though the burn is highly visible and makes an intense impression at the scene, care of the burn itself has low priority. Burn victims should, in general, be managed routinely as trauma patients and have a primary survey performed immediately upon arrival in a safe staging area. Primary survey should follow the standard format described in Chapter 2.

Once it is determined that the patient is stable and "load and go" situations are not involved, attention may be turned to the burn wound itself.

Specific efforts should be made to limit burn wound progression as much as possible. Rapid cooling early in the course of a surface burn injury may help limit progression. Immediately following removal from the source of the burn, the skin is still hot and heat continues to radiate away from the patient and to some degree into the tissues. This will increase burn depth and increase the seriousness of the injury. Cooling halts this process and, if done appropriately, is beneficial. Cooling should be done with any source of water, but this should be undertaken for a maximum of 1 minute since the burn is only 1 or 2 mm thick. Cooling for longer periods is actually detrimental to patients because it will induce hypothermia and subsequent shock.

Following the brief period of cooling, the burns should be managed by the use of clean, dry sheets and blankets to keep the patient warm and prevent hypothermia (it is not necessary to have *sterile* sheets). The patient should be covered even when the environment is not cold because damaged skin loses temperature regulation capacity. Patients should never be transported on wet sheets, wet towels, or wet clothing, and *ice is absolutely contraindicated*. Ice will positively worsen the injury because it causes vasoconstriction and thus reduces the blood supply to already damaged tissue. It is better not to cool the burn wound at all rather than to cool the burn wound improperly and cause hypothermia or additional tissue damage. Initial management of chemical and electrical burn injuries is described in the sections on those injuries.

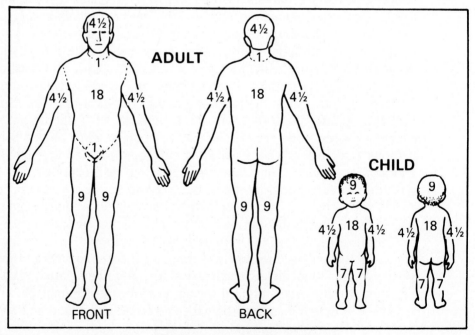

Figure 12–2A. Rule of nines.

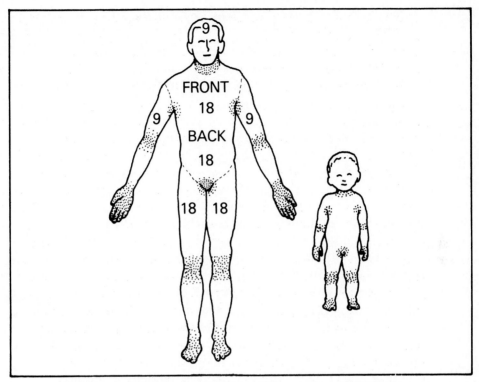

Figure 12–2B. Areas in which small burns are more serious. Second or third degree burns in these areas (shaded portions) should be treated in the hospital.

Assessment should then be made, including a history and physical evaluation. The type of burn mechanism should specifically be noted and the particular circumstances, such as entrapment, explosion, mechanisms for other possible injuries, smoke exposure, chemical/electrical details, and so on, should be recorded. An appropriate past medical history should also be documented in writing.

A standard secondary survey should be performed in stable patients, and this should specifically include an evaluation of the burn, with an estimate of the depth based on appearance and a rough calculation of the burn size. These findings are important in determining the level of medical care that would be appropriate for burn victims. The burn size is best judged by using the rule of nines. The body is divided into areas that are assigned either 9% or 18% sizes, and by roughly drawing in the burned areas, the size can be estimated. There are some differences in body-size proportionality in children. The "rule of nines" is shown in Figure 12–2. For smaller or irregular burns,

Table 12-3   *Injuries that Benefit from Burn Center Care*

A. Second-degree burn greater than 15% of body surface area (BSA)
B. Third-degree burn greater than 5% BSA
C. Significant face, feet, hands, perineal burns
D. High-voltage electrical injury
E. Inhalation injury
F. Chemical burns causing progressive tissue destruction
G. Associated significant injuries

Source: American Burn Association.

the size can be estimated using the surface of the victim's hand as about 1% of the total body surface area.

3. Loose clothing and jewelry should be removed. If burned clothing needs removal for exposure of the patient, cut around that which is adherent.

4. IV line insertion is rarely needed in the field during initial care unless delay in transport to a hospital is unavoidable. It takes hours for burn shock to develop; therefore, *the only reason to initiate IV therapy is if other factors indicate a need for fluid volume or medication administration*. Attempting to start IV therapy in the field in major burn patients is usually difficult and routinely delays initial transport and arrival at the hospital.

5. Medications are rarely needed for the burn itself. Pain medications, if used at all, must be used with extreme caution because the status of associated injuries is unclear and thus medication administration can be dangerous.

It is appropriate that nearly all burn injuries be seen by a physician. This is important since we now have specialized forms of therapy that offer specific advantages to the treatment of first-degree, second-degree, and full-thickness injuries. We have all seen second-degree burns become infected and progress to third-degree burns because of poor care. The sooner that specialized burn therapy can be initiated, the more rapid and satisfactory the results will be. Table 12-3 lists conditions that would benefit from care at a burn center.

Specialized Burn Management Areas

Inhalation Injuries

Inhalation injuries account for more than half of the 12,000 burn-related deaths per year and are classified as carbon monoxide poisoning, heat inhalation injuries, or smoke inhalation injuries. Most frequently, inhalation injuries occur when a patient is injured in a confined space or trapped; however, even victims of fires in open spaces may have inhalation injuries. Flash explosions (no fire) practically never cause inhalation injuries.

Carbon monoxide poisoning and asphyxiation are by far the most common cause of early death associated with burn injury. Carbon monoxide is simply a by-product of combustion and is found as one of the numerous chemicals in common smoke. It is present in high concentrations in auto exhaust fumes and fumes from some types of home space heaters. Since it is colorless, odorless, and tasteless, its presence is virtually impossible to detect. Carbon monoxide binds to hemoglobin (257 times stronger than oxygen), resulting in the hemoglobin being unable to transport oxygen. The patients quickly become hypoxic, even in the presence of very small concentrations of carbon monoxide. Patients exhibit signs of hypoxia with alteration in CNS function being most predominant (see Table 12-4). A cherry-red skin color or cyanosis is virtually *never* present as a result of carbon monoxide poisoning and therefore cannot be used in the assessment of patients for carbon monoxide poisoning. Death usually occurs because of myocardial ischemia and myocardial infarction due to progressive cardiac hypoxia. Patients suspected of having carbon monoxide poisoning should be treated with high-flow oxygen by mask. If such a patient has lost consciousness, advanced life support with intubation and ventilation using 100% oxygen should be undertaken if possible. If a patient is simply removed from the source of the carbon monoxide and allowed to breath fresh air, it takes up to 7 hours to reduce the carbon monoxide–hemoglobin complex to a safe level. Having a patient breathe 100% oxygen decreases this time to about 90–120 minutes (Figure 12-3).

Table 12-4 *Symptoms Associated with Increasing Levels of Carboxyhemoglobin Binding*

Carboxyhemoglobin level (%)	Symptoms
20	Headache common, throbbing in nature; shortness of breath on exertion
30	Headache present; altered CNS function with disturbed judgment; irritability, dizziness, decreased vision
40–50	Marked CNS alteration with confusion, collapse, also fainting with exertion
60–70	Convulsions; unconsciousness; apnea with prolonged exposure
80	Rapidly fatal

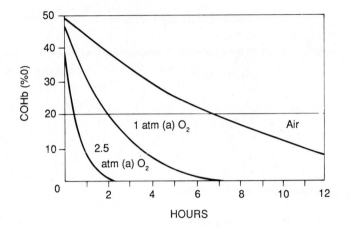

Figure 12-3. Decay curve for disappearance of carboxy-hemoglobin from 50% lethal level to 20% acceptable level in air, 1 atm, O₂ (100% oxygen) and 2.5 atm. O₂ (hypebaric oxygen—100% at 2½ atmospheres).

Heat inhalation injuries selectively damage the upper airway since breathing in flame and hot gases does not result in heat transport down to the lung tissue itself. The water vapor in the air in the tracheal–bronchial tree effectively absorbs this heat. Steam inhalation causes an exception to this rule (since it is already superheated water vapor). As a result of the heat injury, tissue swelling occurs just as it does with surface burns. The vocal cords themselves do not swell because they are dense fibrous bands of connective tissue. The loose mucosa in the supraglottic area (the hypopharynx) is where the swelling occurs, and this can easily progress to complete airway obstruction and death (Figure 12-4). Just as it takes hours for a skin burn to develop swelling, it takes considerable time for airway swelling to develop following heat inhalation. Early signs and symptoms include swollen lips (indicating the presence of hot gases and burn injury at the airway entry) and hoarseness (indicating altered airflow through the larynx area) due to swelling. Stridor (high-pitched breathing, seal-bark cough) indicates severe airway swelling with more than 85% obstruction and represents an immediate emergency. The only appropriate treatment is airway stabilization, preferably via nasotracheal intubation. This procedure may be far more difficult than under other routine circumstances because of significant anatomic alterations due to swelling. Additionally, because of irritation of inflamed damaged tissue, lethal larygospasm may occur when the endotracheal tube first touches the laryngeal area. There-

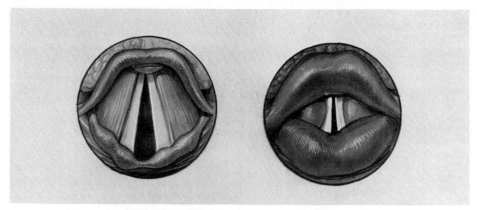

Figure 12–4. Heat inhalation can cause complete airway obstruction by swelling of the hypopharynx. Left side—normal anatomy: Right side—swelling proximal to cords.

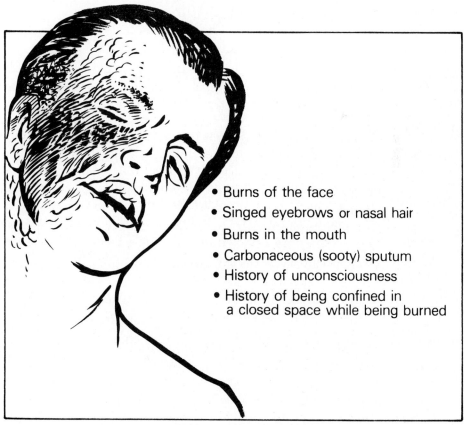

- Burns of the face
- Singed eyebrows or nasal hair
- Burns in the mouth
- Carbonaceous (sooty) sputum
- History of unconsciousness
- History of being confined in a closed space while being burned

Figure 12–5. Danger signs of upper airway injury.

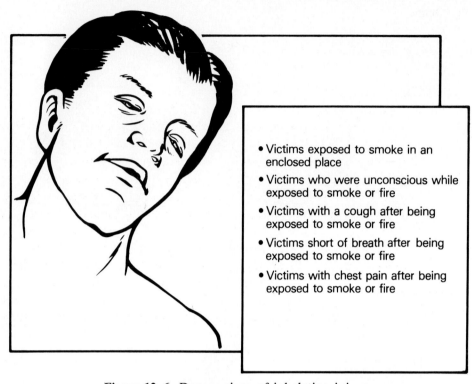

- Victims exposed to smoke in an enclosed place
- Victims who were unconscious while exposed to smoke or fire
- Victims with a cough after being exposed to smoke or fire
- Victims short of breath after being exposed to smoke or fire
- Victims with chest pain after being exposed to smoke or fire

Figure 12–6. Danger signs of inhalation injury.

fore, this procedure is best undertaken in a hospital emergency department and should be done in the field only when *absolutely* necessary.

Smoke inhalation injuries are the result of inhaled toxic chemicals which cause damage to lung cells. Smoke may contain hundreds of toxic chemicals which damage the delicate alveolar cells. Smoke from plastic and synthetic products is the most damaging. This process usually takes days to develop and is virtually never a problem in initial field management.

Patients in whom you should suspect smoke inhalation injury:

1. Patients exposed to smoke in a closed space
2. Patients giving a history of heavy smoke inhalation
3. Patients unconscious during the fire/smoke exposure
4. Patients having an irritative cough or shortness of breath following rescue
5. Patients having chest pain after being exposed to smoke or fire

Chemical Burns

There are virtually thousands of different types of chemicals that can cause burn injuries. Chemicals may not only injure the skin, but may also be absorbed into the body and cause internal organ failure (especially liver and kidney damage). Volatile forms of chemicals may be inhaled and cause lung tissue damage with subsequent severe life-threatening respiratory failure. Chemical injuries are frequently deceiving in that initial skin changes may be minimal even when a severe injury is present. This may cause a secondary problem in that such burns may not be obvious and EMTs can get these chemicals on their own skin unless appropriate precautions are taken. Tissue damage factors include chemical concentration, quantity, manner and duration of skin contact, and the mechanism of action. The pathologic process causing the tissue damage continues until the chemical is either used up in the damage process or is removed. Attempts at inactivation with specific neutralizing chemicals are dangerous because that generates other chemical reactions, which

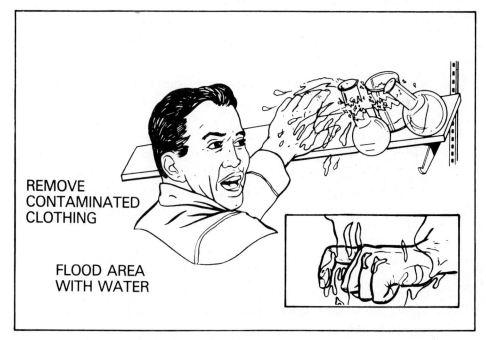

REMOVE
CONTAMINATED
CLOTHING

FLOOD AREA
WITH WATER

Figure 12–7A. Chemical burns of the skin.

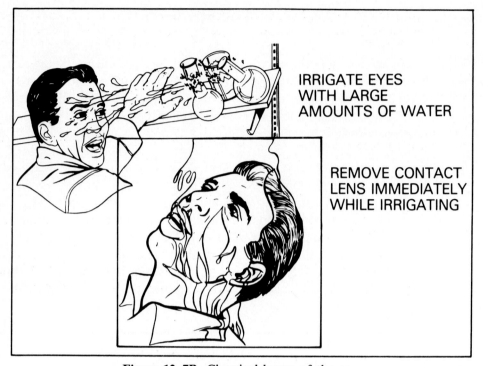

IRRIGATE EYES
WITH LARGE
AMOUNTS OF WATER

REMOVE CONTACT
LENS IMMEDIATELY
WHILE IRRIGATING

Figure 12–7B. Chemical burns of the eye.

may worsen the injury. Therefore, treatment should be aimed at chemical removal, which is done in three steps:

1. All clothing with chemicals on it is removed.
2. Most chemicals are flushed off the body by copious irrigation with any source of available water or other irrigant.
3. Any retained agent adherent to the skin must be removed by any appropriate physical means, such as wiping or scraping. This is followed by further irrigation.

In all but trivial injuries, flushing should be continued for 15 minutes unless a critical or unstable situation warrants transport sooner.

Irrigation of caustic chemicals in the eye is exceptionally important since irreversible damage will occur in a very short period of time (less than the transport time to get to the hospital). Irrigation of injured eyes may be difficult because of pain associated with eye opening. However, irrigation must be undertaken to prevent severe and permanent damage to the corneas. The EMT should check for contact lens and, if present, remove early during irrigation. If dry chemicals are present on the skin, they should first be thoroughly *brushed off* and then copious irrigation performed.

Electrical Burns

In cases of electrical burns, damage is caused by the electricity entering the body and traveling through the tissues. Extremities usually have more significant tissue damage because their small size results in higher local current density. The factors that determine severity of electrical injury include:

1. Type and amount of current
2. Path of the current
3. Duration of contact with the current

The most serious injury that occurs due to electrical contact is immediate cardiac dysrhythmias. *Any patient involved with an electric current injury,*

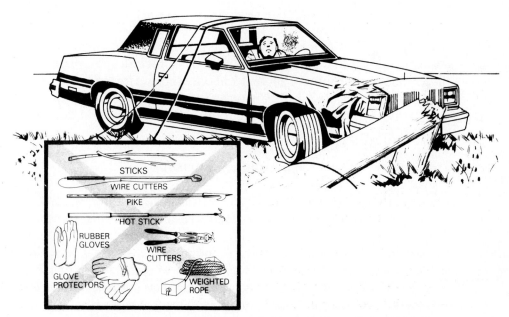

Figure 12-8. Removal of high voltage electrical wires. *Do not* try to remove wires with the safety equipment (or with sticks) unless specially trained. *Do* turn off the electricity at the source of call the power company to remove the wires.

*regardless of how stable they look, should have a careful immediate evalua-
tion of their cardiac status and continuous monitoring of cardiac activity.*
The most common life-threatening dysrhythmias are premature ventricular
contractions, ventricular tachycardia, and ventricular fibrillation. Aggressive
advanced life support management of these dysrhythmias should be undertaken since these patients usually have normal healthy hearts and the chances
for resuscitation are excellent. A patient in ventricular fibrillation with only
basic life support present should have CPR started and immediate transport
to a hospital facility. Most of these victims do not have preexisting cardiovascular disease, and their heart muscle tissue is usually not damaged as a
result of the electricity. Even under circumstances of prolonged CPR, resuscitation is often possible.

Additional electrical injuries include skin burns at entrance and exit sites
because of high temperatures generated by the electric arc (2,500 °C) at the
skin surface. Additional external burns may be present as a result of the patient's clothing being ignited. Fractures may be present due to violent muscle
contractions that electrical injuries cause. Internal injuries usually involve muscle damage, nerve damage, and possible intravascular blood coagulation due
to electrical current passage. *Internal chest or abdominal organ damage is
exceedingly rare.*

In the field it is impossible to tell the total extent of the damage in electrical burns; all electrical burn patients should be transported for hospital
evaluation. The EMT should immediately check for and appropriately manage
the cardiac status (primary survey) and once those efforts are complete, field
care is provided as described previously for thermal burns. Due to the potential for dysrhythmia development, routine IV access should be initiated in
the field for victims with electrical burns.

Secondary Transport

Major burns usually do not occur in locations where immediate transport to
one of the major burn centers is possible. As a result of this, transport from
a primary hospital to a burn center is commonly necessary. During this
transport it is important to be able to continue resuscitation. Evaluation prior
to evacuation should include documentation of stabilization of respiratory
and hemodynamic function. This may necessitate intubation, and certainly
two large-bore IVs for fluid administration are standard. Assessment and
management of associated injuries, review of appropriate lab data (specifically
blood gas analysis), placement of a nasogastric tube in all burns greater than
20% of the body surface area, assessment of peripheral circulation, and appropriate wound management should be completed prior to these secondary

transports. Proper arrangements between the referring physician and receiving physician should be made. After the initial stabilization (which should require between 1 and 3 hours), immediate movement to a major burn center is best for the patient. The EMT should specifically discuss the transport with either the referring or the receiving physician to determine what special functions may need monitoring and to determine the appropriate range for fluid administration since burns often require extremely large hourly IV rates for appropriate cardiovascular support. Careful maintenance of records indicating patient condition and treatment during the transport is important. An in-depth report to the receiving facility should be specifically made.

Important Points to Remember

1. Maintain appropriate safety when removing patients from the source of burn injury.
2. Treat burn patients as trauma patients: primary survey, resuscitation, secondary survey, and treatment.
3. Properly cool surface thermal injury if early after burn event.
4. Almost all types of burns may have inhalation injuries.
5. Chemical injuries, in general, require prolonged and copious irrigation.
6. Immediately check cardiac status of victims of electrical injury.
7. Plan all secondary transports to major burn centers and effectively continue resuscitation during such transports.

Chapter 13

Trauma Cardiorespiratory Arrest

Marlon L. Priest, M.D., F.A.C.E.P

Advanced cardiopulmonary resuscitation has always been directed toward dealing with a cardiac cause for the arrest patient (motionless patient). In the trauma situation cardiorespiratory arrest is usually *not* due to primary cardiac disease, such as coronary artery disease with acute myocardial infarction. Treatment must be directed by identifying the underlying cause of the arrest or success will almost never occur. The primary survey is still utilized to identify the cause.

Hypoxemia

Hypoxemia is the most common cause of the arrest (motionless) trauma patient. Acute airway obstruction and ineffective breathing will be clinically manifested in hypoxemia. Carbon dioxide accumulation from inadequate breathing will play a role in being unable to resuscitate the patient. Airway problems such as those listed in Table 13-1 lead to hypoxemia by preventing the flow of oxygen to the lungs. Drugs and/or alcohol, often in conjunction with minor head trauma, can result in airway obstruction by the tongue. Attention to the intoxicated patient may prevent an arrest situation. The same is true of the patient who is unconscious from a head injury or a cerebral vascular accident (stroke). The lax muscles in the pharynx allow the tongue to fall back and obstruct the airway. Patients without a gag reflex should get at least an oral or nasopharyngeal airway to prevent airway obstruction. Insertion of an endotracheal tube is even better since it will also prevent aspiration if the patient vomits. Patients with cardiorespiratory arrest caused by airway obstruction will respond to advanced life support if the anoxic period was not prolonged.

Patients with hypoxia related to a breathing problem have an adequate airway but are unable to oxygenate their blood because they cannot get oxygen and blood together at the alveolar capillary membrane of the lungs. This could be from:

1. Inability to ventilate as in a tension pneumothorax, sucking chest wound, flail chest, or high spinal cord (C-3 or above) injury.
2. Lung tissue filled with fluid, as in the patient with aspiration of blood or vomitus. Near-drowning victims have hypoxemia early from lack of oxygen, but later their lungs are full of water (like pulmonary edema).
3. Lungs filled with gas (smoke inhalation) that does not contain the appropriate amount of oxygen but instead contains harmful gases such as carbon monoxide or cyanide. In addition, the hot vapor can result in pulmonary edema, further preventing oxygenation.

Patients with breathing problems should have aggressive airway management and ventilation with high-flow oxygen. Many of these victims will respond quickly if they have not been anoxic for too long. A significant number (19% in one study) of near-drowning victims who appear lifeless in the field will eventually have a complete recovery.

Circulatory Problems

Patients with tissue hypoxia because of inadequate blood flow will have one of the causes in Table 13–1. Hemorrhagic shock (empty heart syndrome) is the most common circulatory cause of the trauma cardiorespiratory arrest.

Pericardial tamponade will look like (present as) electromechanical dissociation (EMD) because the cardiac output is so low. The heart is squeezed by the blood in the pericardial sac and cannot fill with blood before each beat because the pressure inside the sac (and thus the heart chambers) is higher than the pressure in the venous system returning blood to the heart. Only a tiny amount of blood flows from the heart with each beat. The main clinical features in isolated tamponade are profound shock with distended neck veins

Table 13-1 *Causes of Cardiac Arrest in the Trauma Situation*

1. Airway problems
   a. Foreign body
   b. Tongue prolapse
   c. Central nervous system depression from drugs/alcohol
   d. Cerebral vascular accident
2. Breathing problems
   a. Tension pneumothorax
   b. Sucking chest wound
   c. Flail chest
   d. High spinal cord injury
   e. Carbon monoxide inhalation
   f. Smoke inhalation
   g. Aspiration
   h. Near-drowning
3. Circulatory problems
   a. Tension pneumothorax
   b. Hemorrhagic shock (empty heart syndrome)
   c. Pericardial tamponade
   d. Myocardial contusion
   e. Electrical shock
   f. Acute myocardial infarction

and normal bilateral breath sounds. In the more typical situation, the patient will have associated blood loss, and the neck veins will not be distended. Patients without distended neck veins will appear to be in EMD but will not respond to ACLS protocols.

Acute myocardial infarction and myocardial contusion can produce inadequate blood flow (circulation) by either or both of two mechanisms. These mechanisms are dysrhythmias or acute pump failure. The victim with a myocardial contusion has usually been in a deceleration accident. There may be a chest wall or sternal contusion.

A full arrest from an electric shock usually presents as ventricular fibrillation. It responds readily to ACLS protocol if you arrive in time. The victim of an electrical shock has suffered severe muscle spasm and may well have been thrown down or fallen a great distance. Thus the same systematic approach to the patient is required to identify all associated injuries and give the patient the best chance for a good outcome. Be sure that the victim is no longer in contact with the electricity source. **Do not become a victim yourself!**

In summary, patients with cardiopulmonary arrest related to inadequate circulation have either:

1. Inadequate return of blood to the heart because of:
   a. Increased pressure in the chest causing increased resistance to the venous return to the heart as in tension pneumothorax or pericardial tamponade
   b. Hemorrhagic shock with inadequate blood volume to be returned to the heart
2. Inadequate pumping of the heart because of:
   a. Rhythm disturbances as in myocardial contusion, acute myocardial infarction, or electrical shock
   b. Acute heart failure with pulmonary edema, as in large myocardial contusion or acute myocardial infarction

Approach to Trauma Victims in Cardiac Arrest

This is a special group of victims. Most are young and do not have preexisting cardiac conditions or coronary disease. These patients should have a good resuscitation rate if attention is paid to the differences from the standard cardiac arrest. The extremely poor resuscitation rate for trauma victims in cardiac arrest is probably due to the fact that we approach these victims in the same way as we do those whose arrests are due to primary heart disease. Patients who suffer cardiorespiratory arrest from isolated head injury usually do not survive, but these patients should be aggressively resuscitated since the extent of injury cannot always be determined in the field and therefore you cannot predict the outcome for the individual patient.

Important Points in the Management of Victims of Trauma Cardiorespiratory Arrest
1. Rapid transport to a surgical facility is necessary.
2. The cause of the arrest must be found and specifically treated utilizing the ABC approach.
3. Three rescuers are needed to treat the arrest:
   a. One to stabilize the neck and ventilate
   b. One to do compressions
   c. One to find and treat the cause of the arrest

General Plan of Action

After determining unresponsiveness, secure the patient's airway and control the cervical spine. Open the airway with the modified jaw thrust; if there are no respirations, give two full breaths. If the airway is obstructed, repeat the jaw thrust and try ventilation again. If the airway is still obstructed by a foreign body, attempt to clear the airway with your fingers or a laryngoscope and suction. You will need assistance to maintain cervical stabilization. If this is unsuccessful, do chest thrusts (the victim must be on a firm surface). If you are still unsuccessful, you may go to cricothyroidotomy or transtracheal jet ventilation (if you are trained and protocols allow). If you are not able to do one of these surgical procedures, you may do the Heimlich maneuver. There is a chance of injuring the spine if there is an associated vertebral injury, but this is of less concern if the patient is dying of an airway obstruction. (Desperate situations often require desperate measures.) Cricothyroidotomy or transtracheal jet ventilation may be necessary if there is airway obstruction from direct trauma.

If the airway is not obstructed, give two full breaths and then check the pulse. *If no pulse is palpable, you must begin cardiopulmonary resuscitation and prepare for immediate transport.* Allow two of your teammates to do the cardiopulmonary resuscitation while you get the monitor and apply the quick-look paddles. If ventricular fibrillation is present, go ahead and defibrillate at 200 W/s. Repeat twice (increasing the charge by 100 W/s each time) if not successful.

If asystole or electromechanical dissociation is present or if the ventricular fibrillation does not immediately convert to a rhythm with a palpable pulse, you must quickly evaluate and treat the patient for the cause of the arrest. This should be done in the ambulance during transport if possible. Follow the ABC primary survey that you follow on every patient.

A.   Establish and control the airway (with an ET tube if possible) and ventilate with 100% oxygen. While the other two rescuers are ventilating and performing chest compressions, you must systematically look for the correctable cause(s) of the arrest.

B.   Look for breathing problems as a cause of the arrest. Answering the questions that follows will allow you to identify any breathing problems that may be the cause or a contributing factor.

Look at the Chest

1.   Does the chest move symetrically with each ventilation?

   2. Are there chest injuries?
       Penetrations?
       Contusions?
       Paradoxical movements?
       Sucking chest wound?

Feel the Chest

   1. Is there any instability?
   2. Is there any crepitation?
   3. Is there any subcutaneous emphysema?

Listen to the Chest

   1. Are breath sounds present on both sides?
   2. Are the breath sounds equal?
       If breath sounds are not equal, percuss the chest.
       Is the side with the absent or decreased breath sounds hyperresonant or dull?
       If intubated, is the endotracheal tube inserted too far?

Look at the Neck

   1. Are the neck veins flat or distended?
   2. Is the trachea midline?
   3. Is there evidence of soft tissue trauma to the neck?

If there are distended neck veins, decreased breath sounds on one side of the chest, the trachea deviated away from the side of the injury, and hyperresonance to percussion of the chest on the affected side, the patient probably has a tension pneumothorax. An improperly positioned endotracheal tube can cause unequal breath sounds and will be harmful to the patient since only one lung can be ventilated. You should always recheck the position of the ET tube before you make a diagnosis of tension pneumothorax; poorly positioned ET tubes are much more common than tension pneumothoraces. A tension pneumothorax requires needle decompression (if trained and protocols allow). Call medical control immediately for permission to decompress. Continue hyperventilation with 100% oxygen. Do not discontinue chest compressions until there is a palpable pulse, even though you have found a cause—there may be other causes for the patient's arrest. Other breathing problems (sucking chest wound, flail chest, simple pneumothorax) will be adequately treated by endotracheal intubation and ventilation with high-flow oxygen. If intubated, you do not have to seal sucking chest wounds or apply external stabilization to flails. It is important to hyperventilate the arrest victim since blowing off carbon dioxide helps protect the brain as well as correct the acidosis.

Now that the patient has both an adequate airway and breathing, you may concentrate on the circulatory system. Apply the quick-look paddles and again determine the rhythm. If ventricular fibrillation is still present, defibrillate once more at 400 W/sec and follow standard ACLS protocols to establish cardiac rhythm while you are continuing your exam. If intravenous access has not been established, you may give epinephrine down the ET tube. If the patient is not intubated, you may squirt the epinephrine into the posterior pharynx so that it is forced into the lungs by your ventilations. The use of the lungs allows for rapid absorption while intravenous access is being established. All of these maneuvers can be done during transport. ACLS protocols are to be used on all patients with ventricular fibrillation or asystole (no matter what the cause), but do not delay at the scene past establishing the airway. As soon as intravenous access is obtained, give 2 L of Ringer's lactate and two ampoules of sodium bicarbonate. *Once again, do not delay at the scene—all treatment past establishing the airway should be done during transport.*

Hemorrhagic shock is the most common circulatory cause of traumatic cardiopulmonary arrest. If there is no external bleeding, the patient must be examined carefully for evidence of internal bleeding.

Once electrical activity is established, the neck veins are reexamined. Flat neck veins with electrical activity favor the presence of hypovolemic shock (empty heart syndrome). Apply the antishock trousers and attempt to start two large-bore intravenous lines while en route.

If during the chest exam there are decreased breath sounds on one side with percussion dullness on the same side, this confirms a hemothorax of such a degree that shock will be present. Obvious bleeding, distended abdomen, multiple fractures, or an unstable pelvis also confirm inadequate volume. If any of these situations exist, you must assume that the arrest is secondary to hemorrhagic shock. Transport rapidly with rapid infusion of 2 to 4 L of Ringer's lactate and two ampules of sodium bicarbonate.

If the neck veins are distended but the trachea is midline and breath sounds are equal, you must suspect pericardial tamponade. Penetrating wounds of the chest or upper abdomen or contusions or the anterior chest are associated with pericardial and/or myocardial contusion. Apply MAST and attempt to start two large-bore intravenous lines. Proceed with all possible haste to the emergency department.

Electrical shock creates a special situation. It usually presents as ventricular fibrillation. Cardiorespiratory arrest secondary to electric shock responds readily to ACLS protocols if you arrive in time. Do not forget to stabilize the spine. A victim of high-voltage electrical shock will often have fallen from a power line or have been thrown several feet by the violent muscle spasm associated with the shock. Be sure that the victim is no longer in contact with the electrical source. Do not become a victim!

All patients suffering a cardiorespiratory arrest related to trauma should receive two ampules of sodium bicarbonate as soon as venous access is obtained.

Important Points to Remember

1. Cardiac arrest following trauma is usually not due to cardiac disease.
2. Do not rely on ACLS protocols alone. They should be modified to provide adequate volume and bicarbonate (and chest decompression when indicated).
3. Transport the patient rapidly. Most procedures should be performed in the ambulance during transport. Do not waste valuable time.
4. The motionless trauma patient requires attention to the ABCs in a systematic fashion to identify treatable problems in the proper priority.
5. You need adequate personnel to handle this situation well: one person to drive the ambulance, one person to stabilize the neck and ventilate, one person to do chest compressions, and one person to diagnose and treat the cause of the arrest.
6. Cardiac arrest in the pregnant victim is treated the same as for other victims. Defibrillation settings and drug dosages are exactly the same. The volume of fluid needed increases, and 4 L of Ringer's lactate or saline should be given as fast as possible during transport.

Chapter 14

Critical Trauma Situations: "Load and Go"

John E. Campbell, M.D.

There are certain situations that require hospital treatment within minutes if the victim is to have any chance for survival. The primary survey is designed to identify these situations. When these situations are recognized, the victim should be loaded immediately onto a backboard, transferred to the ambulance, and transported rapidly with lights and siren. Lifesaving procedures may be needed but should be done during transport. Non-lifesaving procedures (such as splinting and bandaging) must not hold up transport. The following are critical situations that require "load and go."

1. Airway obstruction that cannot be quickly relieved by mechanical methods such as suction, forceps, or intubation
2. Conditions resulting in possible inadequate breathing
   a. Large open chest wound (sucking chest wound)
   b. Large flail chest
   c. Tension pneumothorax
   d. Major blunt chest injury
3. Traumatic cardiopulmonary arrest
4. Shock
5. Head injury with unconsciousness, unequal pupils, or decreasing level of consciousness

Following are assessment findings that should alert you to possible critical trauma conditions.

1. Assess cervical spine control with evaluation of airway and initial level of consciousness.

Critical Findings	*Possible Causes*
a. Unresponsive or poorly responsive	Hypoxia, hypoglycemia, late shock, head injury, cardiac arrest, or drug overdose
b. No movement of air	Airway obstruction or cardiac arrest
c. Respiratory difficulty	Airway obstruction or chest injury

2. Assess breathing and circulation.

Critical Findings	*Possible Causes*
a. No respiration	Cardiac or respiratory arrest
b. Difficulty with rate or depth of respiration	Slow or irregular—head injury Fast, shallow—shock or chest injury
c. No pulse	Cardiac arrest Late shock
d. Pulse at neck but not at wrist	Late shock
e. Slow capillary refill	Early shock
f. Rapid, weak pulse >100 per minute	Shock

3. Examine the neck.

Critical Findings	*Possible Causes*
a. Discoloration and swelling	Developing airway obstruction
b. Distended neck veins and/or deviated trachea respiratory difficulty and shock	Tension pneumothorax
c. Distended neck veins and shock	Pericardial tamponade

4. Examine the chest.

Critical Findings	*Possible Causes*
a. Sucking chest wound	Open pneumothorax
b. Hyperresonant on one side, respiratory difficulty, shock, distended neck veins	Tension pneumothorax
c. Unstable segment of chest wall or sternum, difficulty breathing	Flail chest
d. Difficulty breathing, breath sounds decreased on one side, crepitation	Major blunt chest injury
e. Contusion or puncture wound of anterior chest, shock, distended neck veins	Cardiac tamponade Myocardial contusion
f. Penetrating chest wound, shock	Hemothorax Heart wound Major thoracic vascular injury

5. Control active bleeding.

Critical Findings	*Possible Cause*
Major blood loss or poorly controlled bleeding	Major vascular injury

At this point you should be able to make a decision about critical trauma conditions and who should be in the "load and go" category. Any victim with these symptoms falls in the "load and go" category:

1. Decreased level of consciousness
2. Respiratory difficulty
3. Shock

Any victim with injuries that will rapidly lead to shock or respiratory difficulty should be in the "load and go" category. This includes large flail chest or open pneumothorax even though they may not demonstrate respiratory difficulty at the time of the primary survey. The same is true of massive or poorly controlled bleeding even if shock is not evident at the time of the primary survey.

Secondary Survey

If the victim does not appear to have a critical trauma situation, you may perform the secondary survey before transport. During the secondary survey there are a few conditions that will change the victim's category to "load and go." Be very suspicious of those patients in whom the mechanisms of injury are such that severe injuries could have occurred. These patients may suddenly deteriorate.

1. Development of shock, respiratory difficulty, or decreasing level of consciousness
2. Tender, distended abdomen
3. Bilateral femur fractures
4. Unstable pelvis

Findings 2 to 4 so commonly lead to shock that these victims should be taken to the emergency department without delay. In all "load and go" situations you should call ahead to have the emergency department and possibly the operating room prepared for your arrival. If a specific surgeon is needed, your medical control physician can have him called before you arrive. Rapid transport is not lifesaving if the necessary surgeon is not available to treat the victim when he arrives. The true test of an EMS system is whether every phase of emergency care can work together as a team when a life depends on definitive care within a matter of minutes.

Chapter 15

Fluid Replacement for Shock

Jere F. Baldwin, M.D., and Steve Smit, R.E.M.T.-P

There is some controversy about the use of intravenous fluid replacement therapy by prehospital care providers. Critics have properly pointed out that in some cases victim's on scene times have been so delayed by attempts to start IV therapy that the amount of additional blood loss exceeded the amount of fluid given. It is estimated that 25% of trauma fatalities could be prevented by better trauma care (both prehospital and hospital). The sad fact is that most of these unnecessary fatalities are patients who bleed to death because they are in the field or the emergency department too long before definitive care is provided. Most of these patients could be saved by the efficient use of assessment priorities, critical interventions, and rapid transport to the *operating room*. In spite of efficient use of the "golden hour," some of these victims will still progress to irreversible shock unless fluid replacement is begun in the field. There is a real need for prehospital fluid resuscitation for shock, but in order to "First, do no harm," we must perform this livesaving procedure at the correct time in the correct manner. We must consider the following: (1) the optimum time to begin fluid resuscitation, (2) the optimum fluid for resuscitation, (3) the optimum volume for fluid resuscitation, (4) the optimum site for fluid resuscitation, (5) the optimum equipment for fluid resuscitation, and (6) the optimum techniques for fluid resuscitation.

Optimum Time to Begin Fluid Resuscitation

I.V. Therapy with the Entrapped Victim

For the victim who is entrapped, or for whom transport will be unavoidably delayed, IV therapy should be initiated on scene. The proper time is after the primary survey and during the critical interventions. Many of these victims will eventually be in need of blood transfusion therapy. This is in part because of the prolonged delay in arriving at the hospital, and in part because mechanisms of injury that would cause the victims to be entrapped would also predispose them to significant organ damage. To initiate transfusion therapy sooner, medical control may opt for one of the following. They may suggest that a blood sample be sent ahead by police car to the receiving facility, allowing blood to be typed, crossed, and available at the patient's arrival. In the event of a more prolonged extrication, medical control may elect to send the blood to the scene.

Starting the IV in the Ambulance

The critical patient who is not entrapped should have the primary survey completed, then should be moved to the ambulance for critical interventions (some airway interventions may have to be done on scene). *IV therapy should be begun after transport.* This has several advantages. First, it provides conditions superior to those found outside the ambulance, especially at night or in cold weather. The lighting is better, the equipment is at hand, and the IV solution should be warm. In cold weather the rescuer does not have to hold IV bags under his coat or have to wrap the IV tubing around heat packs. In addition, the initiation of IV therapy in the ambulance eliminates one common problem—the IV that becomes dislodged during the frenzy of transferring the patient from the scene to the ambulance. The most important advantage is that the "golden hour" is not being wasted; thus there is minimal continued blood loss while the IV is being established.

Optimum Fluid for Resuscitation

Before considering the optimum fluid for resuscitation, we must reiterate that the current treatment for blood loss is:

1. Hemostasis for control of major external bleeding
2. Conservation of time for control of internal bleeding

3. Supplemental oxygen and possible assisted ventilation for tissue and cellular oxygenation
4. Volume replacement for tissue perfusion

At the present time, there is a tremendous amount of research into improved resuscitation fluids. The most exciting work is with oxygen-carrying fluids such as PFC (perfluorocarbon) emulsions and SFH (stroma-free hemoglobin). We may soon have prehospital resuscitation fluids that not only expand volume but carry oxygen to tissue. There is also much research into other volume expanders (hypertonic saline, 6% dextran, albumin, and hydroxyethyl starch) as well as drugs that combat the effects of tissue hypoxia (calcium channel blockers, naloxone, thyrotropin-releasing hormone, ATP-MgCl$_2$). In spite of all this work, the optimum fluid for volume replacement is still fresh whole blood and *the optimum fluid for prehospital volume replacement is still Ringer's lactate.* Normal saline is a reasonable substitute but can cause hyperchloremic acidosis if large volumes are used. Vasopressors such as metaraminol (Aramine), norepinephrine (Levophed), and dopamine (Intropin) have no place in the resuscitation of hemorrhagic shock.

Optimum Volume for Fluid Resuscitation

How much is enough? The answer is: the amount required to keep the patient out of irreversible shock until bleeding can be stopped and blood can be replaced. How much is that? Specifically, the volume of fluids infused must exceed the volume of blood lost from the time of the initial IV set up until arrival in the emergency department. Deciding how much to give is based on the patient's clinical condition and on the patient's size. The average sized adult with obvious clinical signs of shock has lost at least 1500 cc (3 pints) of blood. To replace blood with crystalloid (Ringer's lactate or saline) you must give 3 cc of fluid for each cubic centimeter of blood lost. Thus 1500 cc of blood loss requires about 4 L of replacement fluid. Generally, you can blow up the PASG (MAST) and give 2000 cc (or one-half of the estimated total) as quickly as possible. If you have not arrived at the hospital by then, contact medical control about giving another 2000 cc. Remember, patients with head injury, flail chest, and smoke inhalation injury are easily fluid overloaded; they only require "keep open" rates unless they have associated hemorrhagic shock. If you use blood to replace blood, you only have to replace 1 cc for each cc of blood lost, so getting the patient to the hospital rapidly (where internal bleeding can be stopped and blood can be given) is still the most important treatment.

Fluid Resuscitation of the Pediatric Patient

As a general rule, IV therapy is not started on small children in the field (the MAST garment is preferred) unless the situation is desperate and there is a long transport time. Obtaining venous access in infants and small children is fraught with frustration and despair even in the most experienced hands. Their veins are smaller and more effectively hidden from sight and palpation on the upper extremities. If the situation demands IV therapy the amount given depends on body weight. Give 20 cc per kilogram of Ringer's lactate or normal saline rapidly. An additional 20 cc/kg is given (contact medical control) if there is no clinical improvement. Careful attention should be given to the pulse rate since some children respond to hemorrhagic shock with hypotension and *bradycardia* instead of tachycardia. It is mandatory to be able to figure out the weight of the pediatric trauma victim. A table of average weights (Table 15–1) based on age should be posted in the ambulance or in the trauma box. If there is no caretaker to give you the age, you can estimate weight by measuring length.

Table 15–1 *Average Weights for Children*

Age	Weight [lb (kg)]	Length [in. (cm)]	First fluid bolus (cc)
Neonate (term)	7.5 (3.5)	20 (51)	70
6 mo	17 (8)	26 (66)	160
1 yr	22 (10)	30 (75)	200
2 yr	28 (13)	35 (90)	260
3 yr	33 (15)	38 (100)	300
4 yr	37 (17)	41 (105)	340
5 yr	40 (20)	43 (110)	360
6 yr	48 (22)	46 (120)	440
8 yr	60 (27)	51 (130)	540
10 yr	73 (30)	55 (140)	660
12 yr	84 (38)	60 (150)	760
14 yr	110 (50)	64 (165)	1000

Optimum Site for Fluid Resuscitation

Adults

The cephalic vein in the forearm may be the ideal vein to cannulate first. It is large, constant, and straight. The basilic vein in the antecubital space is the next best vein for the second IV since it is equally large and available. However, as with the hand, additional time for armboard stabilization may be necessary. Next, in order of availability, is the external jugular vein. It is constant but may be difficult to cannulate because of poor tissue support and because of interference by the mandible, which cannot be turned out of the way if there is a possible neck injury. In each of these sites, it is important to verify correct catheter placement. IV flow rates will be slowed by more than 50% if the tip of the catheter is against a valve or the wall of the vein.

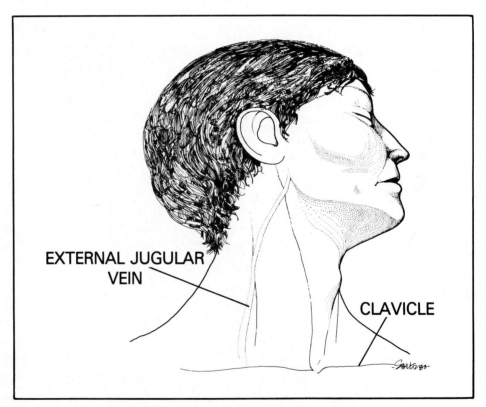

Figure 15–1. Anatomy of external jugular vein.

Pediatric Patients

Veins must be searched for not only in the hands and arms, but also in the scalp (infants may have their scalp veins made available by using a rubber band around the head for a tourniquet) and occasionally in the neck (external jugular vein).

Intraosseous Infusion: Precious time is often lost in attempting to locate a vein in a small infant, especially one in shock. Even in an emergency department it is not uncommon to spend 20 minutes searching for venous access. As a result, recently there has been a renewed interest in the technique of intraosseus infusion, a noncollapsible and easily accessible venous route.

The techniques of IV cannulation are well known. The indications, contraindications, complications, and the anatomy for external jugular venous cannulation and intraosseous infusion are discussed in detail in the Skill Stations.

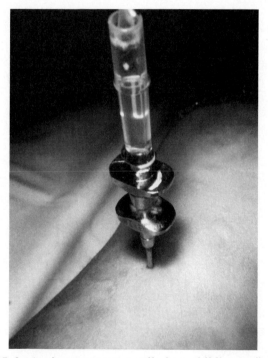

Figure 15–2. An intraosseous needle in a child's proximal tibia being used for intravenous access.

There should be protocols addressing:

1. Appropriate IV site
2. Time spent attempting IV insertion
3. Number of IV insertion attempts

These protocols should include adults and children.

Optimum Equipment for Fluid Resuscitation

The optimum equipment for fluid replacement will deliver the maximum volume of fluid in the shortest time and will require the minimal time of preparation. To give the patient the maximum amount of fluid before he arrives at the hospital, we should use the largest-bore catheter for adults, the shortest catheter and tubing length, the highest position of the IV bag (or better, pressurize the compressible plastic bag with a BP cuff), and the lowest-viscosity fluid (crystalloid at room temperature or body temperature). The size of our catheter is the most important factor, and the length of the catheter is the least important. The presence of extension tubing is somewhat rate limiting for large-bore IVs. The use of the Y-type blood set dramatically improves the rate of administration, more so with the large-bore catheters (the Y-type configuration also saves time in switching bags).

Choosing the proper equipment for pediatric venous access requires different considerations than for the adult. Most often a vein cannot be cannulated a great distance. In addition, the size of the veins is too small to admit the customary large-bore catheters of adults. Thus a large-bore catheter for an infant is a 23-gauge $\frac{3}{4}$ -inch-long butterfly or a 22-gauge 1-inch over-the-needle catheter. A large-bore catheter for the elementary school child is an 18-gauge $1\frac{1}{4}$ -inch over-the-needle catheter.

Optimum Techniques for Fluid Resuscitation

With IV initiation in the ambulance, the transport is begun immediately. The EMT primes the tubing, applies a tourniquet (or better, inflates the BP cuff to 20 mmHg, which is more effective for venous distension than the narrow tourniquet), waits for the venous distension (allowing the arm to dangle for as long as necessary), preps the site, and selects an IV catheter. Once this preparation is completed during transport, the driver can slow down (or even stop momentarily if the hospital is not nearby) while the venipuncture is completed. The ambulance can then resume rapid transport. This method allows transport to occur during the noncritical moments of the IV assembly.

The BP cuff can be placed around the IV bag to improve the rate of flow when necessary. The same cuff can be left applied when the patient is being transported from the ambulance to the hospital. When there is pressure in the cuff, the IV can be placed on the stretcher or the patient and will continue to infuse, even though the hands of the EMTs are busy and cannot hold the bag up. You must be careful to avoid air being infused when using this technique.

In the situation of prolonged scene times in cold climates, the IV fluid may become intolerably cold. One should consider, while waiting for transport, wrapping the IV tubing around a chemical heat pack.

If obvious clinical signs of shock are present, the PASG (MAST) should be inflated before insertion of the IV catheter is attempted. This may make the veins more prominent.

It is customary teaching to examine the distal veins of the forearm before attempting an IV in the antecubital area. However, if these veins are not readily accessible, no time should be expended when the antecubital veins are available. For the patient with an injury to the arm which may possibly impede the venous return, the EMT should avoid cannulating a vein distal to the injury. For the patient in hemorrhagic shock, if only a small catheter can be inserted, a guide wire can be inserted through the catheter and the access can be dilated up to 8 French (kits are available with guide wires that will go through a 20-gauge needle).

The actual venipuncture technique with the large-bore catheter is usually like any other cannulation. But the length of the bevel of the needle (5 mm in some 14-gauge needles) and the distance from the tip of the needle and the tip of the catheter (6 mm in some 14-gauge needles) can cause problems. In the pediatric age group, the length of the bevel of the 23-gauge butterfly is 2 mm. As a result, the tip of the needle can be touching the posterior wall of the vein, while the lumen of the catheter is still occluded by the anterior wall of the vein. This can prevent the flashback. If the catheter is advanced further, there may be flashback, but the tip of the needle may already have penetrated the posterior wall of the vein. To avoid some of the problems inherent with large-bore cannulation, the EMT can turn the needle 180° after penetration through the skin so that the bevel is down. After noting the flashback when the catheter penetrates the vein, the EMT should advance the needle and catheter parallel to the vein to ensure that the tip of the catheter is in the vein. This technique may prove extremely valuable in the pediatric age group. If no flashback occurs after entering the vein, the EMT should try aspirating with a syringe to verify placement. After verifying placement, the catheter may be advanced. The catheter should be taped to the skin, then the tubing is secured to the arm by wrapping the tubing and arm with Kling or Conform. These bandages effectively secure the tubing to the arm, thus preventing traction on the tubing from pulling the catheter out. They are applied as snug as necessary without constricting the arm and preventing venous return.

Summary

We cannot pretend to cover the current treatment of shock completely in this chapter. But a brief review is in order.

When approaching the trauma victim, we need to survey the scene looking for possible mechanism of injury. We need to establish if the patient is conscious or unconscious, and assess and treat any significant airway problem while stabilizing the cervical spine. We need to glance at the neck in our evaluation, noting the color, diaphoresis, coolness, JVD, tracheal position, and carotid pulse. In this way we arrive at the chest, where we assess and treat the significant breathing problems, including the hypoxia, the sucking chest wound, and the tension pneumothorax (if it is significant). At this point we need to check to see if our partners have effectively stopped the major bleeding. Then armed with this information, we need to assess for shock. We have already noted the mechanisms of injury, the level of consciousness, the skin condition, the quality and rate of the carotid pulse, the respiratory rate, and the amount of observed external bleeding. We can compare the quality of the radial pulse to the carotid, and we can note the capillary refill. Considering all this information, we can determine if the patient is critical and needs immediate transfer to a backboard with PASG (MAST) in place. It is only at this point in the stabilization of the trauma patient that we can even consider the use of fluid replacement therapy. If the patient is in shock (early or late) or fits into the "load and go" category, the patient needs to be packaged and transported to the ambulance. The only exception to this is if transport is unavoidably delayed. In the ambulance the primed IV bags/blood tubing need to be simultaneously connected immediately to two 14-gauge catheters and 2 L of fluid should be infused immediately under pressure in the adult victim with any sign of shock. Continued fluid replacement is determined by the estimation of blood loss and the victim's minute-by-minute clinical condition.

Medical control and the appropriate receiving emergency department should be contacted early so that the trauma team (ED nurses, ED physician, trauma surgeon, and appropriate others) can be present in the emergency department when the patient arrives. The operating room team must also be notified. It is only by developing such teamwork in *all* phases of the emergency trauma response that prehospital ALS will have an unquestioned impact in decreasing the morbidity and mortality from trauma.

PART II

Basic Skill Station 1

Primary Survey

Objectives

The objectives of this skill station are:

1. To learn to perform the primary survey correctly.
2. To learn which patients require "load and go."
3. To learn when to perform critical interventions.

Primary Survey

This is a rapid exam to determine the patient's condition. The information that you gather here is used to make decisions about critical interventions and time of transport. This exam should not take over $1\frac{1}{2}$ to 2 minutes. This exam is so important that nothing is allowed to interrupt it except airway obstruction or cardiac arrest. Respiratory distress (other than airway obstruction) is not an indication to interrupt the primary survey because the cause of respiratory distress is frequently found during exam of the chest.

Assessment Priorities

A. Primary Survey

1. Evaluate **airway,** C-spine control, and initial level of consciousness.
2. Evaluate **breathing.**
3. Evaluate **circulation.**
4. Stop major bleeding.

B. Transport Decision and Critical Interventions

C. Secondary Survey

Patient Assessment Using the Priority Plan

Once you approach the victim, your exam should proceed quickly and smoothly. Unless held up by extrication, total on-scene time should be under 10 minutes. *Critical victims should have on-scene times of 5 minutes or less.* Nothing interrupts the primary survey except treatment of airway obstruction or cardiac arrest.

A. *Evaluate airway, C-spine control, initial LOC (level of consciousness).* Assessment begins immediately, even if the victim is being extricated. Extrication should not interfere with patient care. The same priorities apply continually before, during, and after extrication. The team leader should approach the victim from the front (face to face—so the victim does not have to turn his head to see you). A second EMT immediately, gently but firmly, stabilizes the neck in a neutral position. There are times when the team leader may need to stabilize the neck initially. The EMT stabilizing the neck must not release his hold until someone relieves him or a suitable stabilization device is applied. The team leader should say to the patient: "We are EMTs here to help you. What happened?" The patient's reply gives immediate information about both the airway and the level of consciousness. If the patient responds appropriately to your question, you have established that he has an open airway and that his level of consciousness is normal. Your next words should be: "Please do not move until we have checked you for injuries." As you check the conscious victim, you should explain what you are doing and why you are doing it. This has a calming effect on both you and the victim. It also usually ensures the victim's cooperation. If the patient cannot speak or is unconscious, you must evaluate the airway further. Look, listen, and feel for the movement of air. Be sure that both rate and tidal volume are adequate. Open the mouth and clear the airway if necessary. If the airway is obstructed, use an appropriate method to open *before* finishing the primary survey. Because of the ever-present danger of spinal injury, you must never extend the neck to open the airway of a trauma patient. Patients with airway difficulty or decreased level of consciousness are in the "load and go" category. All patients with decreased LOC should be hyperventilated (24 breaths per minute) if they will allow you to do so. Your partner may use his knees to maintain immobilization of the neck, freeing his hands to apply oxygen or use a bag–valve–mask to assist ventilation. This is one reason that all equipment should be within immediate reach. If you assist or control ventilation, be sure that the patient gets not only an adequate ventilatory rate, but also an adequate volume with each breath. *All* victims of multiple trauma should receive oxygen.

B. *Assess breathing and circulation.* It is impractical to separate evaluation of breathing and circulation, since you must check both as you quickly look, listen, and feel the neck and chest. There is much information to be gained when this examination is performed correctly. (Remember: If the patient is not breathing, you must immediately give two full breaths and then check for a carotid pulse. If there is no pulse, you must begin cardiopulmonary resuscitation.) After your partner has immobilized the neck and (if necessary) opened the airway with a modified jaw thrust, you should proceed with evaluation of breathing and circulation in the following manner.

1. Place your face over the patient's mouth so that you can judge both the rate and quality of breathing. Is breathing too fast (>24 breaths per minute) or too slow (<12 breaths per minute)? Is the victim moving an adequate volume of air when he breathes? Any abnormality of breathing signals a search for the cause as well as administration of oxygen and possibly breathing assistance. Your partner can apply the non-rebreather oxygen mask or bag–valve device (while stabilizing the neck with his knees) without interrupting your survey.

2. As your partner holds the neck stable, he will find that it is simple to feel the carotid pulse with his index finger. He should note rate and quality, then compare with your evaluation of the pulse at the wrist. Also evaluate skin color/condition and capillary refill. This information, combined with LOC, is the best early assessment of circulatory status and the presence of shock. If the pulse is present at the neck and the wrist, the blood pressure is greater than 80 mmHg.

(It may be normal; judge by the strength of the pulse—it is not yet time to use the blood pressure cuff.) If a pulse is present at the neck but not at the wrist, the blood pressure is between 60 and 80 mmHg; this means *late* shock. Even if the pulse is present and strong at the neck and wrist, you may be able to diagnose *early* shock by other signs. Other signs of shock include slow capillary refill, rapid heart rate (>100 beats per minute), cold sweaty skin, pale appearance, confusion, weakness, or thirst. Remember, the patient with spinal shock may not be pale, cold, or sweaty and will not have a rapid pulse. He will have low blood pressure and paralysis.

3. As soon as you have noted the breathing and pulse, quickly *look and feel* the neck to see if the trachea is in the midline, if the neck veins are flat or distended, and if there is discoloration, swelling, or subcutaneous emphysema. You may apply a rigid extrication collar at this time. (*Note:* If the team leader elected to stabilize the neck, he should transfer this duty to another EMT at this time.)

4. Now look, feel, and listen to the chest. If there is any difficulty with respiration, the chest must be bared for examination: This is no time for modesty; chest injuries often kill quickly. Look for sucking chest wounds, flail segments, contusions, or deformities. Note if the ribs rise with respiration or if there is only diaphragmatic breathing. Feel for instability, tenderness, or crepitation. Listen for breath sounds. Listen with the stethoscope over the lateral chest about the fourth interspace in the midaxillary line on one side, then immediately compare with the other side. You may also listen to the anterior chest about the second interspace on both sides. The important determination is whether breath sounds are *present and equal* on both sides. If breath sounds are not equal (decreased or absent on one side), you should percuss the chest to see if it is tympanic (pneumothorax) or dull (hemothorax). If abnormalities are found during the chest exam (open chest wound, flail chest, respiratory difficulty), you should make the appropriate intervention (seal open wound, *hand stabilize* flail, give oxygen, assist ventilation, decompress tension pneumothorax).

5. Stop active bleeding. Your other partner should have already done this, or at least begun to do this. Almost all bleeding can be stopped by direct pressure; use gauze pads and bandage or elastic wraps. You may use air splints or antishock garment to tamponade bleeding. Tourniquets may be needed in *rare* situations. If a dressing becomes

blood soaked, you may remove the dressing and redress *once* to be sure you are getting pressure on the bleeding area. It is important that you report such excessive bleeding to the receiving physician. Do not use clamps to stop bleeders; you may cause injuries to other structures (nerves are present alongside arteries).

6. Perform a MAST survey. If your primary survey identified the presence of a critical trauma situation, you should modify the primary survey by adding the MAST survey. Critical conditions require transport before performing the secondary survey. Since you will apply the antishock garment (MAST or PASG) before you do the secondary survey, you need to check quickly the areas of the body that will be hidden by the garment. *You must expose the body to do this.* Quickly cut off the clothes, maintaining body warmth and modesty with a sheet or blanket. The MAST survey consists of a quick examination of the abdomen, pelvis, and legs.

At this point you have enough information to determine critical trauma situations that should be treated by "load and go."

Critical Injuries/Conditions

1. Airway obstruction unrelieved by mechanical methods (i.e., suction, forceps)
2. Conditions resulting in possible inadequate breathing
   a. Large open chest wound (sucking chest wound)
   b. Large flail chest
   c. Tension pneumothorax
   d. Major blunt chest injury
3. Traumatic cardiopulmonary arrest
4. Shock
   a. Hemorrhagic
   b. Spinal
   c. Myocardial contusion
   d. Pericardial tamponade
5. Head injury with decreased level of consciousness.

This can be further simplified into three conditions based on signs and symptoms:

a.   Difficulty with respiration

b.   Difficulty with circulation (shock)

c.   Decreased level of consciousness

Any trauma patient with one or more of these conditions falls into the "load and go" category. When you finish the primary survey, you have enough information to decide if the patient is critical or stable. If the patient has one of the critical conditions, you should immediately transfer him to a long backboard (check his back as you log-roll him), apply MAST and oxygen, load him into an ambulance (if available), and transport rapidly to the nearest appropriate emergency facility. Lifesaving procedure may be needed but should not hold up transport. There are a few brief procedures that are done while at the scene (appropriate airway management, stop major bleeding, seal sucking chest wound, hand stabilize flail, hyperventilate, decompress tension pneumothorax, begin CPR), but most are reserved for transport. *You must weigh every field procedure against the time it will take to perform.* You are spending minutes of the patient's golden hour; be sure the procedure is worth the cost. Nonlifesaving procedures (splinting and bandaging) must not hold up transport. Be sure to call medical control early so that the hospital is prepared for your arrival.

If the primary survey fails to identify a critical trauma situation, you should transfer the victim to the backboard (check the back) and proceed with the secondary survey. (*Note:* You should think of the antishock trousers as a part of the backboard. The trousers are always unfolded on the backboard, ready to be applied if needed.)

Procedure

Short written scenarios will be used along with a model (to act as the victim). You will divide into teams of three to practice performing the primary survey, critical interventions, and transport decisions. The "parrot phrases" are the words you should repeat (like a parrot) at each step of the survey. These represent the answers you should be seeking at each step of the survey. Each member of the team must practice being team leader at least once, and preferably, twice.

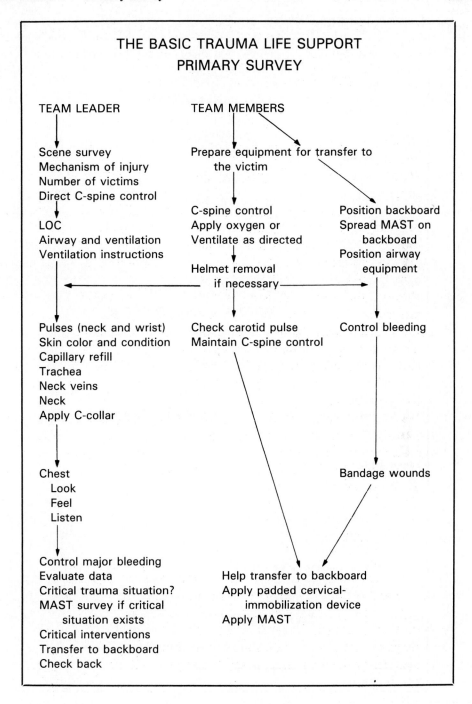

THE BASIC TRAUMA LIFE SUPPORT
PRIMARY SURVEY

TEAM LEADER

Scene survey
Mechanism of injury
Number of victims
Direct C-spine control

LOC
Airway and ventilation
Ventilation instructions

Pulses (neck and wrist)
Skin color and condition
Capillary refill
Trachea
Neck veins
Neck
Apply C-collar

Chest
   Look
   Feel
   Listen

Control major bleeding
Evaluate data
Critical trauma situation?
MAST survey if critical
   situation exists
Critical interventions
Transfer to backboard
Check back

TEAM MEMBERS

Prepare equipment for transfer to
   the victim

C-spine control   Position backboard
Apply oxygen or   Spread MAST on
Ventilate as directed   backboard
                         Position airway
Helmet removal   equipment
if necessary

Check carotid pulse   Control bleeding
Maintain C-spine control

                         Bandage wounds

Help transfer to backboard
Apply padded cervical-
   immobilization device
Apply MAST

This is what should be going through your mind as you perform each step of the survey. They are also the phrases you should repeat (like a parrot) to the instructor as you are being tested on patient evaluation.

SCENE SURVEY

I am surveying the scene: Are there any dangers?
I am surveying the mechanisms of injury.
Are there any other victims?

LEVEL OF CONSCIOUSNESS

We are EMTs here to help you. What happened?
Please do not move until we have checked you for injuries.

AIRWAY

Is the airway clear?
What is the rate and quality of respiration?

VENTILATION INSTRUCTIONS

Order oxygen for any airway difficulty, head injury, or shock.
Assist ventilation if hypoventilating.
Hyperventilate altered level of consciousness.

PULSES

What is the rate and quality of the pulse at the neck and the wrist?

SKIN COLOR AND CONDITION

What is the skin color and condition?

CAPILLARY REFILL

Is the capillary refill normal or delayed?

TRACHEA

Is the trachea midline or deviated?

NECK VEINS

Are the neck veins flat or distended?

NECK

Are there signs of trauma to the neck?

CHEST

I am looking at the chest: Are there any penetrations, contusions, deformities, or paradoxical motions?

I am feeling the chest: Is there any crepitation, tenderness, or instability?

I am listening to the chest: Are the breath sounds present and equal?

IF BREATH SOUNDS ARE NOT EQUAL:

I am percussing the chest. Is there tympany (hyperresonance) or dullness on either side?

BLEEDING

Is there any significant bleeding?

MAST SURVEY

ABDOMEN

Are there any contusions, penetrations, distention, or tenderness of the abdomen?

PELVIS

Is the pelvis tender or unstable?

LOWER EXTREMITIES

Is there any sign of trauma to the legs?

EXAM OF THE BACK
(Done during transfer to the backboard)

Is there any sign of trauma to the back?

Basic Skill Station 2

Secondary Survey

Objectives

The objectives of this skill station are:

1. To learn to perform the secondary survey correctly.
2. To learn which patients require "load and go."
3. To learn how to communicate with medical control.

The secondary survey is a detailed exam to pick up all injuries, both obvious and potential. This exam also establishes the baseline from which many treatment decisions will be made. Critical patients will always have this exam done during transport. If the primary survey has revealed no critical condition, perform this exam while on the scene. It is important to record this exam.

Communications with medical control is a trauma skill that is often performed poorly. Critical patients require early contact with medical control so that the hospital is prepared for your arrival and appropriate surgeons are notified. Most patients are not critical, and communications can wait until you are ready to transport. All communications should be concise and to the point.

Secondary Survey

1. *Vital signs.* Record pulse, respiration, and blood pressure (obtain accurate recordings and use the BP cuff now).

2. *History.* Obtain a history of the injury (your partner may already have done this) via:
    a. Personal observation.
    b. Bystanders.
    c. Victim. In unconscious patients, look for a medic alert tag. Take an *ample* history from conscious patients:
        A   allergies
        M   medications
        P   past medical history (other illnesses)
        L   last meal (when was it eaten)
        E   events preceding the injury

3. *Head-to-toes exam*
    a. Begin at the head examining for contusions, lacerations, raccoon eyes, Battle's sign, and drainage of blood or fluid from the ears or nose. Assess the airway again.
    b. Check the neck again. Look for lacerations, contusions, tenderness, distended neck veins, or deviated trachea. Check the pulse again. If not already done, apply a cervical immobilization device at this time.
    c. Recheck the chest. Be sure that breath sounds are still present and equal on each side. Recheck seals over open wounds. Make sure that flails are well stabilized (hand stabilization is adequate until you are in the ambulance).
    d. Examine the abdomen. Look for signs of blunt or penetrating trauma. Feel for tenderness. Do not waste time listening for bowel sounds. If the abdomen is painful to gentle pressure during examination, you can expect the patient to be bleeding internally. If the abdomen is both distended and painful, you can expect hemorrhagic shock very quickly.
    e. Assess pelvis and extremities. Be sure to check and record distal sensation and pulses on all fractures. Do this before and after straightening any fracture. Angulated fractures of the upper extremities are usually best splinted as found. Most fractures of the lower extremities are *gently* straightened by using traction splints or air splints. *Critical patients have all splints applied during transport.*

Transport immediately if your secondary survey reveals any of the following:

1. Tender, distended abdomen
2. Pelvic instability
3. Bilateral femur fractures

Even though the patient may appear stable at this time, he will probably soon develop shock because of the large blood loss that is associated with these injuries.

4. *Brief neurological exam*
   a. *Level of consciousness*
      A   alert
      V   responds to verbal stimuli
      P   responds to pain
      U   unresponsive
   b. *Motor.* Can he move fingers and toes?
   c. *Sensation.* Can he feel you when you touch his fingers and toes? Does the unconscious patient respond when you pinch his fingers and toes.
   d. *Pupils.* Are they equal or unequal? Do they respond to light?

The neurological exam is very simple but is frequently forgotten. It gives important baseline information that is used in later treatment decisions. Perform and record this exam.

5. If necessary, finish bandaging and splinting.
6. Continually monitor and reevaluate the patient.

If the patient's condition worsens, repeat every step of the primary survey.
Accurately record what you see and what you do. Record changes in the patient's condition during transport. Record the time the antishock garment or tourniquet is applied. Extenuating circumstances or significant details should be recorded in the comments or remarks section of the run report. (Review the documentation in Appendix B.)

Contacting Medical Control

This is important so that the emergency department can be prepared for the arrival of the patient. It is extremely important to do this as early as possible when you have a patient with a critical condition. It takes time to get the appropriate surgeon and the operating room team called in. The critical victim has no time to wait. (Review communications in Appendix A.) The procedure to communicate with medical control is given below.

Phase I: Establishing Contact

1. Initiation of call
    EMS service
    Level of function (basic, paramedic, etc.)
    Unit number
    Medical control facility being contacted
2. Receiving facility response
    Name of facility
    Name and title of radio operator
    Renaming of calling EMS service

Phase II: In-the-Field Report

3. Re-identification
    EMS service
    Level of function
    Unit number
4. Chief complaint/on scene report
    One brief sentence
    Include age, sex, complaint, and/or mechanism of injury
5. Lifesaving resuscitation
    Patient's response to lifesaving interventions
6. Vital signs/primary survey abnormalities
    Vital signs in stable patient or primary survey in unstable patient
7. ETA
8. Request for orders
    State what is desired or state "no orders requested"

Phase III: Hospital-Controlled Activity

9. Physician response
    Physician will agree, deny, or state desired orders
    Physician may request additional history and/or information
10. EMT response
    Clarification or response to requested intervention or therapy

Phase IV: Sign-Off

11. EMS unit sign-off
12. Base station sign-off

Transport the patient to the facility named by medical control. Notify the facility of the estimated time of arrival (ETA), the condition of the patient, and any special needs on arrival.

The following pages contain a brief outline of the secondary survey as well as the thoughts that should go through your mind as you perform the survey.

Procedure

Short written scenarios will be used along with a model (to act as the victim). You will divide into teams of three to practice performing the secondary survey.

THE BASIC TRAUMA LIFE SUPPORT
SECONDARY SURVEY

When performing the secondary survey, you must visualize and palpate from head to toes. Everyone gets a secondary survey: stable patients while at the scene, critical patients during transport. If other team members are available, the blood pressure and accurate pulse and respiratory rates may be taken by one of them.

HEAD

1. Palpate
   Entire scalp for lacerations or contusions
   Face for tenderness or fractures
2. Look
   For Battle's sign
   For blood or fluid in ears
   For raccoon eyes
   For blood or fluid from nose
   For pupil size, equality, reaction to light
   For burns of face, nose hairs, mouth
   For skin changes
   > Pallor
   > Cyanosis
   > Diaphoresis
   > Bruising

---

3. Reassess
   a. Airway
      Recheck patency.
      If burn victim, assess for signs of inhalation injury.
   b. Breathing
      Rate (accurately and record)
      Quality

NECK (If collar has been applied, remove the front)

Reasses circulation
   Pulse rate (accurately and record)
   Pulse quality
   Blood pressure (done by partner if possible)
Signs of trauma?
JVD?
Tracheal deviation?

CHEST

Look for penetrations, contusions, deformities, or paradoxical motions
Feel for instability, tenderness, crepitation.
Listen for breath sounds in all lung fields; if breath sounds unequal:
1. Evaluate for tension pneumothorax and hemothorax.
2. If intubated, check ET tube placement.

ABDOMEN (If MAST has been applied, this has been completed)

Look for penetrations, contusions, distention.
Palpate all four quadrants for tenderness.

PELVIS (If MAST has been applied, this has been completed)

Compress laterally and over symphysis for tenderness or instability.

LOWER EXTREMITIES (If MAST applied, do pulses, neuro, cap refill)

Visualize and palpate for signs of trauma.
Check distal pulses.
Do neurological
   sensory (pinch toes)
   motor (move toes)
Check range of motion.
Repeat capillary refill.

UPPER EXTREMITIES

Visualize and palpate for signs of trauma.
Begin at the midline, checking clavicles, shoulders, arms, and hands.

Check distal pulses.
Do neurological
    sensory (pinch fingers)
    motor (move fingers)
Check range of motion.
Repeat capillary refill (unless you have already made the diagnosis of shock).

PARROT PHRASES—SECONDARY SURVEY

HEAD

I am feeling the scalp: Are there lacerations, contusions, or deformity?
I am feeling the face: Are there contusions or deformity?
Are Battle's sign or raccoon eyes present?
Is blood or fluid draining from the ears or nose?
What is pupil size? Are the pupils equal? Do they react to light?
Is there pallor, cyanosis, diaphoresis, or bruising?
Are there burns of the face, nose hairs, or inside the mouth?

AIRWAY

Is the airway clear?
What is the rate and quality of respiration?
Are there signs of burns in the mouth or nose (if a burn victim)?

CIRCULATION

What is the rate and quality of the pulse?
What is the blood pressure?
Is the capillary refill normal or delayed? (Not done if a diagnosis of shock has already been made.)

NECK

Are there signs of trauma to the neck?
Are the neck veins flat or distended?
Is the trachea midline or deviated?

CHEST

I am looking at the chest: Are there any penetrations, contusions, deformities, or paradoxical motion?
I am feeling the chest: Is there any crepitation, tenderness, or instability?
I am listening to the chest: Are the breath sounds present and equal?
I am percussing the chest: Is it hyperresonant or dull? (Do only if breath sounds are unequal.)

ABDOMEN (If MAST has been applied, this has been completed)

I am looking at the abdomen: Are there penetrations, contusions, or distention?
I am feeling the abdomen: Is there any tenderness?

PELVIS (If MAST has been applied, this has been completed)

Is the pelvis tender or unstable?

LOWER EXTREMITIES (If MAST has been applied, do pulses, neuro, and capillary refill)

Are there any signs of trauma to the legs?
Are pulses present?
Can he feel me touch his toes?
Can he move his toes?
Is range of motion normal?
Is capillary refill normal or delayed? (Not done if a diagnosis of shock has already been made.)

UPPER EXTREMITIES

Is there any sign of trauma to the arms?
Are pulses present?
Can he feel me touch his fingers?
Can he move his fingers?
Is range of motion normal?
Is capillary refill normal or delayed? (Not done if a diagnosis of shock has already been made.)

Basic Skill Station 3

Rapid Patient Assessment

Objective

The objective of this skill station is to practice the proper organized sequence of evaluation and management of the multiple-trauma victim.

Procedure

Short written trauma scenarios will be used along with a model (to act as the victim). Students will be divided into three-member teams to practice the management of simulated trauma situations using the principles and techniques taught in the course. You will be tested in the same manner on the second day of the course. You will be expected to use all the principles and techniques taught in this course while managing these simulated victims. Review Chapters 2 and 14 and Basic Skill Stations 1 and 2.

Ground Rules for Teaching and Testing

1. You will be allowed to stay together in three-member groups throughout the practice and testing.

2. You will have three practice scenarios. This allows each member of the team to be team leader once.

3. You will be tested as team leader once.

4. You will assist as a member of the rescue team during two scenarios in which another member of your team is being tested as team leader. You may assist, but all assessment must be done by the team leader. This gives you a total of six scenarios from which to learn: three practice, one test, and two assists while others are tested.

5. Wait outside the door until the instructor comes out and gives you your scenario.

6. You will be allowed to look over your equipment before you start your exam.

7. Be sure to ask about scene hazards if not already given in the scenario.

8. If you have a live model for a victim, you must talk to that person just as you would a real victim. It is best to explain what you are doing as you examine the victim. Be confident and reassuring.

9. You must ask your instructor for things you cannot find out from your model. *Example:* blood pressure, pulse, breath sounds, etc.

10. Wounds must be dressed just as if they are real. Procedures must be done correctly (blood pressure, log-rolling, strapping, splinting, etc.)

11. If you need a piece of equipment that is not available, ask your instructor. He may allow you to simulate the equipment.

12. During practice and testing, you may go to any station, but you cannot go to the same station twice.

13. You will be graded on:
    a. Assessment of the scene   e. Leadership
    b. Assessment of the victim   f. Judgment
    c. Management of the victim   g. Problem-solving ability
    d. Efficient use of time   h. Patient interaction

14. When you finish your testing scenario, there is to be *no* discussion of the case. If you have any questions, they will be answered after the faculty meeting at the end of the course.

Patient Assessment Pearls

1. Do not approach the victim until you have done a scene survey.

2. Do not interrupt the primary survey except for:
    a. Airway obstruction or near obstruction
    b. Cardiac or respiratory arrest

3. Give ventilation instructions as soon as you assess airway and breathing.

4. Hyperventilate (~24 breaths per minute) all victims with decreased level of consciousness.

5. Assist ventilation on anyone who is hypoventilating (8 or less per minute).

6. Give oxygen to all victims of multiple trauma. If in doubt, give oxygen.

7. Endotracheal tubes are the best method to protect the airway and ventilate the patient.

8. If the primary survey reveals that the patient has a critical trauma situation, complete the MAST survey.

9. If absolutely necessary, certain interventions may have to be done before transport. Remember that you are trading minutes of the patient's "golden hour" for those procedures. Use good judgment.

10. Indications to decompress a tension pneumothorax:
    a. Loss of radial pulse (obvious shock)
    b. Loss of consciousness or obviously decreasing level of consciousness
    c. Cyanosis

11. Start IVs in the ambulance en route unless the patient is entrapped or the ambulance has not arrived on scene.

12. Transfer the patient to the backboard as soon as the primary survey (and MAST survey if indicated) is completed.

13. When primary survey is completed, decide if the patient is critical or stable. Critical trauma situations:
    a. Decreased level of consciousness
    b. Difficulty with breathing
    c. Shock

14. Critical patients get a secondary survey en route to the hospital.

15. Stable patients get a secondary survey at the scene.

16. Transport immediately if your secondary survey reveals any of the following:
    a. Tender, distended abdomen
    b. Pelvic instability
    c. Bilateral femur fractures

17. Critical patients should not have traction splints applied at the scene (it takes too long).

18. Call medical control early if you have a critical patient (other physicians may have to be called in to treat the patient).

19. Anytime the patient's condition worsens, repeat the primary survey.
20. Anytime you make an intervention, repeat the primary survey.
21. When you repeat the primary survey, repeat *every* step.
22. Unconscious patients cannot protect their airways.
23. Transport pregnant victims with the backboard tilted slightly to the left. Do not let them roll over onto the floor.
24. Remain calm and *think*. Your knowledge, training, and concern are the most important tools you carry.

Example of a Teaching Scenario

This is to give you an idea of what is expected and how you will be graded. (You will practice a different scenario in the skill station.)

Situation

A young male was driving through an intersection. His automobile was hit in the driver's side by another vehicle. (This is all you would be told; you must obtain all other information by observation or by asking the instructor.)

Injuries

This is what you are expected to identify (or at least suspect, such as spinal injuries). In the *teaching* stations you will be told the injuries when you finish your assessment. In the *testing* stations there is no discussion of the case—questions will not be answered until after the faculty meeting.

1. Fracture of C-7, but no spinal cord injury yet
2. Flail chest on the left.
3. Ruptured spleen (abdominal injury)
4. Multiple fractures of pelvis

Patient Instructions

These are instructions given to the patient in order for him to correctly portray his injuries. *You will not be aware of his instructions.*

Patient: You are awake and alert. If asked, you complain of pain in the left chest and "hip." Do not complain of abdominal or neck pain. If the abdomen or neck is checked, you admit to a "little" tenderness. If your neck is not immobilized or if your neck is allowed to move, become paralyzed.

Instructions to Faculty

The faculty member is expected to know this, so he can answer your questions as you perform the survey.

Primary Survey

Airway is open, initial respiratory rate 24 per minute and shallow.
Pulse rapid but strong, present at neck and wrist.
Capillary refill is delayed.
The patient is diaphoretic.
Neck veins are flat, trachea midline.
There is an unstable rib segment on the left.
Breath sounds are bilateral and equal.

Mast Survey

Slight LUQ tenderness of abdomen
Pelvis tender and unstable
Legs normal

Secondary Survey

Head normal.
Patient still alert, pupils midposition, equal, and reactive to light.
Airway is open, respiratory rate 24 per minute and shallow.
Pulse 120 per minute and strong, present at neck and wrist.
Capillary refill delayed.
Blood pressure 120/90.
Neck veins flat.
Trachea midline.
Chest unchanged.
Arms normal, pulses normal, sensation and motor normal.
Abdomen is slightly more tender.
Pelvis should not be examined again (would cause further internal bleeding).
Legs unchanged, pulses present, sensation and motor normal, capillary refill delayed.

During Transport There Will Be a Condition Change

Patient becomes poorly responsive (verbal stimuli).

Pulse 150 per minute, respiration 30 per minute, and shallow, BP 70/40.

Grade Sheet

A sheet such as this will be used by the instructor to grade you.

Student's Name _____

Practice ____ Test _____

Time began evaluation _____

Surveys scene and notes mechanisms of injury _____

Has partner immobilize the neck (team leader may elect to do this) _____

Talks to victim—notes normal level of consciousness _____

Checks airway _____

Checks breathing _____

Checks pulse at the wrist, has partner check at the neck _____

Checks capillary refill _____

Checks neck veins _____

Checks trachea _____

Checks chest _____

Recognizes flail _____

Stabilizes flail (may wait until victim is extricated) _____

Extricates properly onto long backboard _____

Stabilizes flail if not already done (KED will stabilize) _____

Orders oxygen by non-rebreathing mask (may do earlier) _____

Completes MAST survey _____

Recognizes abdominal tenderness ____

unstable pelvis _____

Checks for bleeding _____

Time primary survey completed _____

Makes decision to "load and go" _____

Knows why—respiratory problem and probable early shock _____

Applies padded cervical-immobilization device _____

Applies MAST (may inflate to stabilize the pelvis) _____

Securely straps patient to the spine board _____

Transports _____

Time of transport _____

Calls medical control and correctly describes situation _____

Monitors vital signs _____

Recognizes change in condition (shock) _____

Repeats the primary survey _____
Inflates MAST if not already inflated _____
Calls medical control and advises of change in condition _____

Performed organized primary survey   yes_____   no_____
Interacted well with victim   yes_____   no_____
Performed organized secondary survey   yes_____   no_____
Efficient utilization of time   yes_____   no_____
Displayed leadership and teamwork   yes_____   no_____
Overall Grade
Excellent—instructor potential _____
Good _____
Adequate _____
Inadequate _____

Comments _____
_____

Instructor _____

Basic Skill Station 4

Spinal Immobilization Using a Short Backboard and Emergency Rapid Extrication

Skill 4A: Spinal Immobilization—Short Backboard

Objectives

The objectives of this skill station are as follows:

1. To learn when to use spinal immobilization.
2. To learn the correct technique of spinal immobilization with a short backboard.

Who Should Have Spinal Immobilization?

1. Any victim of trauma with obvious neurological deficit, such as paralysis, weakness, or paresthesia (numbness or tingling)
2. Any victim of trauma who complains of pain in the head, neck, or back
3. Any victim of trauma who is unconscious
4. Any victim of trauma who may have injury to the spine but in whom evaluation is difficult due to altered mental status (e.g., drugs, alcohol)
5. Any unconscious patient who may have been subjected to trauma

271

6. Any trauma victim with facial or head injuries
7. Any trauma victim subjected to deceleration forces

When in doubt, immobilize.

When to Immobilize

Patients requiring immobilization must have it done *before* they are moved. In the case of an automobile accident, the victim must be immobilized before he is removed from the wreckage. More movement is involved in extrication than at any other time, so immobilization of neck and spine must be accomplished before beginning extrication.

Technique of Spinal Immobilization Using the Short Backboard

This device is for use on the patient who is in a position (such as an automobile) that does not allow use of the long backboard. There are several different devices of this type; some devices have different strapping mechanisms from the one explained here. You must become familiar with the equipment you will employ before using it in the field.

1. Remember that the routine priorities of evaluation and management are done before the immobilization devices go on.
2. One EMT must, if possible, station himself behind the victim, place his hands on either side of the victim's head, and immobilize the neck in a neutral position. This step is part of the ABCs of evaluation. It is done at the same time that you begin evaluation of the airway.
3. When you have the patient stable enough to begin splinting, you must apply a rigid extrication collar. If you have enough people, this can be done while someone else is doing the ABCs of evaluation and management.
4. Position the backboard behind the victim. The first EMT continues to immobilize the neck while the short backboard is being maneuvered into place. The victim may have to be moved forward to get the backboard in place; great care must be taken that moves are coordinated so as to support the neck and back.
5. Secure the victim to the board: there are usually two straps for this. Bring each strap over a leg, down between both legs, back around the outside of the same leg, and then across the chest, then attach them to the opposite upper straps that were brought across the shoulders.

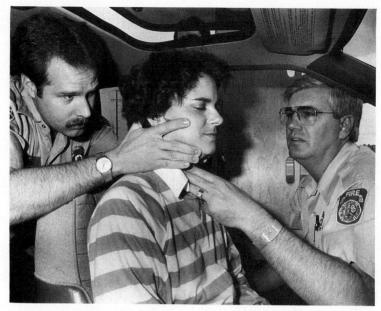

Figure S4–1. Stabilize the neck and perform the primary survey.

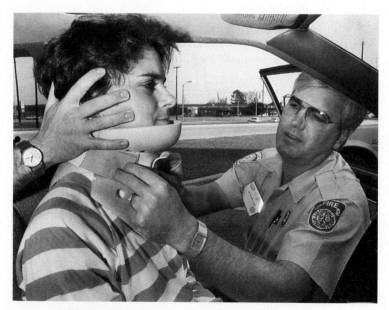

Figure S4–2. Apply a rigid extrication collar.

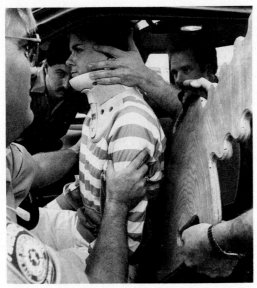

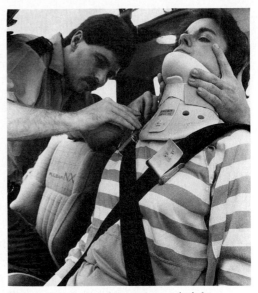

Figure S4–3. Position the short backboard behind the victim. Coordinate all movement so that the spine is kept immobile.

Figure S4–4. Apply straps and tighten securely.

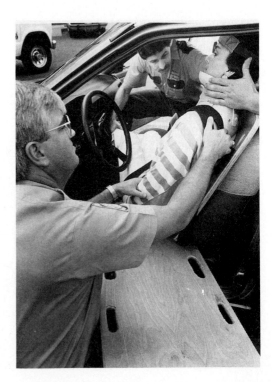

Figure S4–5. Turn the victim carefully then lower onto the long backboard.

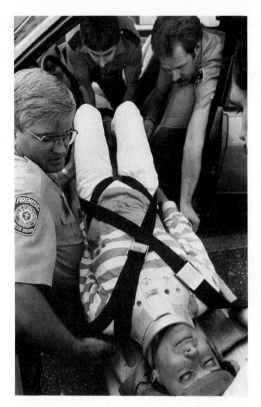

Figure S4-6. Slide the victim and the short backboard up into position on the long backboard. Loosen the straps and allow the legs to extend out flat then retighten the straps. Secure the victim and the short backboard to the long backboard. Apply padded immobilization device to secure the victim's head and neck.

6. Tighten the straps until the victim is held securely.

7. Secure the victim's head to the board by wide tape or elastic wraps around the forehead. Apply padding under the neck and head as needed to maintain a neutral position.

8. Transfer the victim to a long backboard. Turn the victim so that his back is to the opening through which he is to be removed. Someone must support his legs so that the upper legs remain at a 90°-angle to the torso. Position the long backboard through the opening until it is under the victim. Lower the victim back onto the long backboard and slide the victim and the short backboard up into position on the long backboard. Loosen the straps on the short board and allow the patient's legs to extend out flat and then retighten the straps. Now secure him to the long board with straps, and secure his head with a padded immobilization device. When he is secured in this way, it is possible to turn the whole board up on its side if the victim has to vomit. The patient should remain securely immobilized.

Points to Remember

1. When you are placing the straps around the legs on a male, do not catch the genitals in the straps.
2. Do not use the short board as a "handle" to move the victim. Move both victim and board as a unit.
3. When you are applying the horizontal straps (long backboard) around a woman, place the upper strap above her breasts, not across them.
4. When you are applying the lower horizontal strap on a pregnant woman, see that it is low enough so as not to injure the fetus.
5. Injuries may force you to modify how you attach the straps.
6. The victim must be secured well enough to have no motion of the spine if the board is turned on its side.

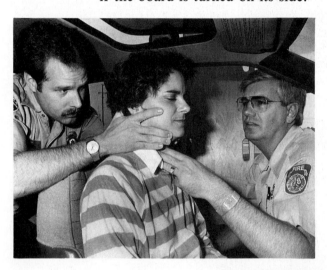

Figure S4–7. Kendrick Extrication Device (K.E.D.). Stabilize the neck and perform the primary survey.

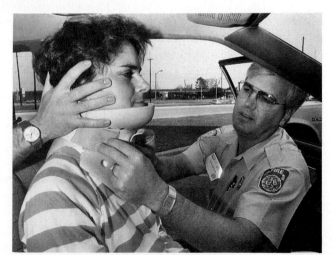

Figure S4–8. Apply a rigid extrication collar.

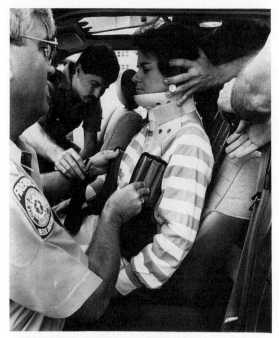

Figure S4–9. Position the device behind the victim. Coordinate all movements so that the spine is kept immobile. Position the chest panels up well into the armpits.

Figure S4–11. Loop each leg strap around the ipsilateral (same side) leg and back to the buckle on the same side. Fasten snugly.

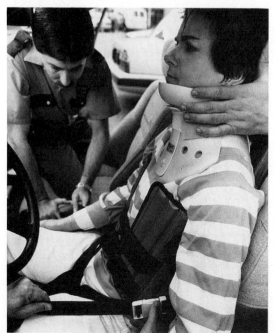

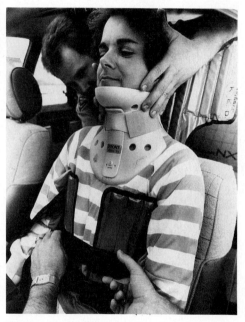

Figure S4–10. Tighten the chest straps.

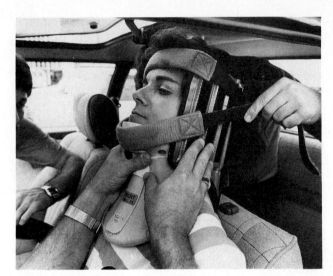

Figure S4–12. Apply firm padding as needed between the head and the headpiece to keep the head in a neutral position. Bring the head flaps around to the side of the head and secure firmly with straps, tape, or elastic wrap.

Figure S4–13. Turn the patient and the device as a unit, then lower onto a long backboard. Slide the patient and the device up into position on the board. Loosen the leg straps and allow the legs to extend out flat, then retighten the straps. Secure the patient and the device to the backboard.

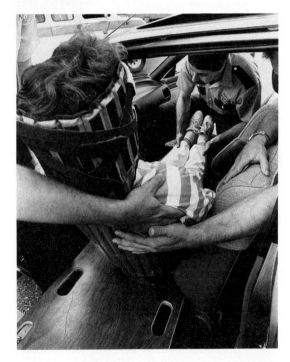

Skill 4B: Emergency Rapid Extrication

Victims left inside vehicles after an accident are usually stabilized on a short backboard (or extrication device) and then transferred onto a long backboard. Although this is the best way to extricate anyone with a possible spinal injury, there are certain situations where a more rapid method must be used.

Objective

The objective of this skill station is to learn indication and technique of emergency rapid extrication.

Situations Requiring Emergency Rapid Extrication

Scene survey identifies a condition that may *immediately* endanger the victim (and the EMTs).

Examples

1. Fire or immediate danger of fire
2. Danger of explosion
3. Rapidly rising water
4. Structure in danger of collapse

Primary survey of the victim identifies a condition that requires immediate intervention that cannot be done in the vehicle.

Examples

1. Airway obstruction that is not relieved by jaw thrust or finger sweep
2. Cardiac or respiratory arrest
3. Chest or airway injuries requiring ventilation or assisted ventilation
4. Deep shock or bleeding that cannot be controlled

This procedure is to be used *only* in a situation where the victim's life is in *immediate* danger. Any time that you use the procedure it should be noted in the run report and you should be prepared to defend your actions at a run review by your medical control physician. This is an example of "desperate situations often demand desperate measures."

Procedure

1. One rescuer must, if possible, station himself behind the victim, place his hands on either side of the victim's head, and stabilize the neck in a neutral position. This step is part of the ABCs of evaluation. It is done at the same time that you begin evaluation of the airway.

2. Do a rapid survey as you quickly apply a cervical collar. You should have the collar with you when you begin.

3. If your scene survey or your primary survey of the victim reveals an immediate life-threatening situation, go to the emergency rapid extrication technique. This requires at least four and preferably five or six persons to perform well.

4. Immediately slide the long backboard onto the seat and, if possible, at least slightly under the victim's buttocks.

5. A second EMT stands close beside the open door of the vehicle and takes over control of the cervical spine.

6. EMT 1 or another EMT is positioned on the other side of the front seat ready to rotate the victim's legs around.

7. Another EMT is also positioned at the open door by the victim. By holding the upper torso, he works together with the EMT, holding the legs to turn the victim carefully.

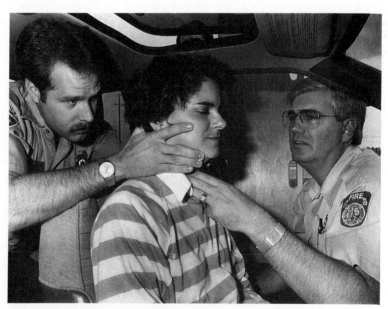

Figure S4–14. Stabilize the neck and perform the primary survey.

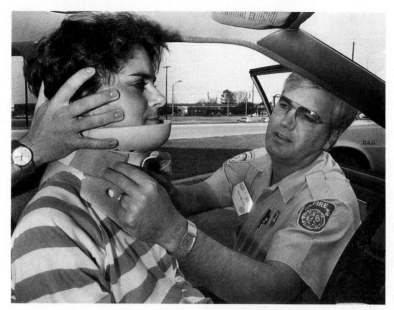

Figure S4–15. Apply a rigid extrication collar.

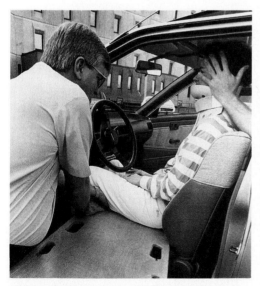

Figure S4–16. Slide the long backboard onto the seat and slightly under the patient.

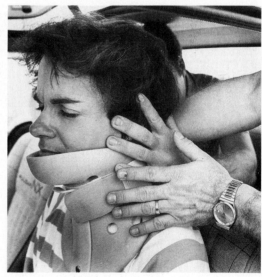

Figure S4–17. A second EMT stands close beside the open door of the vehicle and takes over control of the cervical spine.

8. The victim is turned so that his back is toward the backboard. His legs are lifted and his back is lowered to the backboard. The neck and back are not allowed to bend during this maneuver.

9. Using teamwork, the victim is carefully slid to the full length of the backboard and his legs are carefully straightened.

10. The victim is then moved immediately away from the vehicle (to the ambulance if available) and resuscitation is begun. He is secured to the backboard as soon as possible.

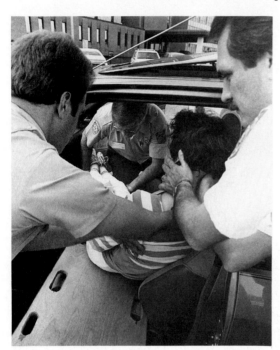

Figure S4-18. Carefully supporting the neck, torso, and legs, the EMTs turn the patient.

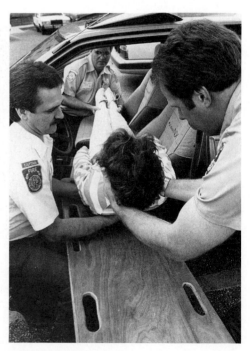

Figure S4-19. The legs are lifted and the back is lowered to the backboard.

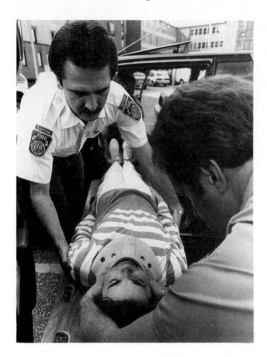

Figure S4–20. Carefully slide the patient to the full length of the backboard.

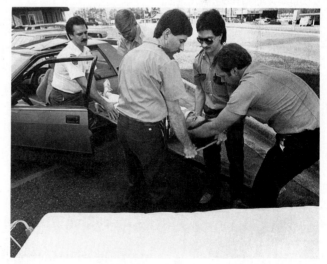

Figure S4–21. The patient is immediately moved away from the vehicle and into the ambulance, if available. Secure the patient to the backboard as soon as possible.

Basic Skill Station 5

Using a Long Backboard

Objectives

The objectives of this skill station are as follows:

1. To learn and practice log-rolling a victim onto a long backboard.
2. To learn and practice securing a victim to a long backboard.
3. To learn and practice immobilizing a victim from a standing position.
4. To learn and practice immobilizing the head and neck when a neutral position cannot safely be attained.

Procedures

Log-rolling the Supine Victim

1. EMT 1 maintains the spine immobilized in a neutral position. A rigid extrication collar is applied. Even with the collar in place, EMT 1 maintains the head and neck in a neutral position until the log-rolling maneuver is completed.

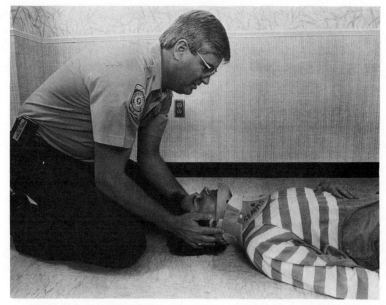

Figure S5-1. EMT #1 maintains the neck immobilized in a neutral position.

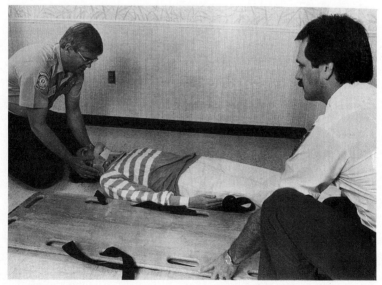

Figure S5-2. The long backboard is positioned beside the victim. Note that the straps are already laced into the correct holes in preparation for securing the victim.

2. The victim is placed with his legs extended in the normal manner and his arms (palms inward) extended by his sides. The victim will be rolled up on one arm with that arm acting as a splint for the body.

3. The long backboard is positioned next to the body. If one arm is injured, place the backboard on the injured side so that the victim will roll upon the uninjured arm.

4. EMTs 2 and 3 kneel at the victim's side opposite the board.

5. EMT 2 is positioned at the midchest area and EMT 3 is by the upper legs.

6. With his knees, EMT 2 holds the victim's near arm in place. He then reaches across the victim and grasps the shoulder and the hips, holding the victim's far arm in place. Usually, it is possible to grasp the victim's clothing to help with the roll.

7. With one hand, EMT 3 reaches across the victim and grasps the hip. With his other hand, he holds the feet together at the lower legs.

8. When everyone is ready, EMT 2 gives the order to roll the victim.

9. EMT 1 carefully keeps the head and neck in a neutral position (anteroposterior as well as laterally) during the roll.

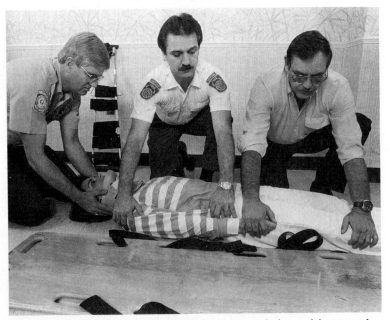

Figure S5–3. EMT #2 and EMT #3 assume their positions at the victim's side opposite the board.

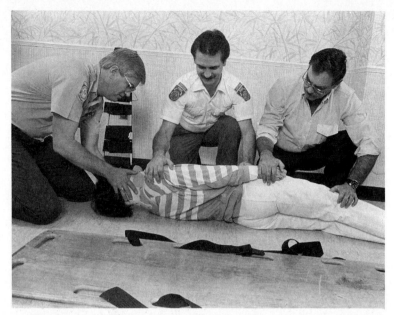

Figure S5-4. The victim is carefully rolled upon her side.

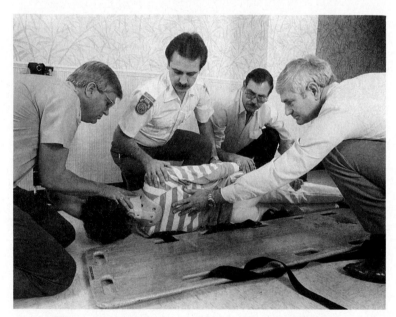

Figure S5-5. Quickly examine the back for injuries.

10. EMTs 2 and 3 roll the victim up on his side toward them. The victim's arms are kept locked to his side to maintain a splinting effect. The head, shoulders, and pelvis are kept in line during the roll.

11. When the victim is on his side, EMT 2 (or EMT 4 if available) quickly examines the back for injuries.

12. The backboard is now positioned next to the victim and held at a 30 to 45° angle by EMT 4. If there are only three EMTs, the board is pulled into place by EMT 2 or 3. The board is left flat in this case.

13. When everyone is ready, EMT 2 gives the order to roll the victim onto the backboard. This is accomplished keeping the head, shoulders, and pelvis in line.

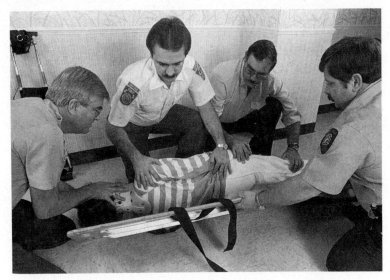

Figure S5-6A. If another EMT is available, he positions the backboard next to the victim at a 30-45 degree angle.

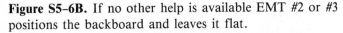

Figure S5-6B. If no other help is available EMT #2 or #3 positions the backboard and leaves it flat.

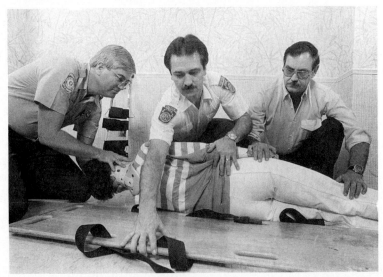

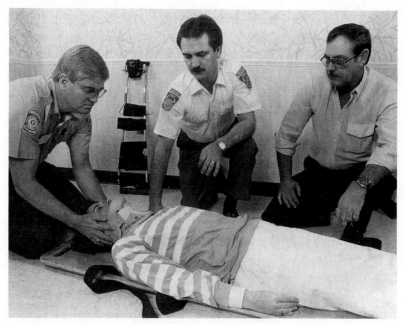

Figure S5–7. At EMT #2's order, the victim is rolled onto the backboard. All movements are coordinated so that the spine is kept straight at all times.

Log-rolling the Prone (Face-Down) Victim

The status of the airway is critical for decisions concerning the order of the log-rolling procedure. There are three clinical situations that dictate how you should proceed.

1. The victim who is not breathing or who is in severe respiratory difficulty must be log-rolled immediately in order to manage the airway. Unless the backboard is already positioned, you must log-roll the victim, manage the airway, then transfer the victim to the backboard (in a second log-rolling step) when ready to transport.

2. The victim with profuse bleeding of the mouth or nose must not be turned to the supine position. Profuse upper-airway bleeding in a supine victim is a guarantee of aspiration. This victim will have to be carefully immobilized and transported prone or on his side, allowing gravity to help keep the airway clear.

3. The victim with an adequate airway and respiration should be log-rolled directly onto a backboard.

Log-rolling the Supine Victim Who Has an Adequate Airway

1. EMT 1 immobilizes the neck in a neutral position. When placing the hands on the head and neck, the EMT's thumbs always point toward the victim's face. This prevents having the EMT's arms crossed when the victim is log-rolled. A rigid extrication collar is applied.

2. A rapid survey is done (including the back) and the victim is placed with his legs extended in the normal manner and his arms (palms inward) extended by his sides. The victim will be rolled up on one arm with that arm acting as a splint for the body.

3. The long backboard is positioned next to the body. The backboard is placed on the side of EMT 1's lower hand (if EMT 1's lower hand is on the victim's right side, the backboard is placed on the victim's right side). If the arm next to the backboard is injured, carefully raise the arm above the victim's head so that he does not roll on the injured arm.

4. EMTs 2 and 3 kneel at the victim's side opposite the board.

5. EMT 2 is positioned at the midchest area and EMT 3 is by the upper legs.

6. EMT 2 grasps the shoulder and the hip. Usually, it is possible to grasp the victim's clothing to help with the roll.

7. EMT 3 grasps the hip (holding the near arm in place) and the lower legs (holding them together).

8. When everyone is ready, EMT 2 gives the order to roll the victim.

9. EMT 1 carefully keeps the head and neck in a neutral position (anteroposterior as well as laterally) during the roll.

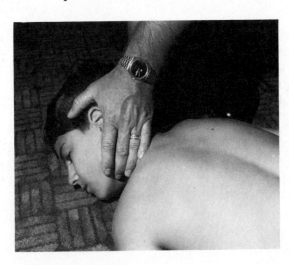

Figure S5–8. When immobilizing the neck of the prone (or supine) victim, your thumbs always point toward the face (not the occiput). This prevents having your arms crossed when the victim is rolled over.

10. EMTs 2 and 3 roll the victim up on his side away from them. The victim's arms are kept locked to his side to maintain a splinting effect. The head, shoulders, and pelvis are kept in line during the roll.

11. The backboard is now positioned next to the victim and held at a 30 to 45° angle by EMT 4. If there are only three EMTs, the board is pulled into place by EMT 2 or 3. The board is left flat in this case.

12. When everyone is ready, EMT 2 gives the order to roll the victim onto the backboard. This is accomplished keeping the head, shoulders, and pelvis in line.

Securing the Victim to the Backboard

There are several different methods of securing the victim using straps. Two of the best commercial devices for full-body immobilization are the Reeves Sleeve and the Miller Body Splint. The Reeves Sleeve is a heavy-duty sleeve that a standard backboard will slide into. Attached to this sleeve are:

1. Head-immobilization device
2. Heavy vinyl-coated nylon panels that go over the chest and abdomen and are secured with seat-belt-type straps and quick release connectors
3. Two full-length leg panels to secure the lower extremities
4. Straps to hold the arms in place beside the victim
5. Six handles for carrying the victim
6. Metal rings (2500-pound strength) for lifting the victim by rope

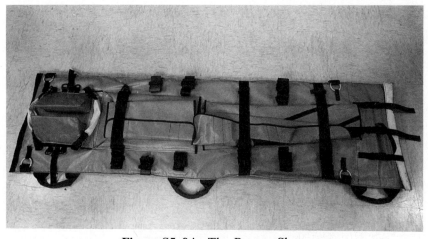

Figure S5–9A. The Reeves Sleeve.

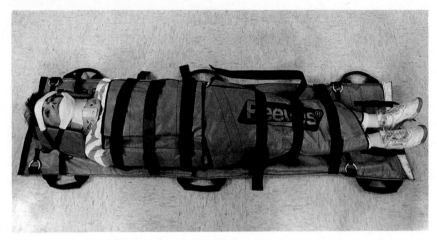

Figure S5–9B. A victim immobilized on a Reeves Sleeve. The arms can be positioned inside the vinyl panels, between the panels and the straps, or outside the panels and the straps.

When the victim is in this device, he remains immobilized when lifted horizontally, vertically, or even carried on his side (like a suitcase). This device is excellent for the confused, combative victim who must be restrained for his safety.

The Miller Body Splint is a combination backboard, head immobilizer, and body immobilizer. Like the Reeves Sleeve, it does an excellent job of full-body immobilization with a minimum of time and effort.

Securing the Victim to the Long Backboard Using Straps (Straps 12 feet in Length Are Preferred)

1. The head and neck are held in a neutral position (a rigid collar should already be in place) while padding is placed behind the head to maintain this position. A blanket roll or a commercial head immobilizer are applied and strapped into position using elastic wraps or wide tape. Do not use chin straps unless they can be applied to the chin portion of the extrication collar itself. Chin straps that hold the victim's mouth closed guarantee aspiration if the victim vomits.

2. Two straps are laced through the top two lateral holes of the backboard. Apply them so that they connect together across the chest below the armpits.

3. Bring the other ends of the straps over the shoulders and across the chest.

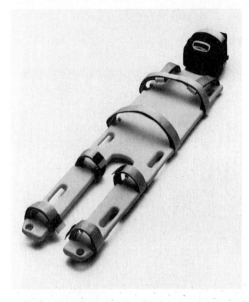

Figure S5–10. The Miller Body Splint.®

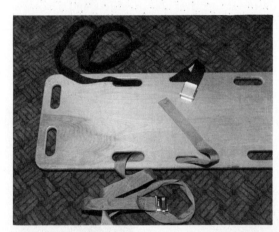

Figure S5–11A & B. Victim on backboard with lower end of straps connected below the armpits. The upper ends of the straps are pulled over the shoulders. Note that the victim should have his neck immobilized either manually or by an immobilization device.

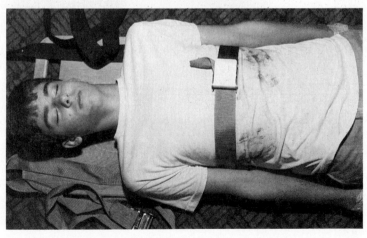

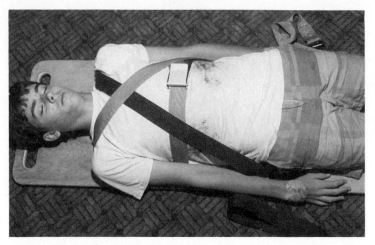

Figure S5–12. Bring the straps over the shoulders and across the chest. Lace the straps through the lateral holes at the level of the pelvis.

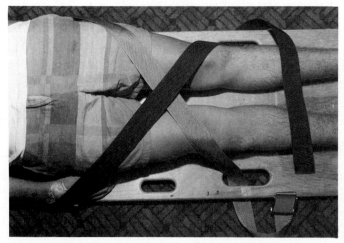

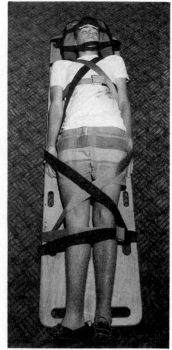

Figure S5–13A. Bring the straps back across the lower pelvis and upper legs, then lace through the lateral holes and connect below the knees.

Figure S5–13B. The straps should be tight enough to prevent any movement in case the board has to be tilted. Note that the chin strap should not be applied as shown here.

4.   Lace the straps through the lateral holes at the level of the pelvis.

5.   Bring the straps back across the lower pelvis and upper legs, then lace through the lateral holes and connect below the knees. The straps must be applied quite snug so that the body does not move if the board has to be turned to allow the victim to vomit.

Nine-foot straps will work, but are usually too short to go below the knees. If you use two 9-foot straps, most adults will require another strap below the knees.

Applying and Securing a Long Backboard to a Standing Victim

Method I

1.   One EMT stands behind the victim and immobilizes the head and neck in a neutral position. A rigid extrication collar is applied. The EMT continues to maintain stabilization in a neutral position.

2.   A long backboard is placed on the ground behind the victim.

3.   Other EMTs stabilize the shoulders and trunk and allow the victim to sit down carefully on the backboard.

4.   The victim is carefully lowered back onto the backboard, maintaining stabilization of the head, neck, and trunk.

5.   The victim is centered on the backboard and secured.

Method II

1.   EMT 1 stands in front of the victim and immobilizes the head and neck in a neutral position. A suitable cervical collar is applied. EMT 1 continues to maintain stabilization in a neutral position.

2.   EMT 2 places a long backboard against the victim's back.

3.   EMT 3 secures the victim to the board using nylon straps. These must cross over the shoulders and the pelvis and legs to prevent movement when the board is tilted down.

4.   Padding is placed behind the head to maintain a neutral position and a blanket roll or commercial head immobilizer is applied and secured using elastic wraps or wide tape.

5.   The board is carefully tilted back onto a stretcher and the legs secured and feet tied together.

Immobilizing the Head and Neck
When a Neutral Position Cannot Safely Be Attained

If the head or neck is held in an angulated position and the victim complains of pain upon any attempt to straighten it, you should immobilize it in the position found. The same is true of the unconscious victim whose neck is held to one side and does not easily straighten with gentle traction. You cannot use a cervical collar or commercial head immobilizer in this situation. You must use pads or a blanket roll and careful taping to immobilize the head and neck in the position found.

Basic Skill Station 6

Using Traction Splints

Objectives

The objectives for this skill station are as follows:

1. To learn when to use a traction splint.
2. To learn the possible complications of using a traction splint.
3. To learn how to apply the most common traction splints:
   a. Thomas splint
   b. Hare splint
   c. Klippel splint
   d. Sager splint
   e. Donway splint

Traction splints are designed to immobilize fractures of the lower extremities. They are useful for fractures of the femur or upper tibia. They are not useful for fractures of the hip, knee, ankle, or foot. Applying firm traction to a fractured or dislocated knee may tear the blood vessels behind the knee. If there appears to be a pelvic fracture, you cannot use a traction splint because it may cause further damage to the pelvis. Fractures below the midthigh that are not angulated or severely shortened may just as well be immobilized by air splints or the antishock garment. Traction splints work by applying a padded device to the back of the pelvis (ischium) or to the groin. A hitching device is then applied to the ankle and countertraction is applied until the limb is straight and well immobilized. The splints must be applied to the pelvis and groin very carefully to prevent excessive pressure on the genitalia. Care must also be used when attaching the hitching device to the foot and ankle so as not to interfere with circulation. To prevent any unnecessary movement, traction splints should not be applied until the victim is on a long backboard. If the splint extends beyond the end of the backboard, you must be very careful when moving the victim and when closing the ambulance door. You must check the circulation in the injured leg, so remove the shoe before attaching the hitching device. In every case at least two EMTs are needed. One must hold steady, gentle traction on the foot and leg while the other applies the splint. When dealing with "load and go" situations, the splint should not be applied until the victim is in the ambulance (unless the ambulance has not arrived).

Procedures

Applying a Thomas Splint (Half-Ring Splint)

1. The first EMT supports the leg and maintains gentle traction while the second EMT cuts away the clothing and removes the shoe and sock to check pulse and sensation at the foot.
2. Position the splint under the injured leg. The ring goes down and the short side goes to the inside of the leg. Slide the ring snugly up under the hip, where it will be pressed against the ischial tuberosity.
3. Position two support straps above the knee and two below the knee.
4. Attach the top ring strap.
5. Apply padding to the foot and ankle.
6. Apply the traction hitch around the foot and ankle.
7. Maintain gentle traction by hand.
8. Attach the traction hitch to the end of the splint.
9. Increase traction by Spanish windlass action using a stick or tongue depressors.
10. Release manual traction and reassess circulation and sensation.
11. Support the end of the splint so that there is no pressure on the heel.

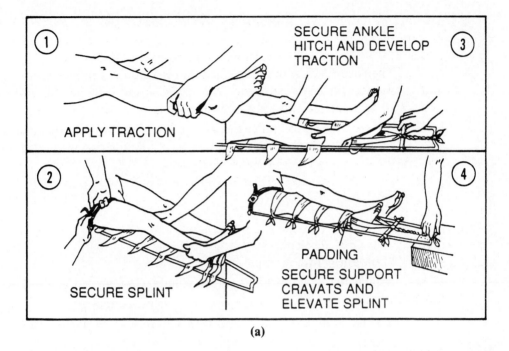

APPLY TRACTION

SECURE ANKLE HITCH AND DEVELOP TRACTION

SECURE SPLINT

PADDING

SECURE SUPPORT CRAVATS AND ELEVATE SPLINT

(a)

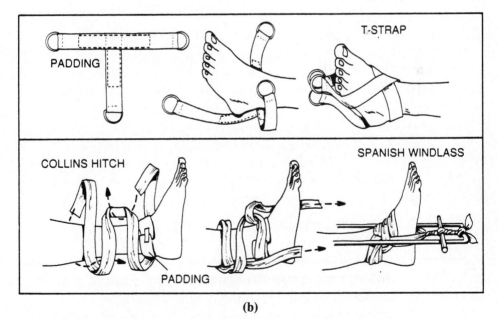

PADDING

T-STRAP

COLLINS HITCH

SPANISH WINDLASS

PADDING

(b)

Figure S6–1A. Applying a traction (Thomas) splint.

Figure S6–1B. Applying a traction hitch to the ankle.

Applying a Hare Splint

1. Position the victim on the backboard or stretcher.
2. The first EMT supports the leg and maintains gentle traction while the second EMT cuts away the clothing and removes the shoe and sock to check pulse and sensation at the foot.
3. Position the splint under the injured leg. The ring goes down and the short side goes to the inside of the leg. Slide the ring up snugly under the hip against the ischial tuberosity.
4. Position two support straps above the knee and two below the knee.
5. Attach the heel rest.
6. Attach the top strap.
7. Apply the padded traction hitch to the ankle and foot.
8. Maintain gentle manual traction.
9. Attach the traction hitch to the windlass by way of the S-hook.
10. Turn the ratchet until the correct tension is applied.
11. Release manual traction and recheck circulation and sensation.
12. Attach support straps around the leg with Velcro straps.
13. To release traction, pull the ratchet knob outward and then slowly turn to loosen.

Applying a Klippel Splint

1. Position the victim on the long backboard or stretcher.
2. The first EMT supports the leg and maintains gentle traction while the second EMT cuts away the clothing and removes the shoe and sock to check the pulse and sensation at the foot.
3. Using the uninjured leg as a guide, pull the splint out to the correct length.
4. Turn the footplate up by pushing to the side and then turning.
5. Turn the heel rest down by pushing in both knobs simultaneously and then turning.
6. While maintaining gentle traction and support, slide the splint under the leg (ring turned down) until the ring is snugly under the hip and against the ischial tuberosity.
7. Position two support straps above the knee and two below the knee.
8. Attach the top ring strap.

9. Push the footplate up against the sole of the foot. Push the two release levers to shorten the splint.

10. Apply padding to the foot and ankle.

11. Bring the traction hitch up under the ankle and then cross the two straps over the foot, around the footplate, and back over the foot where they attach by Velcro fasteners.

12. While maintaining manual traction, extend the splint by pulling on the two rails until correct tension is obtained.

13. Release manual traction and recheck circulation and sensation.

14. Attach support straps around the leg with Velcro fasteners.

Applying a Sager Splint

This splint is different in several ways. It works by providing countertraction against the pubic ramus and the ischial tuberosity medial to the shaft of the femur, thus does not go under the leg. The hip does not have to be slightly flexed as with the Hare and Klippel. The Sager is also lighter and more compact than other traction splints. You can also splint both legs with one splint if needed. The new Sagers are significantly improved over older models and may represent the "state of the art" in traction splints.

1. Position the victim on a long backboard or stretcher.

2. The first EMT supports the leg and maintains gentle traction while the second EMT cuts away the clothing and removes the shoe and sock to check the pulse and sensation at the foot.

3. Using the uninjured leg as a guide, pull the splint out to the correct length.

4. Position the splint to the inside of the injured leg with the padded bar fitted snugly against the pelvis in the groin. The splint can be used on the outside of the leg, using the strap to maintain traction against the pubis. Be very careful not to catch the genitals under the bar (or strap).

5. While maintaining gentle manual traction, attach the padded hitch to the foot and ankle.

6. Extend the splint until the correct tension is obtained.

7. Release manual traction and recheck circulation and sensation.

8. Apply elastic straps above and below the knee.

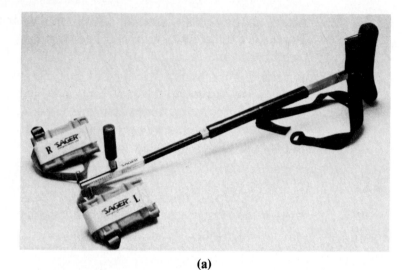

(a)

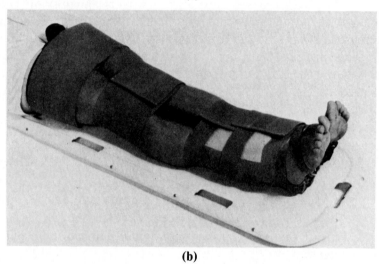

(b)

Figure S6–2A. Sager Traction Splint.

Figure S6–2B. Patient with both legs splinted with Sager Traction Splint.

Applying a Donway Splint

This is a fairly new variation of the Thomas half-ring splint. The ischial ring removes for easier attachment and traction is applied by a pneumatic pump. This splint can be applied by a single person if necessary.

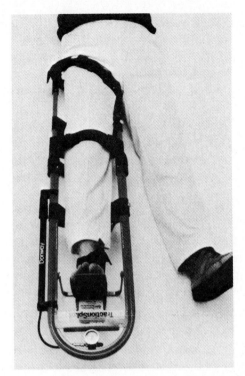

Figure S6-3. Donway Traction Splint.

1. Position the victim on a long backboard or stretcher.

2. The first EMT supports the leg and maintains gentle traction while the second EMT cuts away the clothing and removes the shoe and sock to check the pulse and sensation at the foot.

3. Feed the ischial ring under the knee, adjust around the thigh, and fasten the buckle to achieve a loose fit.

4. Depress the air release valve to ensure that no excess pressure is retained in the system.

5. Unlock the collets, raise the footplate into the upright position, and place the splint over the leg.

6. Adjust the sidearms of the splint to the desired length, attach to the ischial ring pegs, and lock by turning the side arms.

7. Open the ankle strap and employing the necessary support, place the patient's heel in the padded portion of the strap with the foot against the footplate.

8. Maintaining the heel against the footplate, adjust the lower Velcro attachment to ensure that the padded support member is positioned high on the ankle.

9. Crisscross the top straps tightly over the instep, starting with the longest strap.

10. Tighten the straps around the footplate and secure with the Velcro attachments.

11. Apply pneumatic pressure with the pump, up to the desired level of traction (15 lbs maximum), and upon completion, moderately tighten the strap to secure the ring in the ischial load-bearing position. The operating range of the splint is 10 to 40 pounds of traction. Safety pressure relief valves operate automatically if this range is exceeded. In this event, the collets should be locked, the air released, and the normal procedure for application of traction is repeated.

12. Release manual traction and recheck circulation and sensation.

13. Align the opened leg supports with the calf and thigh. Feed the leading tapered edge under the leg, over the top of the opposite sidearm, and back under the leg. Adjust the tension to provide the required support and secure with the button fastener.

14. Feed the knee strap under the leg and secure above the knee with the buckle fastener.

15. As the injured leg is under traction and adequately supported, the heel stand can be raised. Recheck the traction level and adjust where necessary.

16. Turn the collets until hand tight and apply a further quarter-turn to lock the position of the sidearms, and release the pneumatic pressure by depressing the air release valve until the gauge reads zero.

Basic Skill Station 7

Antishock Garment Application and Helmet Removal

Basic Skill 7A: Application of the Antishock Garment*

Objectives

The objectives of this skill station are as follows:

1. To learn and practice the proper method of applying and inflating the antishock garment.
2. To learn and practice the proper method of deflating and removing the antishock garment.
3. To learn the indications and contraindications for use of the antishock garment.

Caution: If these trousers are applied to live models, do not inflate them; they may cause elevations in the blood pressure.

*Also known as military antishock trousers (MAST) or pneumatic antishock garment (PASG).

Procedure

Application

1. Evaluate the victim through at least the primary survey. Apply a blood pressure cuff to his arm.
2. Have the second EMT unfold the trousers and lay them flat on a long backboard and place the backboard beside the victim.
3. If shock is present, cut the clothing from the lower body and perform the MAST survey.
    a. Quickly examine the abdomen.
    b. Feel the pelvis for stability.
    c. Check the legs for injury.
4. Maintaining immobility of the spine, log-roll the victim (check the back quickly as you do this) onto the backboard. The top of the antishock garment should be just below the lowest rib.
5. Wrap the trousers around the left leg and fasten the Velcro strips.
6. Wrap the trousers around the right leg and fasten the Velcro strips.
7. Wrap the abdominal compartment around the abdomen and fasten the Velcro strips. Be sure the top of the garment is below the bottom ribs.
8. Attach the tubes from the foot pump to the connections on the trousers.

Inflation of Trousers

Indications for inflation of trousers:

1. Systolic blood pressure less than 80 mmHg
2. Systolic blood pressure of 100 or less with other symptoms of shock
3. Spinal shock
4. Pelvic fractures
5. Fractures of legs
6. Massive abdominal bleeding

Procedure for inflation of trousers:

1. Recheck and record the vital signs.
2. Inflate the leg compartments while monitoring the blood pressure. If the blood pressure is not in the range 100 to 110 mmHg, inflate the abdominal compartment.

3. When the patient's blood pressure is adequate (100 to 110 mmHg), turn the stopcocks to hold the pressure.

4. Remember, it is not the pressure in the trousers you are monitoring but the pressure in the patient.

5. Continue monitoring the patient's blood pressure, adding pressure to the trousers as needed.

Deflation of Trousers: Before deflation occurs, two large-bore IVs must be inserted and sufficient volume of fluids and/or blood given to replace the volume lost from hemorrhage. The antishock garment is usually deflated only at the hospital. The only reason to deflate them in the field is if they cause difficulty with breathing (pulmonary edema).

1. Record the patient's vital signs.

2. Obtain permission to deflate the trousers from a physician knowledgeable in their use.

3. Slowly deflate the abdominal compartment while monitoring the patient's blood pressure.

4. If the blood pressure drops 5 mmHg or more, you must stop deflation and infuse more fluid or blood until the vital signs stabilize again (this usually requires at least 200 cc).

5. Proceed from the abdominal compartment to the right leg and then left leg with your deflation, continuously monitoring the blood pressure and stopping to infuse fluid when a drop of 5 mmHg occurs.

6. If the patient experiences a sudden precipitous drop in blood pressure while you are deflating, stop and reinflate the garment.

Application of Antishock Trousers to a Victim Requiring a Traction Splint

1. Have your partner hold traction on the fractured leg.

2. Unfold the trousers and lay them flat on a long spine board.

3. Log-roll the victim, holding traction on the injured leg and keeping the neck stabilized.

4. Slide the spine board and the victim so that the top of the trousers is just below the lowest rib. If the victim is already on a spine board, you may simply unfold the trousers and slide them under the victim while maintaining traction on the injured leg.

5. Wrap the trousers around the injured leg and fasten the Velcro strips.

6. Wrap the trousers around the other leg and fasten the Velcro strips.

7. Wrap the abdominal compartment around the abdomen and fasten the Velcro strips. Make sure that the top of the garment is below the bottom ribs.

8. Apply a traction splint (Thomas, Hare, Sager, or Klippel) over the trousers. Attach the straps and apply traction.

9. Inflate the trousers in the usual sequence.

Critical Points

1. Remove the trousers only in the hospital setting unless pulmonary edema is precipitated by application.

2. Inflate the trousers until a systolic blood pressure of 100 to 110 mmHg is obtained.

3. Monitor vital signs frequently.

Figure S7–1. Application of the MAST.

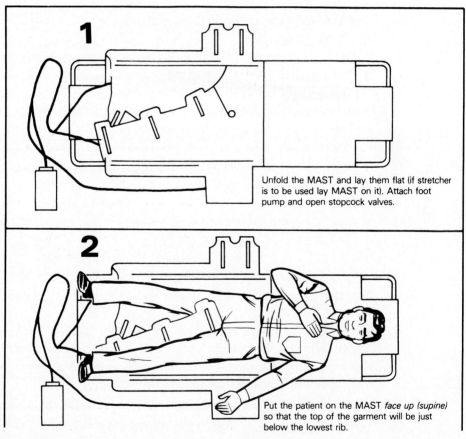

1

Unfold the MAST and lay them flat (if stretcher is to be used lay MAST on it). Attach foot pump and open stopcock valves.

2

Put the patient on the MAST *face up (supine)* so that the top of the garment will be just below the lowest rib.

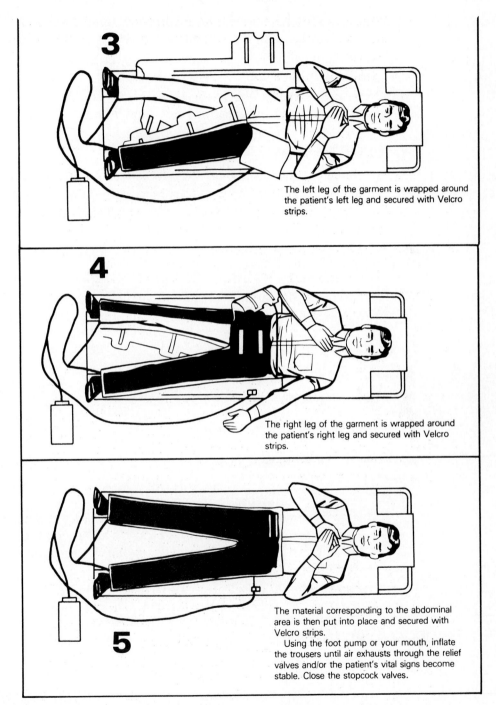

3

The left leg of the garment is wrapped around the patient's left leg and secured with Velcro strips.

4

The right leg of the garment is wrapped around the patient's right leg and secured with Velcro strips.

The material corresponding to the abdominal area is then put into place and secured with Velcro strips.
    Using the foot pump or your mouth, inflate the trousers until air exhausts through the relief valves and/or the patient's vital signs become stable. Close the stopcock valves.

5

Figure S7-1. Cont.

4. During deflation, a blood pressure drop of 5 mmHg signals that deflation must stop until more fluids are replaced.

5. Never allow deflation of the antishock garment by personnel inexperienced in their use.

6. Never deflate the antishock trousers without adequate volume replacement and a good intravenous route established.

7. Never deflate the entire garment at once.

8. Never deflate the legs before the abdomen.

9. Do not allow anyone to cut the garment.

10. If necessary, patients may go to surgery with the garment in place.

Review

Indications for Use of Antishock Trousers

1. Systolic blood pressure less than 80 mmHg
2. Systolic blood pressure of 100 or less with other symptoms of shock
3. Spinal shock
4. Pelvic fractures
5. Fractures of legs
6. Massive abdominal bleeding

Contraindications for Use of Antishock Trousers

1. *Absolute:* pulmonary edema.
2. *Conditional:*
    a. *Pregnancy.* May use leg compartments.
    b. *Abdominal injury with protruding viscera.* Use leg compartments.
    c. *Penetrating chest wounds with shock.* Do not attempt to raise the blood pressure above 100 mmHg systolic. You may increase intrathoracic bleeding.
    d. *Diaphragmatic hernia.* Use leg compartments.

Basic Skill 7B: Helmet Removal

Objective

The objective of this skill station is to learn and practice how to remove a helmet without injuring the spine.

Procedures

Removing a Helmet from a Victim with a Possible Cervical Spine Injury

1. The first EMT positions himself above or behind the victim, places his hands on each side of the helmet, and immobilizes the head and neck by holding the helmet and the victim's neck.
2. The second EMT positions himself to the side of the victim and removes the chin strap. Chin straps can usually be removed easily without cutting them.
3. The second EMT then assumes the stabilization by placing one hand under the neck at the occiput and the other hand on the anterior neck with the thumb pressing on one angle of the mandible and the index and middle fingers pressing on the other angle of the mandible.
4. The first EMT now removes the helmet by pulling out laterally on each side to clear the ears and then up to remove. Full-face helmets will

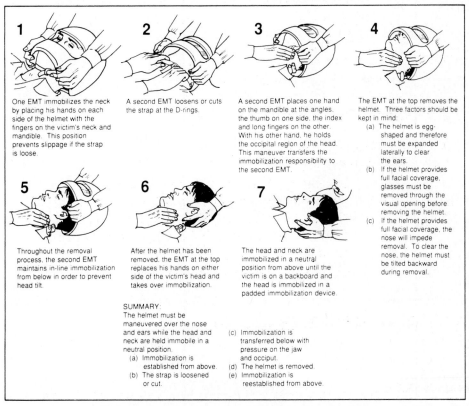

1
One EMT immobilizes the neck by placing his hands on each side of the helmet with the fingers on the victim's neck and mandible. This position prevents slippage if the strap is loose.

2
A second EMT loosens or cuts the strap at the D-rings.

3
A second EMT places one hand on the mandible at the angles. the thumb on one side. the index and long fingers on the other. With his other hand. he holds the occipital region of the head. This maneuver transfers the immobilization responsibility to the second EMT.

4
The EMT at the top removes the helmet. Three factors should be kept in mind:
  (a) The helmet is egg-shaped and therefore must be expanded laterally to clear the ears.
  (b) If the helmet provides full facial coverage, glasses must be removed through the visual opening before removing the helmet.
  (c) If the helmet provides full facial coverage, the nose will impede removal. To clear the nose, the helmet must be tilted backward during removal.

5
Throughout the removal process. the second EMT maintains in-line immobilization from below in order to prevent head tilt.

6
After the helmet has been removed. the EMT at the top replaces his hands on either side of the victim's head and takes over immobilization.

7
The head and neck are immobilized in a neutral position from above until the victim is on a backboard and the head is immobilized in a padded immobilization device.

SUMMARY:
The helmet must be maneuvered over the nose and ears while the head and neck are held immobile in a neutral position.
  (a) Immobilization is established from above.
  (b) The strap is loosened or cut.
  (c) Immobilization is transferred below with pressure on the jaw and occiput.
  (d) The helmet is removed.
  (e) Immobilization is reestablished from above.

Figure S7–2. Helmet removal from injured patient.

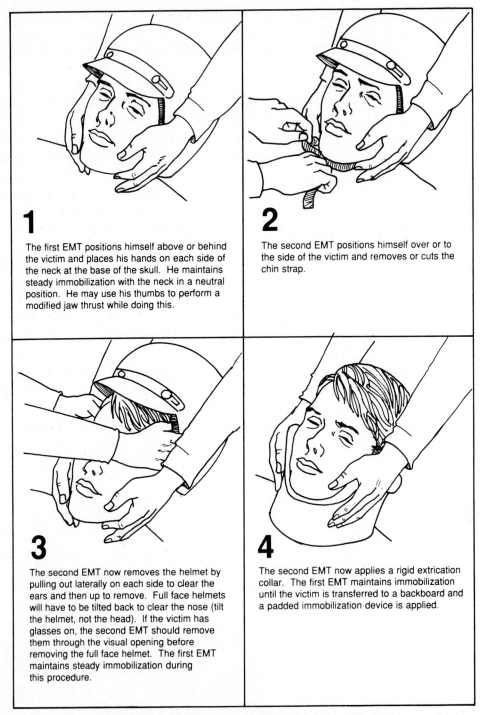

1

The first EMT positions himself above or behind the victim and places his hands on each side of the neck at the base of the skull. He maintains steady immobilization with the neck in a neutral position. He may use his thumbs to perform a modified jaw thrust while doing this.

2

The second EMT positions himself over or to the side of the victim and removes or cuts the chin strap.

3

The second EMT now removes the helmet by pulling out laterally on each side to clear the ears and then up to remove. Full face helmets will have to be tilted back to clear the nose (tilt the helmet, not the head). If the victim has glasses on, the second EMT should remove them through the visual opening before removing the full face helmet. The first EMT maintains steady immobilization during this procedure.

4

The second EMT now applies a rigid extrication collar. The first EMT maintains immobilization until the victim is transferred to a backboard and a padded immobilization device is applied.

Figure S7–3. Alternate method for removal of helmet.

have to be tilted back to clear the nose (tilt the helmet, not the head). If the victim is wearing glasses, the first EMT should remove them through the visual opening before removing the full-face helmet. The second EMT maintains steady immobilization of the neck during this procedure.

5. After removal of the helmet, the first EMT takes over the neck immobilization again by grasping the head on either side with his fingers holding the angle of the jaw and the occiput.

6. The second EMT now applies a suitable cervical-immobilization device.

Alternative Procedure for Removing a Helmet: This has the advantage of one EMT maintaining immobilization of the neck throughout the whole procedure. This procedure does not work well with full-face helmets.

1. The first EMT positions himself above or behind the victim and places his hands on each side of the neck at the base of the skull. He immobilizes the neck in a neutral position. If necessary, he may use his thumbs to perform a modified jaw thrust while doing this.

2. The second EMT positions himself over or to the side of the victim and removes the chin strap.

3. The second EMT now removes the helmet by pulling out laterally on each side to clear the ears and then up to remove. The first EMT maintains immobilization of the neck during the procedure.

4. The second EMT now applies a suitable cervical-immobilization device.

Basic Skill Station 8

Basic Airway Management

Objectives

The objectives of this skill station are as follows:

1. To learn how to suction the airway.
2. To learn how to insert a nasopharyngeal and oropharyngeal airway.
3. To learn how to use the pocket mask.
4. To learn how to use the bag-valve mask.

Procedures

Suctioning the Airway

1. Attach the suction tubing to the portable suction machine.
2. Turn the device on and test it.
3. Insert the suction tube through the nose or mouth without activating the suction.
4. Activate the suction and withdraw the suction tube.
5. Repeat the procedure as necessary.

Inserting Pharyngeal Airways

Nasopharyngeal airway

1. Choose the appropriate size. It should be the largest that will fit easily through the external nares.
2. Lubricate the tube.
3. Insert it straight back through the right nostril with the beveled edge of the airway toward the septum.
4. To insert it in the left nostril, turn the airway upside down so that the bevel is toward the septum, then insert straight back through the nostril until you reach the posterior pharynx. At this point, turn the airway over 180° and insert it down the pharynx until it lies behind the tongue.

Oropharyngeal airway

1. Choose the appropriate size.
2. Open the airway:
    a. Scissor maneuver
    b. Jaw lift
    c. Tongue blade

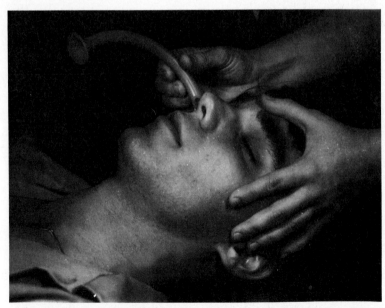

Figure S8-1. The nasopharyngeal airway is inserted with the bevel slid along the septum or floor of the nasal cavity.

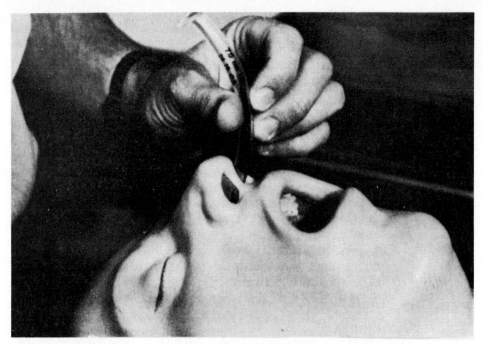

Figure S8–2A. Insertion of nasopharyngeal airway into left nostril. Insert upside down so bevel is toward the septum.

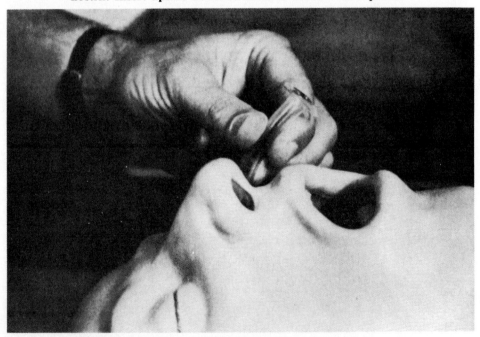

Figure S8–2B. When tip is to the back of the pharynx, rotate airway 180 degrees.

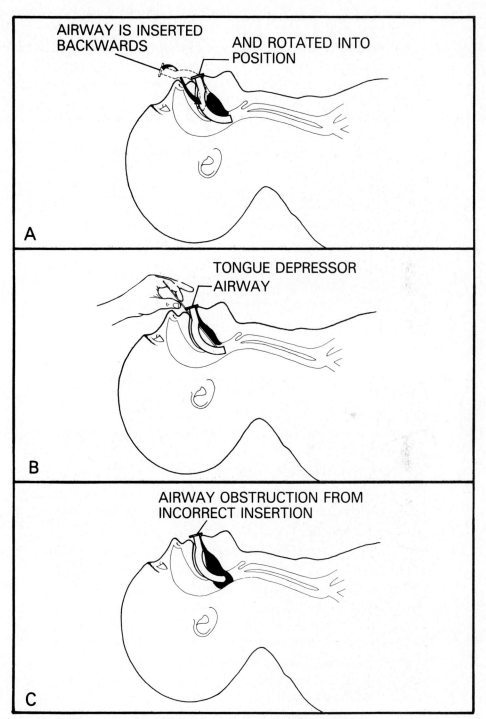

Figure S8–3. Insertion of oral airway.

3. Insert the airway gently without pushing the tongue back into the pharynx.

    a. Insert the airway upside down and rotate into place. This method should not be used in children.

    b. Insert the airway under direct vision using the tongue blade.

Using a Pocket Mask with Supplemental Oxygen

1. Have your partner stabilize the neck in a neutral position (or apply a good stabilization device).
2. Connect the oxygen tubing to the oxygen cylinder and the mask.
3. Open the oxygen cylinder and set the flow rate at 12 L/min.
4. Open the airway.
5. Insert the oral airway properly.
6. Place the mask on the face and establish a good seal.
7. Ventilate mouth-to-mask with enough volume (about 800 to 1000 cc) to cause the green light to come on in the recording mannequin.

Using the Bag–Valve Mask

1. Stabilize the neck with a suitable device.
2. Connect the oxygen tubing to the bag–valve system and oxygen cylinder.
3. Attach the oxygen reservoir to the bag–valve mask.
4. Open the oxygen cylinder and set the flow rate at 12 L/min.
5. Select the proper size mask and attach it to the bag–valve device.
6. Open the airway.
7. Insert the oral airway properly (do not insert if the patient has a gag reflex).
8. Place the mask on the face and have your partner establish and maintain a good seal.
9. Ventilate with enough volume (about 800 cc) to cause the green light to come on in the recording mannequin. Use both hands.
10. If you are forced to ventilate without a partner, use one hand to maintain a face seal and the other to squeeze the bag. This decreases the volume of ventilation because less volume is produced by only one hand squeezing the bag.

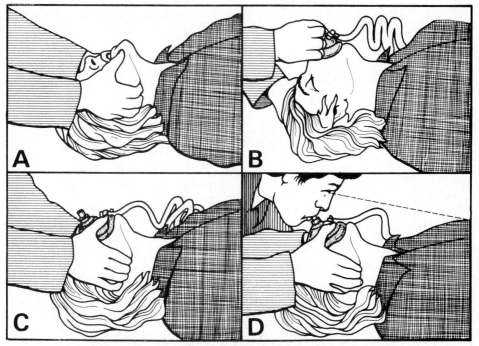

Figure S8–4. Pocket mask.

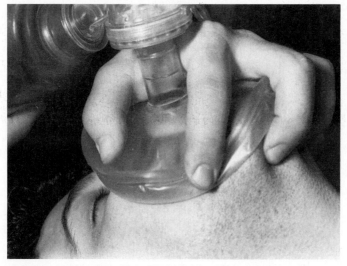

Figure S8–5. The Seal Easy™ balloon mask has been shown to reduce mask leak and provide greater volumes during ventilation with bag/mask devices.

11. Hyperventilation. All trauma victims who have a decreased level of consciousness should be hyperventilated with 100% oxygen at a rate of one ventilation about every 2 seconds (24 to 30 breaths per minute). Using procedure steps 1–9 above, practice hyperventilation until you feel comfortable with the rhythm of ventilating at the rate of 24 to 30 breaths per minute.

──Advanced Skill Station 9──

Advanced Airway Management

Preparations

Whatever the method of intubation used, both patients and rescuers should be prepared for the procedure. The following are considered basic to all intubation procedures:

1. *Oxygenation.* All patients should be ventilated, or should breathe high-flow oxygen (12 L/min) for several minutes prior to the attempt.
2. *Gloves.* Rubber examining gloves (not necessarily sterile) should be worn for all intubation procedures.
3. *Equipment.* All equipment should have been checked and should be kept at hand in an organized kit. For laryngoscopic intubation, the endotracheal tube should be held in a "hockey stick" shape by a malleable stylet that is first lubricated and inserted until the distal end is just *proximal* to the side hole of the endotracheal tube. The cuff of the endotracheal tube should be checked by inflating it with 10 cc of air. The air should then be *completely* removed and the syringe filled with air left attached to the pilot tube. The cuff and distal end of the tube is then lubricated.

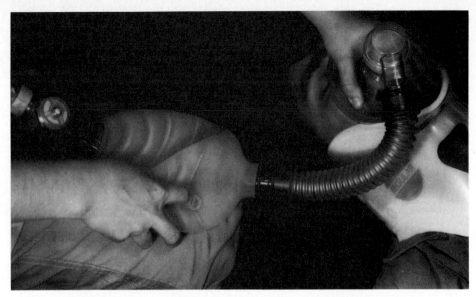

Figure S9-1. A ventilating port extension attached to a ventilating bag permits a better mask seal and therefore greater delivered volumes. When the bag is compressed against the rescuer's thigh as shown, delivered volumes may be further increased.

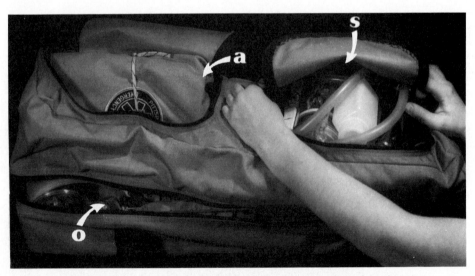

Figure S9-2a. An airway kit containing the essentials for airway management. Note that portable suction is included in this design(s). The total weight (with aluminum "D" oxygen cylinder) is approximately 10Kg. (22 lbs), about the same as a steel "E" oxygen cylinder. a-airway wrap; o-oxygen cylinder.

4. *Suction.* Suction must be immediately at hand.

5. *Assistant.* An assistant should be available to help in the procedure, and Sellick's maneuver should be applied during ventilation and the subsequent intubation attempt. The assistant may also aid in holding the head and neck immobile and counting aloud to 30.

6. *Lidocaine.* Intravenous lidocaine HCl, given 4 to 5 minutes before intubation is attempted, has been shown to decrease the adverse cardiovascular and intracranial pressure effects of the intubation procedure. *If time permits,* an IV bolus of 100 to 125 mg may be given to all adult patients prior to intubation or suctioning.

Advanced Skill 9A: Laryngoscopic Orotracheal Intubation

In this method, the upper airway and the glottic opening are visualized and the tube is slipped gently through the cords. Its advantages include the ability to see obstructions and to visualize accurate placement of the tube. It has the disadvantage of requiring a relatively relaxed patient without anatomic distortion, and with minimal bleeding or secretions.

Equipment

1. Straight (Miller) or curved (MacIntosh) blade and laryngoscope handle
2. Transparent endotracheal tube, 28 to 33 cm in length and 7.0, 7.5, or 8.0 mm in internal diameter
3. Stylet to help mold the tube into a "hockey stick" shape
4. Water-soluble lubricant (there is no need for it to contain a local anesthetic)
5. 10- or 12-cc syringe
6. Magill forceps
7. Tape/tincture of benzoin or endotracheal tube holder

Procedure

Following ventilation and initial preparations, the following steps should be carried out:

1. An assistant holds the head, performs Sellick's maneuver, and counts slowly *aloud* to 30.

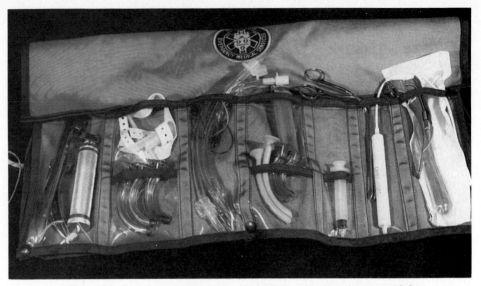

Figure S9-2b. An "Intubation WRAP" contains the essentials for carrying out endotracheal intubation. The kit folds on itself and is compact and portable (A). When opened (B), it provides a clean working surface. Note the transparent pockets.

2. The intubator pulls down on the chin and slides the blade into the right side of the patient's mouth, pushing the tongue to the left and "inching" the blade down along the tongue in an attempt to see the epiglottis. A key maneuver must be performed here; the blade must pull forward on the tongue to lift up the epiglottis and bring it into view (Figure S9A-1).

3. The laryngoscope blade is used to lift the tongue and epiglottis up and forward in a straight line. "Levering" the blade is a common error with novices and can result in broken teeth and other trauma. The laryngoscope is essentially a "hook" to lift the tongue and epiglottis up and out of the way so that the glottic opening can be identified.

4. The tube is advanced along the right side of the oropharynx once the epiglottis is seen. When the glottic opening (or even just the arytenoid cartilages) is identified, the tube is slipped through to a depth of about 5 cm beyond the cords.

5. Should visualization be difficult, an assistant can put posteriorward pressure on the laryngeal prominence to bring the cords into view.

6. While the tube is still held firmly, the cuff is inflated and ventilation begun.

7. The tube is then checked for placement by the confirmation protocol (page 334).

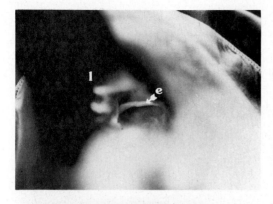

Figure S9A-1A. LANDMARKS DURING INTUBATION—View looking into the oropharynx during the act of direct laryngoscopy. A—the laryngoscope (l) is inserted into the vallecula and the tongue is pulled forward to expose the epiglottis (e).

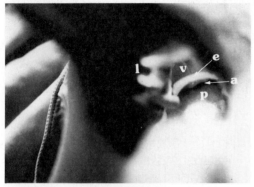

Figure S9A-1B. B—pulling forward further (not levering) in a straight line allows the arytenoid cartilages (a) to become into view; l-laryngoscope; p-posterior pharyngeal wall; v-vallecula; e-epiglottis.

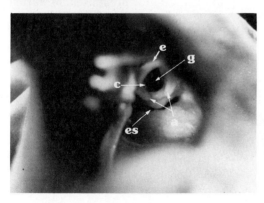

Figure S9A-1C. C—intubator's view of larynx. e—epiglottis; g—glottic opening; c—cords; a—arytenoids; es—esophagus.

Advanced Skill 9B: Nasotracheal Intubation

The nasotracheal route of endotracheal intubation in a field setting may be justified when the patient's mouth cannot be opened because of clenched jaws and when the patient cannot be ventilated by other means. The great disadvan-

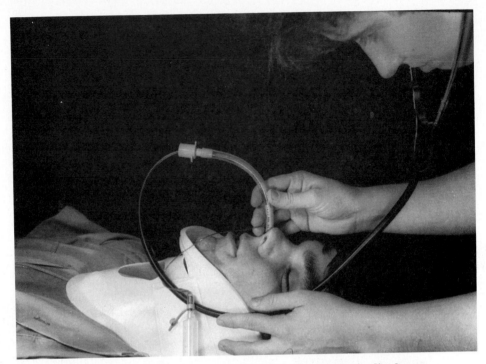

Figure S9B-1. Following removal of the stethoscope's diaphragm and bell, the tubing can be squeezed into the adapter of the endotracheal tube as an aid to listening for breath sounds during nasotracheal intubation.

tage of this method is its relative difficulty, depending as it does on an appreciation of the intensity of the breath sounds of spontaneously breathing patients. It is a blind procedure and as such requires extra effort to demonstrate proper intratracheal placement.

Guidance of the tube through the glottic opening is a question of the intubator perceiving the intensity of the sound of the patient breathing out. The tube can, with some difficulty, be guided toward the point of maximum intensity and slipped through the cords. Breath sounds can be better heard and felt with the ear placed against the proximal opening of the tube or, even better, the bell of a single-tube stethoscope can be removed and the tube inserted into the endotracheal tube (Figure S9B–1).

The success of this method will also depend on an anterior curve to the tube that will prevent its passing into the esophagus. This may better be achieved by preparing two tubes prior to carrying out the intubation attempt. The distal end of the 33-cm tube is inserted into its proximal opening, thus molding it into a formed circle. Preparing two tubes permits the immediate use of a second, more rigid tube should the first plastic tube become warm with body temperature, thus losing its anterior curve. The Endotrol, a directional-tip tube, has been introduced to help in achieving an anterior curve, but this has not been shown to be extremely helpful. Displacing the tongue and jaw forward may also be helpful in achieving placement, since this maneuver lifts the epiglottis anteriorly out of the way of the advancing tube.

Procedure

1. Perform routine preparation procedures (page 321).
2. Following lubrication of its cuff and distal end, a 7.0- or 7.5-mm endotracheal tube with the bevel against the floor or septum of the nasal cavity is slipped distally through the largest naris.
3. When the tube tip reaches the posterior pharyngeal wall, great care must be taken on "rounding the bend" and then directing the tube toward the glottic opening.
4. By watching the neck at the laryngeal prominence the intubator can judge the approximate placement of the tube; tenting of the skin on either side of the prominence indicates catching up of the tube in the pyriform fossa, a problem solved by slight withdrawal and rotation of the tube to the midline. Bulging and anterior displacement of the laryngeal prominence usually indicates that the tube has entered the glottic opening and has been correctly placed. At this point the patient, especially if not deeply comatose, will cough, strain, or both. This may be alarming to the novice intubator, who might interpret this as laryngospasm or misplacement of the tube. The temptation may be to pull the tube and ventilate, since the patient may not breathe immediately. Holding the hand or ear over the opening of the tube to detect airflow may reassure the intubator that the tube is correctly placed, and the cuff may be inflated and ventilation begun.
5. Confirm placement by the confirmation protocol (page 334).

Advanced Skill 9C: Digital Intubation

The original method of endotracheal intubation, quite widely known in the eighteenth century, was the "tactile" or "digital" technique. The intubator merely felt the epiglottis with the fingers and slipped the endotracheal tube distally through the glottic opening. Recently, the technique has been refined and demonstrated to be of use in the field for a wide variety of patients.

Indications

Tactile orotracheal intubation is particularly useful for deeply comatose or cardiac arrest patients who:

1. Are difficult to position properly
2. Are somewhat inaccessible to the full view of the rescuer
3. May be at risk of cervical spine injury
4. Have facial injuries that distort anatomy
5. Have copious oropharyngeal bleeding or secretions that render visualization difficulty

Personnel may prefer to perform tactile intubation when they are more confident in their ability with the technique, or when a laryngoscope fails or is not immediately available. We have found the technique most valuable in those patients in difficult positions (e.g., extrications) and in those who have copious secretions despite adequate attempts at suctioning.

Equipment

This method of intubation requires the following:

1. Endotracheal tube, 7.0-, 7.5-, or 8.0-mm internal diameter
2. Malleable stylet (*Note:* Some prefer to perform the procedure without a stylet)
3. Water-soluble lubricant
4. 12-cc syringe
5. Dental prod, mouth gag, or other device for placing between the teeth
6. Rubber examining gloves

Technique

1. Perform routine preparation procedures (page 321).
2. The tube is prepared by inserting the lubricated stylet and bending the tube into an "open J" configuration. The stylet should *not* protrude beyond the tip of the tube, but it should come to at least the side hole.
3. A water-soluble lubricant is used liberally on the tip and cuff of the tube.

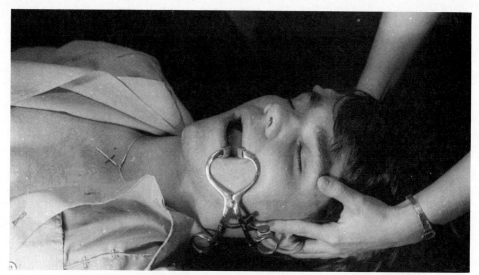

Figure S9C-1. DIGITAL INTUBATION—A: preparing patient with use of mouth (dental) prod to protect the intubator against being bitten.

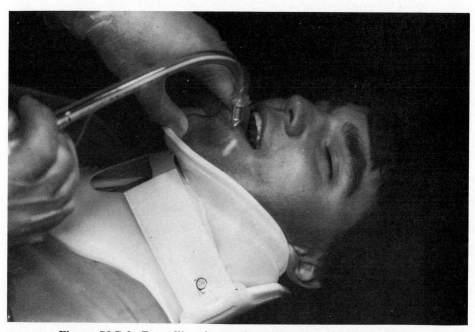

Figure S9C-2. B: pulling forward on the tongue and jaw lifts the epiglottis and allows for intubation with the stylet. The bend in the stylet must not be too far proximal so that it will not strike against the posterior pharyngeal wall. Note gloves are worn.

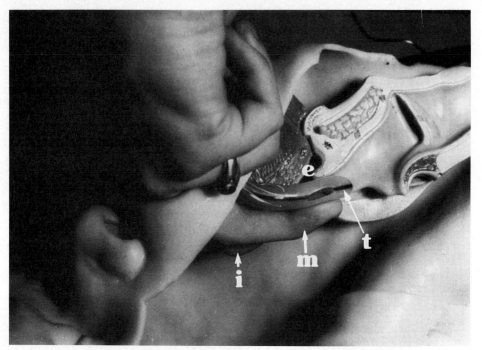

Figure S9C–3. B: the fingers are slid down the tongue and the tube guided towards the epiglottis (e) by the long (m) and index (i) fingers.

4. Gloves are used for protection.

5. The intubator kneels at the patient's left shoulder facing the patient and places a dental prod or mouth gag between the patient's molars (Figure S9C-1).

6. The intubator then "walks" the index and middle fingers of his left hand down the midline of the tongue, all the while pulling forward on the tongue and jaw. *This is a most important maneuver and serves to lift the epiglottis up within reach of the probing fingers (Figure S9C-2).*

7. The middle finger palpates the epiglottis; it feels much like the tragus of the ear.

8. The epiglottis is pressed forward and the tube is slipped into the mouth at the left labial angle anterior to the palpating fingers (Figure S9C-3). The index finger is used to keep the tube tip against the side of the middle finger (that is still palpating the epiglottis). This guides the tip to the epiglottis. The side hole of the tube can also be used as

a landmark to ensure that the intubator is always aware of the position of the tip of the endotracheal tube. *This is a crucial principle of this technique.*

9. The middle and index fingers guide the tube tip to lie against the epiglottis in front and the fingers behind. The right hand then advances the tube distally through the cords as the index and middle fingers of the left palpating hand press forward to prevent the tube from slipping posteriorward into the esophagus. (*Note:* At this point the tube–stylet combination may encounter resistance, especially if the distal curve of the tube is sharp. This usually means that the tube tip is impinging on the anterior wall of the thyroid or cricoid cartilage. Pulling back slightly on the stylet will allow the tube to conform to the anatomy, and the tube should slip distally.)

10. Confirm placement by the confirmation protocol (page 334).

Advanced Skill 9D: Transillumination (Lighted Stylet)

The transillumination or lighted stylet method of endotracheal intubation is based on the fact that a bright light inserted inside the upper airway can be seen through the soft tissues of the neck when inside the larynx or trachea. This permits the intubator to guide the tube tip through the glottic opening without directly visualizing the cords. This has been called the "indirect visual" method, and has been shown in several studies to be reliable, quick, and atraumatic. It is particularly attractive in trauma patients since it appears to move the head and neck less than do conventional orotracheal methods.

Equipment

1. *Stylet.* The lighted stylet (Figure S9D-1) is a malleable wire connecting a proximal battery housing to a distal light bulb, covered with a tough plastic coating that prevents the light from being separated from the wire. The wire stylet part is 25 cm in length. An on/off switch is located at the proximal end of the battery housing.

2. *Endotracheal tubes.* All tubes should be 7.5 to 8.5 mm in (internal diameter), and should be cut to 25 cm to accommodate the stylet. [*Note:* A longer (33-cm) stylet will soon be commercially available.]

3. Other equipment will be standard to any intubation procedure: suction, oxygen, gloves, lubricant, and so on.

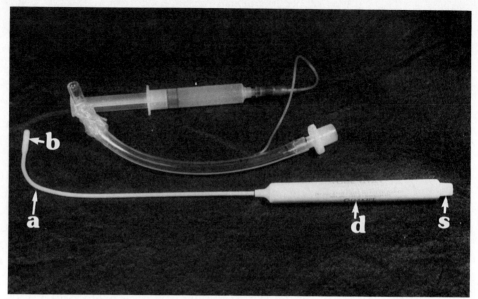

Figure S9D-1. THE LIGHTED STYLET: A: S- on/off switch; d—battery housing; a—diotal bend; b—bulb.

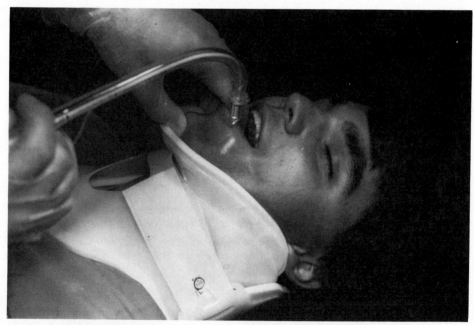

Figure S9D-2. B: pulling forward on the tongue and jaw lifts the epiglottis and allows for intubation with the stylet. The bend in the stylet must not be too far proximal so that it will not strike against the posterior pharyngeal wall. Note gloves are worn.

332

Technique

The success of this method of intubation will depend on several factors:

1. Level of ambient light
2. Pulling forward on the patient's tongue, or tongue and jaw
3. Bend of the stylet–tube

The light should be cut down to about 10% of normal, or the neck should be shielded from direct sun or bright daylight. While the transilluminated light can be perceived in thin patients even in daylight, success will be more likely the darker the surroundings.

Pulling forward on the tongue—or tongue and jaw—lifts the epiglottis up out of the way. This is *essential* to this method (Figure S9D-2).

The stylet–tube combination should be bent just proximal to the cuff—a bend that is too far proximal will cause the tube to strike against the posterior pharyngeal wall and prevent the tube from advancing anteriorly through the glottic opening (Figure S9D-2). The lubricated stylet is slipped into the tube and held firmly against the battery housing while the tube–stylet is bent. Bend more sharply if the patient is not in the sniffing position.

Procedure

1. Perform routine preparation procedures (page 321).
2. The intubator stands or kneels on either side facing the patient's head. Gloves are worn for the procedure. The light is turned on.
3. The patient's tongue—or more easily, the tongue and jaw—is grasped by the intubator and drawn gently forward while the liberally lubricated tube-stylet combination is slipped down the tongue.
4. Using a "soup ladle" motion, the epiglottis is "hooked" up to the tube-stylet and the transilluminated light can be seen in the midline. Correct placement at or beyond the cords is indicated by the appearance of a circumscribed, easily perceived light at the level of the laryngeal prominence (Figure S9D-3). A dull glow, diffuse and difficult to see, indicates esophageal placement.
5. When the light is seen, the stylet is held firmly in place and the fingers of the other hand support the tube lying along the tongue as they advance the tube off the stylet more distally into the larynx.
6. Confirm placement of the tube with the confirmation protocol (page 334).

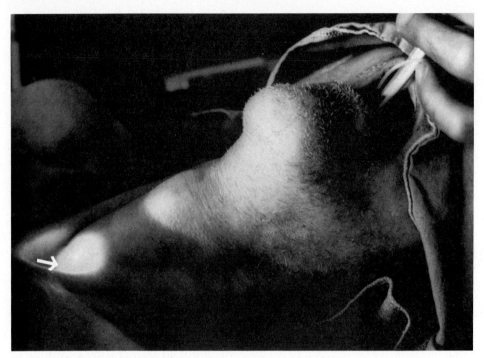

Figure S9D-3. B: Dim ambient lighting will assist in identifying the bright circumscribed glow of correct intratracheal placement.

Advanced Skill 9E: Confirmation of Tube Placement

One of the greatest challenges of intubation facing prehospital care providers is ensuring correct intratracheal placement of endotracheal tubes. An unrecognized esophageal intubation is a lethal complication of a lifesaving procedure, and is, even in the context of field care, inexcusable. Every effort must be made to avoid this catastrophe, and a strict protocol must be followed to reduce the risk.

Although the most reliable method of ensuring proper placement is actually visualizing the tube passing through the glottic opening, this is often a luxury that we cannot always count on in field care of the trauma patient. Visualization of the arytenoids is perhaps as much as we can expect, especially in a patient whose head and neck are immobilized and at risk if moved.

A simple, yet effective protocol for tube confirmation is possible and practical for the field setting. Such a protocol should recognize the unreliable nature of auscultation as a sole method of confirming intratracheal placement. Correct intratracheal placement should be suspected from the following signs:

1. An anteriorward displacement of the laryngeal prominence as the tube is passed distally.

2. Coughing, bucking, or straining on the part of the patient. [*Note: Phonation* (any noise made with the vocal cords) is *absolute evidence that the tube is in the esophagus and should be removed immediately.]*

3. Breath condensation on the tube with each ventilation—not 100% reliable, but very suggestive of intratracheal placement.

4. Normal compliance with bag ventilation. The bag does not suddenly "collapse," but rather, there is some resiliance to it and resistance to lung inflation.

5. No cuff leak after inflation—persistant leak indicates esophageal intubation until proven otherwise.

The following procedure should then be carried out to prove correct placement:

1. *Auscultation* of six sites:
   a. Right and left apex
   b. Right and left midaxillary lines
   c. The epigastrium—perhaps the most important; it should be silent, with no sounds heard
   d. The sternal notch—"tracheal" sounds should readily be heard here

2. *Palpation* of the chest wall to feel the ribs parting and the chest wall moving and gentle palpation of the tube cuff in the sternal notch while the pilot balloon is compressed between the index finger and thumb; a pressure wave should be felt in the pilot balloon.

3. *Inspection* for full movement of the chest with ventilation; watch for any change in the patient's color or in the ECG reading.

4. *Transillumination.* A flexible lighted stylet designed for nasotracheal intubation is available and can readily be passed distally after lubrication into the tube (Figure S9E-1). A bright glow first in the oropharynx, then at the laryngeal prominence (the light in the oropharynx disappears as the bulb passes the cords), is almost absolute evidence of intracheal placement (Figure S9E-2). It is essential that the ambient lighting be as low as possible for this procedure to be successful. Covering the neck to shield it from light will help. In the ambulance, the lights in the patient's compartment can be turned out.

The protocol for confirmation of tube placement should be applied following intubation only after several minutes of ventilation. Thereafter the pro-

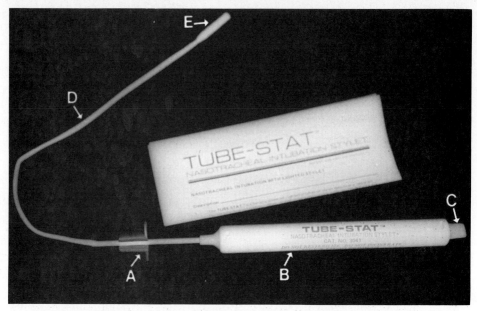

Figure S9E–1. A: The soft flexible stylet can be slipped distally into an in-place tube to prove intratracheal placement.
A—adapter; B—battery housing; C—on/off switch; E—bulb; D—soft wire stylet.

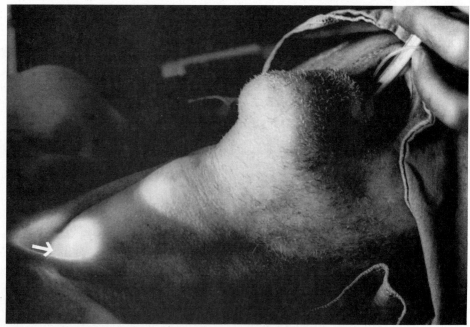

Figure S9E-2. Dim ambient lighting will assist in identifying the bright circumscribed glow of correct intratracheal placement.

tocol should be followed after movement of the patient from the floor to the stretcher, after loading into the ambulance, and immediately prior to arrival at the hospital. If at any time placement is in doubt, *visualize directly or remove the tube*. Never *assume* that the tube is in the right place—always be *sure* and *record* that the protocol has been followed carefully.

Advanced Skill 9F: Anchoring the Tube

Anchoring the tube can be a frustrating exercise. Not only does it require some fine movements of the hands when we appear to be all thumbs, but it is difficult to perform this task when ventilation, movement, or extrication is being carried out. There is one thing to keep in mind; there is no substitute for the human anchor. That is, one person should be held responsible for ensuring that the tube is held fast and that it does not migrate in or out of the airway. To lose a tube can be a catastrophe, especially if the patient is rather inaccessible or the intubation was a difficult one to begin with.

Fixing the endotracheal tube in place is important for several reasons. First, movement of the tube in the trachea will produce more mucosal damage and may increase the risk of post-intubation complications. In addition, movement of the tube will stimulate the patient to cough, strain, or both, leading to cardiovascular and intracranial pressure changes that could be detrimental. Most of all, there is a greater risk in the field of dislodging a tube and losing control of the airway if it is not anchored solidly in place.

The endotracheal tube can be secured in place either by tape or by a commercially available holder. Although taping a tube in place is convenient and relatively easily done, it is not always effective, since there is often a problem with the tape sticking to skin, which is often wet with rain, blood, airway secretions, or vomitus. If tape is to be used, several principles should be followed:

1. An oropharyngeal airway should also be in place to prevent the patient from biting down on the tube.
2. The patient's face should be dried off and tincture of benzoin applied to ensure proper adhesion of the tape.
3. The tape should be carried right around the patient's neck in anchoring the tube. The neck must not be moved.
4. The tube should be anchored at the labial angle, not in the midline.

Because of the difficulty of fixing the tube in place with tape, we prefer to use a commercial endotracheal tube holder that uses a small rubber strap to fix the tube in a plastic holder that acts as a bite block (Figure S9F-1).

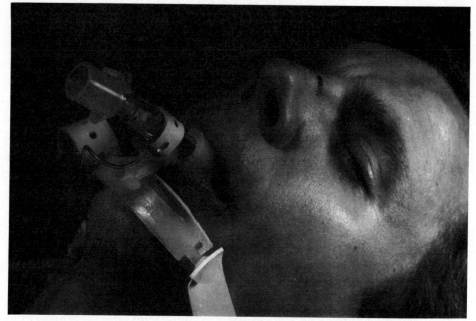

Figure S9F-1. A commercial endotracheal tube holder. Note the
two separate rubber straps holding the tube around the neck
and in a bite block.

A second rubber strap passes around the patient's neck. Although this is not
an ideal solution, it is easier to use and more quickly applied. If tube holders
with Velcro are used, care must be taken not to get the small hooks embedded
in the fingers or in the patient's lips.

Since flexion or extension of the patient's head can move the tube in or
out of the airway by 2 or 3 cm, it is a good practice to restrict head and neck
movement of any patient who has an endotracheal tube in place. If the patient is immobilized because of the risk of cervical spine injury, we need not
worry about this. However, in those who do not have a collar or other device
in place, we prefer to tape the head to the longboard or stretcher in order
to restrict movement. Failing this, the airway manager is required to ensure
that the head and neck are kept in a neutral position.

Advanced Skill 9G: Esophageal Gastric Tube Airway

Several essentials must be remembered about the use of the EGTA:

1. It is used only in patients who are unresponsive and without protec-
    tive reflexes.

2. It should *not* be used in patients with upper-airway or facial trauma, where bleeding into the oropharynx is a problem. It must *not* be used in any patient with injury to the esophagus (e.g., caustic ingestions) or in children who are below the age of 15 and are of average height and weight.

3. Adequate mask seal must be ensured; this means appropriate lifting forward of the jaw, with careful attention to keeping the neck immobile.

4. Great attention must be paid to proper placement. Unrecognized *intratracheal* placement is a lethal complication that produces complete airway obstruction. Such an occurrence is not always easy to detect, and the results are catastrophic. One of the great disadvantages of this airway is the fact that correct placement can be determined only by auscultation and observation of chest movement—both may be quite unreliable in a field setting.

5. Insertion must be gentle and without force.

6. The EGTA is not recommended *in place of* the endotracheal tube, but rather, can be used for patients in whom attempts at endotracheal intubation have been unsuccessful. Even in these, careful attempts at intubation should be continued despite the successful insertion of an EGTA.

7. The EGTA should not be removed from an unconscious patient without first inserting an endotracheal tube to protect the airway. Patients almost always vomit when the EGTA is removed.

Insertion

The airway is relatively easily inserted and must never be forced. In the supine patient the following procedure is followed:

1. Ventilation should be carried out with mouth-to-mask or bag–valve–mask, and suctioning performed prior to insertion of the airway.

2. After liberal lubrication, the airway, with mask attached, is slid into the oropharynx while the tongue and jaw are pulled forward.

3. The airway is advanced along the tongue and into the esophagus. Care should be taken to observe the neck. "Tenting" of the skin in the area of the pyriform fossae, or anterior displacement of the laryngeal prominence, indicates that misplacement has occurred. The airway should be repositioned by pulling back and reinserting.

4. Following gentle insertion (without force) so that the mask now rests easily on the face, the mask is sealed firmly on the face as the jaw is pulled forward to ensure a patent airway.

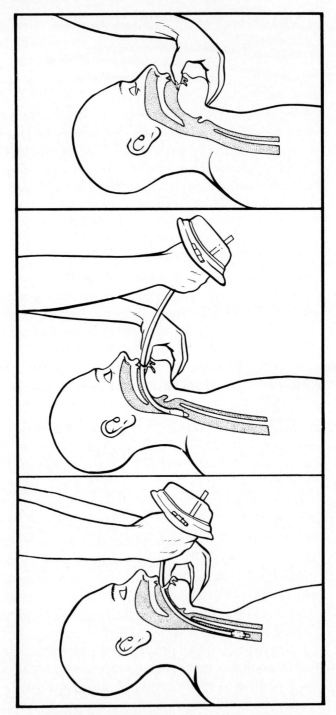

Figure S9G-1. Insertion of esophageal airway.

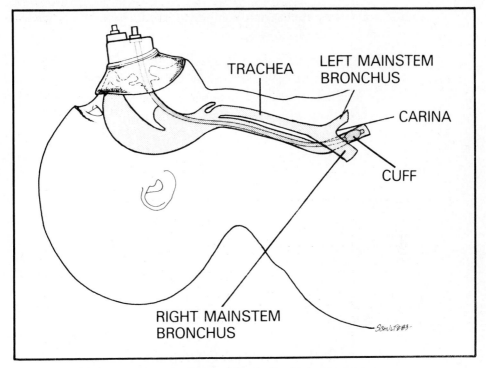

Figure S9G-2. Final position of EGTA.

5. Prior to inflating the cuff, ventilation is attempted with mouth-to-mask or a bag–valve device. If the chest is seen to rise, breath sounds are heard, and compliance appears good, the cuff of the airway is inflated with 35 cc of air.

6. Following inflation, the lung fields are auscultated again and the chest wall is felt as well as observed for movement. The epigastrium should not distend.

If there is any doubt about placement of the airway, remove it and reinsert.

Advanced Skill 9H: Translaryngeal Jet Ventilation

When access below the level of the cords is sought, translaryngeal jet ventilation (TLJV) provides a quick, reliable, and relatively safe method of adequate oxygenation and ventilation, especially in the trauma patient. Many misconceptions and erroneous impressions persist about this technique, and the medical literature is in a state of confusion on the subject. Clinical experience and studies done using appropriate equipment in both animals and patients would clearly indicate the following:

1. Patients can be both oxygenated and ventilated with this technique, which delivers 100% oxygen in volumes exceeding 1 L per second.
2. Ventilation can proceed indefinitely, provided that the correct-size cannula is used with the proper driving pressure.
3. Cannulae of 14 gauge or larger, with side holes, must be used.
4. Driving pressures of at least 50 psi (30 psi in a small child) must be used to deliver sufficient volumes to ensure adequate ventilation.

Patients cannot be ventilated using small-bore cannulae with continuous-flow oxygen attached; the principles listed above must be adhered to if this technique is to be used safely and effectively.

Equipment

The tools needed for TLJV should be prepared well in advance and stored in a small bag or kit:

1. *14- or 13-gauge cannula, with side holes.* These sizes are the *minimum* necessary for adequate ventilation. Side holes are especially important, since they prevent the cannula from remaining against the tracheal wall and subjecting it to sudden pressures that could rupture it. A cannula, recently designed especially for TLJV, has proven particularly useful in field practice (Figure S9H-1). This 13-gauge ventilating cannula, with side holes and a slight curve that allows for ease of insertion, has as a major feature an around-the-neck tie that fixes it in place very conveniently. A patently unattractive feature of this cannula is the 15-mm connector at the ventilating port, since its presence suggests that the patient could be ventilated through the cannula with demand valve or resuscitator bag. It is *absolutely impossible* to ventilate a patient using this technique; the developers of this cannula themselves recognize this.
2. *Manual jet ventilator device* (Figure S9H-2). These are commercially available and are merely valves that allow high-pressure oxygen to flow through them when a button is depressed. They should have high-pressure tubing attached solidly with special fasteners and tape.
3. *Wrench.* A small wrench should be *attached* to the jet ventilator tubing so that no time will be lost looking for a way to tap into the oxygen tank, or turn it on.

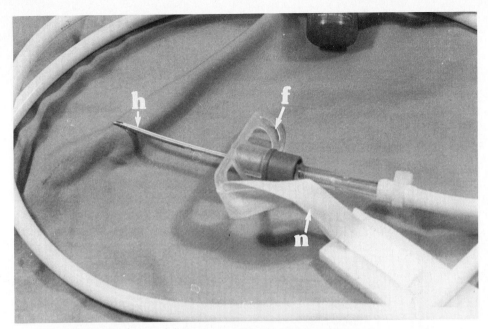

Figure S9H-1. A specially—designed 13 G cannula for translaryngeal jet ventilation. Note side-holes (n), flange (f), and neck strap (n). This is hooked into a 50 psi oxygen source for adequate ventilation and oxygenation.

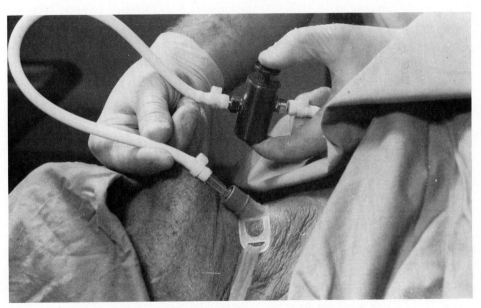

Figure S9H-2. Patient is ventilated indefinitely with 1 to 1.5 second bursts of oxygen from a 50 psi source at a rate of 15-20/min.

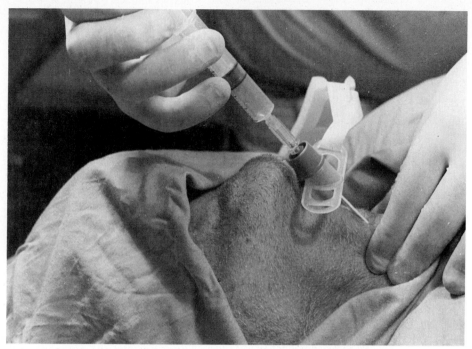

Figure S9H-3. Puncture of cricothyroid membrane with jet ventilator cannula. Note syringe in place filled with saline—bubbles on aspiration indicate correct intratracheal placement.

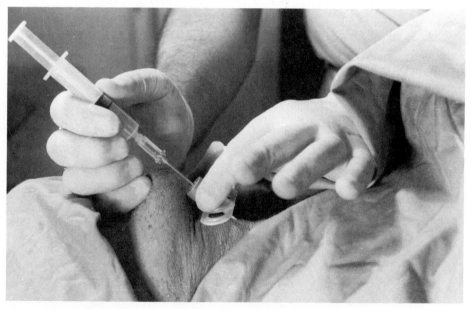

Figure S9H-4. Cannula is slid distally off the needle when membrane is punctured.

Technique

Identification of the cricothyroid membrane is essential to this technique, although placement between the tracheal rings would probably not result in major complications.

1. With continued attempts at ventilation and oxygenation, the cricothyroid membrane is punctured by the cannula firmly attached to a 5-cc syringe filled with 1 to 2 cc of saline (Figure S9H-3). (*Note:* Several cubic centimeters of 2% lidocaine can be used instead of saline, to produce local anesthesia of the mucosa in the area of the distal port of the cannula.

2. The cannula is directed downward, with continual aspiration to demonstrate prompt entry into the larynx, identified when bubbles of air are readily aspirated. At this point, if lidocaine is contained in the syringe, it can be injected to provide some anesthesia and prevent the coughing that sometime occurs in those patients who are somewhat responsive.

3. On entry into the larynx, the cannula is slid off the needle trochar and is held in place while the TLJV is connected to the proximal port of the cannula (Figure S9H-4).

4. The patient is immediately ventilated using 1-second bursts of oxygen from the 50-psi manual source. The rate used is at least 20 per minute (i.e., an inspiratory/expiratory ratio of 1:2; Figure S9H-2).

5. If a tie is available, the cannula is fixed in place. Tape can also be used, but it must be fastened firmly to the cannula and then around the patient's neck. Firm pressure at the site of insertion can reduce the small amount of subcutaneous emphysema that usually occurs with this technique.

─Advanced Skill Station 10─

Chest Decompression

Objectives

The objectives for this skill station are as follows:

1. To learn the indications for emergency decompression of a tension pneumothorax
2. To learn the technique of needle decompression of a tension pneumothorax
3. To learn the complications of needle decompression of a tension pneumothorax

Indications

As with all advanced procedures, this technique must be accepted local protocol and you must obtain medical control permission before performing it. The conservative management of tension pneumothorax is oxygen, ventilatory assistance, and rapid transport. The indication for performing emergency field decompression is the presence of a tension pneumothorax and any one of the following:

1. Respiratory distress and cyanosis
2. Loss of the radial pulse
3. Loss of consciousness

Complications

1. Laceration of intercostal vessel with resultant hemorrhage. The inter-costal artery and vein run around the inferior margin of each rib. Poor needle placement can lacerate one of these vessels.
2. Creation of a pneumothorax if not already present. If your assessment was not correct, you may give the patient a pneumothorax when you insert the needle into the chest.
3. Laceration of the lung. Poor technique or inappropriate insertion (no pneumothorax present) can cause laceration of the lung, causing bleeding and more air leak.
4. Infection. Adequate skin preparation with an antiseptic will usually prevent this.

Procedure

1. Assess the patient to make sure that his condition is due to a tension pneumothorax:
    a. Poor ventilation despite an open airway
    b. Neck vein distention (may not be present if there is associated severe hemorrhage)
    c. Tracheal deviation away from the side of the injury (may not always be present)
    d. Absent or decreased breath sounds on the affected side
    e. Tympany (hyperresonance) to percussion on the affected side
    f. Shock
2. Give the patient high-flow oxygen and ventilatory assistance.
3. Determine that one of the indications for emergency decompression is present; then obtain medical control's permission to perform the procedure.
4. Identify the fourth or fifth intercostal space in the midaxillary line (the nipple is usually over the fifth rib) on the same side as the pneumothorax.*

*An alternate site is the second intercostal space in the midclavicular line.

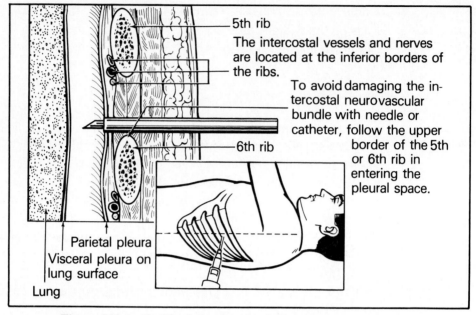

5th rib

The intercostal vessels and nerves are located at the inferior borders of the ribs.

To avoid damaging the intercostal neurovascular bundle with needle or catheter, follow the upper border of the 5th or 6th rib in entering the pleural space.

6th rib

Parietal pleura
Visceral pleura on lung surface
Lung

Figure S10-1. Needle decompression of tension pneumothorax.

5. Quickly prepare the area with a Betadine swab.

6. Make a one-way valve by inserting a 13- or 14-gauge over-the-needle catheter through a condom (the finger of a rubber glove will not work).

7. Insert the catheter into the skin over the fifth or sixth rib and direct it just over the top of the rib (superior border) into the interspace (Figure S10-1).

8. Insert the catheter through the parietal pleura until air escapes. It should exit under pressure.

9. Remove the needle and leave the plastic catheter in place until it is replaced by a chest tube at the hospital.

Advanced Skill Station 11

Fluid Resuscitation

It is expected that all students of this course are familiar with the technique of inserting an intravenous cannula in the veins of the lower arm or antecubital space, so only other sites will be discussed here.

Advanced Skill 11A: Cannulation of the External Jugular Vein

Objective

The objective of this skill station is to learn the technique of cannulation of the external jugular vein.

Indication

The pediatric or adult patient who needs IV access and in whom no suitable peripheral vein is found.

Surface Anatomy

The external jugular vein runs in a line from the angle of the jaw to the junction of the medial and middle third of the clavicle. This vein is usually easily

349

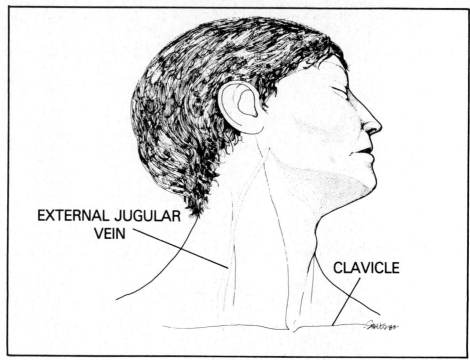

Figure S11-1

visible through the skin and can be made more prominent by pressing on it just above the clavicle. It runs into the subclavian vein.

Procedure

1. The patient must be in the supine position, preferably head down, to distend the vein and prevent air embolism.

2. If there is no danger of cervical spine injury, you should turn the patient's head to the opposite side. If there is a danger of cervical spine injury, the head must not be turned but rather, must be stabilized by one rescuer while the IV is started.

3. Quickly prepare the skin with an antiseptic and then align the cannula with the vein. The needle will be pointing at the clavicle at about the junction of the middle and medial thirds.

4. With one finger, press on the vein just above the clavicle. This should make the vein more prominent.

5. Insert the needle into the vein at about the midportion and cannulate in the usual way.

6. If it was not done already, draw a 30-cc sample of blood and store it in red and purple stoppered tubes.
7. Tape down the line securely. If there is a danger of a cervical spine injury, a cervical collar can be applied over the IV site.

Advanced Skill 11B: Intraosseous Infusion

Objectives

The objectives of this skill station are as follows:

1. To learn the indications for the use of intraosseous infusion
2. To learn the proper techniques for performing intraosseous infusion

Discussion

The technique of bone marrow infusion of fluid and drugs is not new. It was first described in 1922 and was used commonly in the 1930s and 1940s as an alternative to intravenous infusion of crystalloids, drugs, and blood. The technique was recently "rediscovered" and studies have confirmed that it is a fast, safe, and effective route to infuse medications, fluids, and blood. Because the flow is not as rapid as peripheral venous infusions, it is limited to volume resuscitations of children. Intraoseous infusion has the advantage of being quick and simple to perform while providing a stable (anchored in bone) access that is not easily dislodged during transport.

Indications

1. A pediatric or adult patient who is in cardiac arrest and in whom you cannot quickly obtain peripheral venous access
2. Hypovolemic pediatric patients who have a prolonged transport and in whom you are unable to quickly obtain peripheral venous access

Procedure

1. Determine the need for this procedure and obtain permission from medical control.
2. Have all IV equipment ready prior to bone penetration.

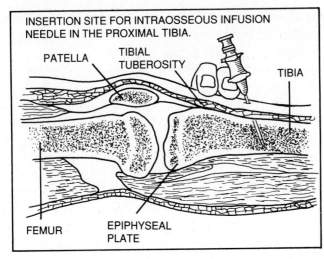

Figure S11B-1

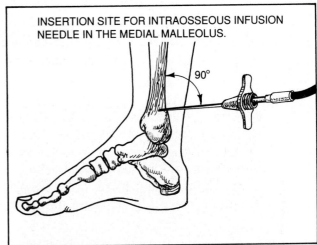

Figure S11B-2

3. Select the site (the preferred site will depend on local protocol):
   a. *Proximal tibia:* one fingersbreath below the tibial tuberosity either midline or slightly lateral to the midline (Figure S11B-1).
   b. *Distal tibia:* midline just above the medial malleolus (Figure S11B-2).
4. Prep the skin with Betadine.
5. Obtain the proper needle. The needle must have a stylet to prevent becoming plugged with bone. While 13-, 18-, and 20-gauge spinal needles will work, they are difficult and uncomfortable to grip during the insertion process. Long spinal needles tend to bend easily, so if you use spinal needles; try to obtain the short ones. The preferred needle is

a 14 to 18-gauge bone marrow needle. The 13 gauge needle can break a bone in a small child so use a smaller needle with smaller patients.

6. Insert the needle into the bone marrow cavity.

    a. Tibial technique. Place sand bags or rolled towels under the knee. Insert the needle perpendicular to the skin directed away from the epiphyseal plate, and advance to the periosteum. The bone is penetrated with a slow boring or twisting motion until you feel a sudden "give" (decrease in resistance) as the needle enters the marrow cavity. This can be confirmed by removing the stylet and aspirating blood and bone marrow.

    b. Medial malleolus technique. Insert the needle at a 90° angle to the bone using a slow boring or twisting motion until you feel a sudden "give" (decrease in resistance) as the needle enters the marrow cavity. This can be confirmed by removing the stylet and aspirating blood and bone marrow.

7. Attach standard IV tubing and infuse fluid and/or medications.

8. Tape the tubing to the skin and secure the bone marrow needles as if to secure an impaled object (4 × 4's taped around insertion site).

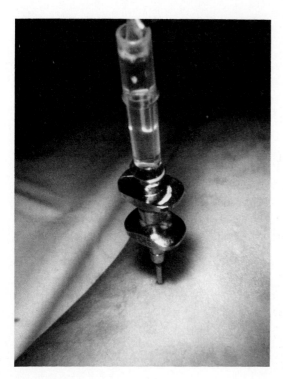

Figure S11B-3 An intraosseous needle in a child's proximal tibia being used for intravenous access.

Important Points

1. As with all advanced procedures, this technique must be accepted local protocol and you must obtain medical control permission before performing.

2. If infiltration occurs (rare), do not reuse the same bone. Another site must be selected, as fluid will leak out of the original hole made in the bone.

3. Never place an intraosseous line in a fractured extremity. If the femur is fractured, use the opposite leg.

4. Potential complications:
   a. Subperiosteal infusion due to improper placement
   b. Osteomyelitis
   c. Sepsis
   d. Fat embolism
   e. Marrow damage

   Studies have proven all of these complications to be rare; however, good aseptic technique is important, just as with intravenous therapy.

Appendix A

Radio Communications

Corey M. Slovis, M.D., F.A.C.P., F.A.C.E.P.

It is imperative that the EMT/paramedic provide his or her hospital base station physician with an accurate, succinct, on-the-scene assessment. This can be very difficult, as there are potentially thousands of bits of information that could be relayed. In the field EMS personal do not have the luxury of giving a long and complete history and physical to the physician at the other end of the radio. The purpose of radio communication is not to give all available information to the medical control physician but to transmit only the information needed for appropriate care. Due to his responsibilities to patients already in the emergency department, the physician receiving the call would like to spend a minimum of time on the radio.

When speaking over the radio, no matter how emergent the situation, the EMT should speak clearly and avoid speaking rapidly in an emotional, high-pitched voice. However, using a slow monotone voice in reporting a cardiac arrest would be inappropriate as well. The EMT/paramedic should try to convey the urgency of the situation in a professional manner. The radio microphone should be held a few inches from the mouth to allow accurate voice transmission but not so far (greater than 6 inches) as to allow interference from other noises at the scene.

The following format for communications is designed to maximize the efficient transfer of information. It may also be used for calls not involving trauma.

355

Four-Phase Communication Policy

The BTLS communications policy is divided into four parts. The first of these phases is devoted to the EMS unit confirming radio contact with a specific hospital or base station.

Phase 1: Contact Phase

Step 1—Identification: In attempting to establish radio contact, the EMT/paramedic should state what EMS service is calling, the unit's level of function (i.e., basic, paramedic, etc.), and the unit's identification number: for example, "This is "County Advanced Unit 501 calling County Hospital." It is important for the unit to identify its level of function so that the physician knows which procedures and medications to consider. The EMS service should be identified, because different services operating in the same area may function with different protocols. The EMS unit's own identification number needs to be included for later contacting and tape audit purposes. As different hospitals may have the same radio frequency, the specific facility being called should be stated each time contact is initiated.

Step 2—Facility Response: The base station or receiving hospital should now respond by identifying the facility, which person is on the radio, and to what EMS unit they are responding. An example might be: "This is Dr. Thomas Smith at County Hospital. Go ahead County Advanced Unit 501." By restating the EMS unit's service and number, confusion will be minimized when multiple units are involved with a single receiving facility. It is recommended that the hospital-based radio operator identify himself. This is important because often the initial response is not by a physician. It is just as important that the physician identify himself or herself so that an EMS unit may record who is giving them orders.

Phase II: In-the-Field Report

The second phase of communications is the most important. Here the EMT/paramedic should give all important primary survey information and request appropriate orders. This phase of communications is divided into the six steps listed below.

Step 3—Re-identification: Once contact has been confirmed, the in-the-field report begins by the EMT/paramedic reidentifying his EMS service its level of function and unit number. This information may not yet have been recorded or even heard by the physician who has probably just arrived at the radio console.

Step 4—Chief Complaint/On-scene Report: After the EMT has identified his level of function and unit number, the next sentence should provide the physician with the most complete picture of the patient possible. This sentence should include the patient's approximate age, sex, complaint, and/or mechanism of injury. Having information such as the victim's approximate age and sex allows the physician to get a mental picture of the patient. Similarly, by knowing the chief complaint and/or type of injury, the physician has an idea of the type of emergency call with which he or she is now involved. An example of this part of the communication might be: "We are on the scene with a 23 YO female who has a gunshot wound to the chest" or "We are at the scene where a 78 YO male involved in an MVA is now complaining of chest pain." The patient's medications, additional complaints, or more complete description of injuries should not be given at this time.

Step 5—Lifesaving Resuscitation: If any emergency maneuvers or lifesaving therapy has been performed during the primary survey, it should be reported next. Thus, if an airway maneuver has been performed or CPR started, it should be reported at this point. Examples of this include: "The patient's sucking chest wound has been sealed" or "We have begun CPR and defibrillated the patient." Results of a fingerstick glucose, if already performed on a comatose patient, should be reported during this phase.

Step 6—Vital Signs/Primary Survey Abnormalities: In the next sentence, the EMT should give vital signs and/or primary survey abnormalities. In stable patients with a normal primary survey, a complete set of vital signs are blood pressure, pulse, respiratory rate, and skin temperature (if pertinent). A typical communication might be "The patient has a normal primary survey with vital signs of blood pressure 130/90, pulse 90, respiration 16." If, however, there is an abnormal primary survey, a full set of vital signs would not be reported. In this type of unstable patient, problems with airway, breathing, cardiovascular stability, and screening neurologic exam would be reported to the physician. In this so-called "load and go" type of call, no additional physical findings, historical facts, or medication usage would be reported at this time. A typical communication would be: "Primary survey as follows: no palpable pulses present, respiration are 40; chest exam reveals a sucking chest wound; patient is confused and combative."

Step 7—Estimated Time of Arrival (ETA):   The EMT/paramedic should now state how much time it will take to get to the hospital from the present location. If they are en route, this should be reported. If however, significant additional time is required to extricate or load the patient into the EMS vehicle, this should be specifically stated. Examples of the ETA phase of communication include: "We are en route to your location, our ETA is less than

4 minutes" or "We are still on the scene and will require 10 to 15 minutes before we begin transport to the hospital."

Step 8—Request for Orders: Prior to relinquishing radio control to the base station, the EMT should state what orders are desired, that no orders are desired, or that he or she is requesting the base station physician's help in determining what to do for their patient. Examples of these respective situations include: "Requesting MAST trousers legs only and two large-bore IVs of lactated ringers wide open" or "No orders requested" or "Base station, how do you advise?"

Phase III: Base-Station-Controlled Activity

In this phase of communication the EMT is no longer in charge of the radio. He or she should now respond to the physician's approval or denial of orders. In other cases there may be talk back and forth between the physician and EMT/paramedic.

Step 9—Physician's Response: It is now up to the physician to determine how to proceed with management of the patient. The physician may merely agree with your request by stating, "Go ahead with your requested therapy" or might completely disagree: "Orders denied, transport the patient as soon as possible." In complicated patients, the physician may need more information than you have transmitted. This is *not* a criticism of the EMT's radio abilities, but merely a need for the physician to obtain additional information. For example, "Are the patient's neck veins up or down?" or "Does the patient seem to improve in Trendelenberg position?" EMTs should be prepared to answer routine questions readily and to perform requested maneuvers.

Step 10—EMT Response: The EMT should confirm any given orders by repeating them. If the base station has given orders that are either incomplete or with which the EMT disagrees, it is now appropriate for the EMT to give additional history or rerequest an order. Examples of these problems include: "Be advised the patient has a long cardiac history and is on multiple medications" or "Base station, did you copy that the patient is hypotensive and that we are requesting an IV of lactated ringers and inflation of MAST trousers?" If the questions cannot be answered by the EMT, the physician should be told. Examples of this type of exchange would be, "We don't have any available information on downtime" or "We are unable to attempt this, the patient is still trapped inside the vehicle."

Table A-1 *BTLS Communications Format*

Phase I: Establishing Contact
  1. Initiation of call
     EMS service
     Level of function (basic, paramedic, etc.)
     Unit number
     Medical control facility being contacted
  2. Receiving facility response
     Name of facility
     Name and title of radio operator
     Renaming of calling EMS service

Phase II: In-the-Field Report
  3. Re-identification
     EMS service
     Level of function (basic, paramedic, etc.)
     Unit number
  4. Chief complaint/on-scene report
     One brief sentence
     Includes age, sex, complaint, and/or mechanism of injury
  5. Lifesaving resuscitation
     Patients response to lifesaving maneuvers
  6. Vital signs/primary survey abnormalities
     Vital signs in stable patient
     or
     Primary survey in unstable patient
  7. ETA
     State ETA
  8. Request for orders
     State what is desired
     or
     State "no orders desired"

Phase III: Hospital-Controlled Activity
  9. Physician response
     Agree or deny or state desired orders
     Request for additional history and/or information
  10. EMT response
     Clarification or response to requested maneuver or therapy

Phase IV: Sign-Off
  11. EMS unit sign-off
  12. Base station sign-off

Phase IV: Sign-Off

The final phase of EMS–base station communications is the sign-off. The EMT should make it very clear that the unit is leaving the medical frequency and returning to a dispatch frequency.

Step 11—EMS Unit Sign-Off: The EMT should now advise the base station that it is ending communications. Although each EMT seems to favor a different phrase to end with, each EMS service should agree on a common sign-off phrase. The use of a time signal at the end of a comment is recommended but is optional. Acceptable closings include "Advanced Unit 501 is clear" or "Unit 501 is out at 13:59 hours."

Services should avoid using code numbers, as many physicians may not understand them or may use similar codes for different purposes; thus "Unit 501 is 10-8 your location code 3" is not recommended, nor is "501, 10-8, 1359."

Step 12—Base Station Closing: The base station physician should similarly end his communication with the same agreed upon phrase: for example, "County Hospital clear."

Summary

This chapter is designed to facilitate rapid accurate communications between EMS units and their base stations. A copy of Table A-1 should be kept by the EMS radio in the hospital. EMTs should try to concentrate on transmitting the most information with the least amount of words.

Appendix B

Documentation: The Written Run Report

Arlo F. Weltge, M.D., F.A.C.E.P.

With the recognition of the important and increasing role of the EMT-P in the prehospital setting has come deserved respect. However, with this recognition comes the expectation of a standard of care and resultant liability when the care does not meet that standard.

In this chapter we address the tool that chronicles the medical care, communicates medical information, and provides a permanent record that can be used as evidence that the standard of care was delivered. That tool is the written documentation in the medical record.

The Written Report

The EMS system run report can vary dramatically from primarily a billing form to an excellent narrative medical record. In most EMS systems the run report will usually provide enough space for medical documentation to be adequate for the majority of transports, since most runs do not require much more than a simple transport.

It is important to use the system run report effectively. There should be enough space for a chief complaint, simple history and assessment, and space for other comments. All run reports should be filled out completely. Even though the transport may have been "simple," failure to document vital signs, complete check-off boxes for the history and physical, and enter times, events, and other "simple" information may reflect poorly on the care delivered if the report is ever reviewed.

If the system report does not provide adequate space for a reasonable history and assessment, or if the case is more difficult, for example, requiring intervention, long transport times, or involving potential patient complications, it may be necessary to include a continuation sheet. The continuation sheet can be a simple form. It does require some basic identification, including the patient's name, date, identification of the EMS system, and the run identification number. The report should be written at or near the time of the run, and the original must be signed and kept as a regular part of the system's medical records and attached to the regular run report. A simple form is shown in Figure B–1.

A simple continuation sheet allows it to be used for almost any situation or problem. The written, or narrative report, using the continuation sheet, requires much more effort, however, since there are not a host of "fill-in-the-blank" or "check-off" boxes when writing the report. To document a complex case adequately using the continuation sheet, one needs to be familiar with the general form or sequence of a written narrative report. The form is dictated by convention (or otherwise known as a generally agreed-upon habit or standard in the medical community). Effective documentation requires using this convention, as well as skill and practice to yield a useful record.

The written report should be brief, yet like the verbal report, relevant and focused. There are times when the clinical problem is confusing and the report must be more lengthy, but length does not necessarily reflect accuracy or relevancy.

The report should document relevant events and discrepancies, and should be written so that another reader can reconstruct the events. The report should also justify the action, even if one's impression at the time was wrong. A "mistake" may have been entirely justified given the circumstances at the time, but that mistake can be justified only if the circumstances are clearly and honestly documented as part of the record.

The report contains the following information, but rarely will include all the information. In fact, it is more important to treat the patient effectively and document that treatment than to get all the information while the patient suffers because of lack of treatment or delay in transport. It is reasonable to take brief notes and fill out the run report at the hospital before returning to service. Taking care of the patient is the first goal.

1. Run Call: One should note how the call was dispatched, particularly if there is a discrepancy between the dispatch description and the actual find-

THIS MUST BE ATTACHED TO CORRESPONDING EMS REPORT

DATE _____   HO NO: _____

NAME _____

ATTENDANT: _____

EMT REPORT:	TIME	B.P.	PULSE	RESP. RATE	TEMP.

SIGNATURE
X

EMS CONTINUATION

P & S AMBULANCE TEXAS, INC.
7849 ALMEDA
HOUSTON, TEXAS 77054

WHITE—FINANCE, CANARY—HOSPITAL, PINK—SUPERVISOR

Figure B-1.   Example of a Continuation Sheet.

ings. It is helpful, for example, to explain delays in transport if a call came in as a sick party when actually it was a motor vehicle accident with multiple victims. Time should be documented whenever possible, but the dispatch time is important because realistically it may be the last documented time until arriving at the hospital.

2. Scene Description: One should document any scene hazards that delay or affect patient treatment or transport. It is easy to forget some hazards, but delays may affect patient outcomes, and the mention of scene hazards may help jog the memory of the run when reading the report at a later time.

The mechanisms should be noted as well, and often most effectively by stick figures (see Figure B–2). The EMT is often the only source of the mechanism of injury for subsequent treatment providers. Clear simple drawings of mechanisms are quick and easy, useful for communicating mechanism and suspicion of occult injuries, and can help jog the memory of the event at a later time.

3. Chief Complaint: Record age, sex, mechanism, chief complaint or injury, and time. These identifiers focus the thought process. If mentioned previously, the mechanism does not have to be documented here.

4. History of the Present Illness/Injury or Symptoms: Record relevant positives and negatives. If the patient is talking, any relevant history should be documented. If the history does not come from the patient but from another witness, it is important to note clearly the source and the specific information from that person, especially when it conflicts with other history.

Additional useful information includes the patient's recollection of the events immediately prior to the accident (e.g., did the patient faint first and then

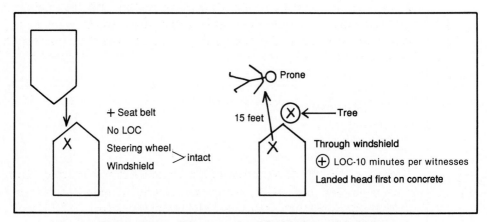

Figure B–2.   Diagrams for Mechanism of Injuries.

fall?), prior injuries to the same location (e.g., fractured the same leg last year), and any treatment prior to your arrival (e.g., patient pulled from car by bystanders).

5. Past Medical History: Record previous illness, medications, recent surgery, and allergies. The EMT is usually not responsible for getting a complete medical history. However, in acutely sick and injured victims, the EMT may be the last person able to get this information before the patient loses consciousness. Again, treating the patient is the most important priority, but a little bit of useful information may save a lot of complications. The priorities include current or chronic illnesses, current regular medications, any recent or major surgery, and allergies.

Other information that can be useful may include the last meal (if the patient may need surgery) and relevent family history (any relevant diseases that run in the family) and social history (use of alcohol or other drugs) may also be included in this section.

If the time is available, this can be documented as the *ample* history:

A   allergies
M   medications
P   past medical history (other illnesses)
L   last meal
E   events preceding accident

6. Physical Exam: Record appearance, vital signs, level of consciousness, primary survey, and secondary survey. A general statement of the appearance helps focus the reader on urgencies (e.g., the patient appeared alert and in no distress, or appeared in extreme pain and was ashen and short of breath). The level of consciousness should be documented with the vital signs. This is best done using stimulus and response (responds to voice/pain with moan, decerebrate posturing). The best method is to note the stimulus that provokes a response or the AVPU method:

A   alert
V   responds to verbal stimuli
P   responds to pain
U   unresponsive

The exam should document that a complete exam was done. Simply stating the body part (back, abdomen, upper extremity) with a zero or slash afterward can be used to indicate that the part was examined and there were no significant findings.

One of the easiest and best way to document the exam in a seriously injured patient is to note the findings and procedures sequentially as one did the primary and secondary survey. It can be helpful to write "Primary Survey:", note findings, describe the resuscitation, then start the rest of the exam with "Secondary Survey:". By doing this, anyone reviewing the record should immediately recognize the paramedic as being oriented to trauma assessment, and by assumption, as having performed an organized primary survey.

One picture is worth a thousand words and may aid the memory at a later date. Diagrams of injuries for locations or for severity (like cuts) should be simple, yet contain enough detail to locate site of injury, that is, identify if it right or left, volar (palmar) or dorsal part of an extremity, front or back trunk (see Figure B-3).

7. Procedures (Indication, Procedure, Result): All invasive procedures should have documented need, description of the procedure, ideally with time, and response to the procedure. Any procedure potentially can have a harmful effect, sometimes delayed, so all procedures should be documented (e.g., stating that an IV was started in the right forearm on the second stick protects you from charges of improper technique when the patient later develops a thrombophlebitis from an IV in the left arm). It may not be possible to document every IV attempt; however, invasive treatment procedures such as needle decompressions and needle cricothyroidotomies should document the need, the confirming evidence, the procedure, and the effect—even if the effect is a negative result.

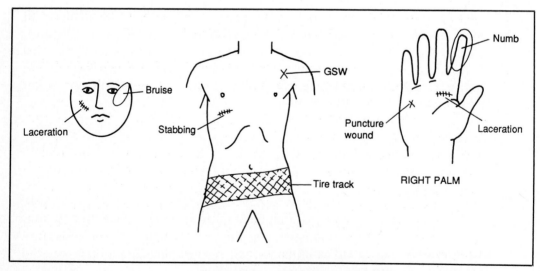

Figure B-3.   Diagrams of Injuries.

EXAMPLE: Properly Documented Field Procedure "Patient was pale, short of breath, lost the radial pulse (hypotensive), and had decreased breath sounds on right side (the suspicion). The right chest was tympanic and the trachea was deviated to the left, but neck veins were not distended (confirming findings present or absent). A 14-gauge needle was inserted over the top of the fifth rib in the midaxillary line with a rush of air. The patient's radial pulse returned and color improved, but respirations were still labored."

8. Monitoring (Recheck, Changes, Condition on Arrival): Documenting the initial findings establishes a baseline, but reevaluations during long transports, changes while the patient is still in your care, and condition on or just prior to arrival should be written as necessary to establish that decompensation did not occur while in your care. It is important to remember that as soon as the patient arrives, other people will perform an exam and record their findings. Any discrepancies or findings documented in their report will be presumed to have occurred while in your care unless documented by you as having existed prior to your intervention. The burden for documentation is then on the paramedic to show that complications did not occur while in transport but at the scene prior to one's arrival.

9. Impression: May be included to summarize the significant findings. However, care must be taken not to overdiagnose. A tender forearm does not necessarily mean fracture any more than shortness of breath must mean a tension pneumothorax. Impressions should be as "generic" as possible, noting the actual finding, such as pain or bruising (not the diagnosis, such as fracture or "pulmonary contusion") and include relevant information such as distal pulse. Suspicions should be noted as such:

Shortness of breath, decreased breath sounds on right, and tender right chest
Tender right forearm, possible fracture, sensation/pulse intact

10. Documenting the Priorities: The detailed description is designed for the occasion when events allow time for gathering of the information and completion of the secondary survey. There are times when urgent priorities limit the evaluation to treating the immediate complications, and the exam never gets past the primary survey. Taking care of the patient is the first priority. Often the best way to document this is to describe the sequence as it occurs, using the primary and secondary surveys.

EXAMPLE: Documenting the Priorities (Just the Facts)
Call: single MVA

Scene: one victim in roadway, car head-on into pole, patient through windshield supine in roadway

Diagram (see Figure B–2)

Primary assessment: mid-20s unresponsive male, ashen, grunting respiration with contusions to face, neck, and anterior chest. Rapid, thready carotid pulse, absent radial pulse, sucking wound right chest. C-spine controlled manually, no change in respiration with jaw thrust, chest wound covered.

Patient log-rolled onto long board, no obvious back injuries. Loaded and transported.

En route: patient's right pupil fixed and dilated, left midposition. Respirations remained rapid and shallow. Patient given oxygen and hyperventilated by B-V-M. One 14-gauge IV RL right anticub started, arrived at city hospital in 3 minutes, patient still with rapid thready carotid pulse.

Summary of the Narrative Report

1. Run call
2. Scene description
3. Chief complaint
4. History
5. Past medical history
6. Physical exam
7. Procedures
8. Monitoring
9. Impression

Improving Documentation Skills

Documentation reflects on the quality of clinical practice. Like clinical care, one can improve skills by practice, as well as by observing the better qualities of others. Some of the following are suggestions to help improve the quality of documentation.

Practice documentation with critique. Have somebody else try and reconstruct the events based on your narrative and evaluate what comments were useful and what comments were left out. Sometimes the most obvious events are the easiest to forget to document.

Read others' narrative reports and try to reconstruct the events.

Practice anticipating problems and criticisms. A fractured bone needs to have distal pulse and sensation checked and documented. Invasive procedures, complications, unusual events, or anticipated patient complaints can be noted and justification written. Many complications of invasive procedures, such as infections, may not be discovered for days or weeks. Anticipation of these delayed complications can be an important part of the documentation process.

Write to remind yourself. If there are specific events unique to this run, or which will help you distinguish this run from other similar runs, note it in the record.

Be professional. People's lives depend on your care. Your records should reflect that you take your responsibility seriously. The medical record is not a place for humorous or derogatory comments. Use caution when describing the patient. Do not use words that could indicate that your care was prejudiced by the patient's presentation. Words like "the patient was hysterical" would be better written as "the patient was very excited and upset."

Be concise. Longer is not necessarily better. If it is of interest, write it down, but get to the point and write what is important.

Review your own records. Can you reconstruct the events, and were complications anticipated? Would this record be a friend in court?

Practice good-quality care, including caring for the patient. A patient is a potential adversary or advocate. The excitement of the minute often results in a brusque attitude. Ask yourself if you would have been happy with the way you were treated had you been the patient.

Important Points about the Narrative Report: The run sheet with attached narrative report should be kept as a regular part of the patient's record and be considered a legal document. There are some basic rules to follow:

1. Keep the report legible.
2. If there are blanks, fill them in. Empty boxes imply that the question was not asked. Open spaces leave the implication that information might be added after the fact.
3. Never alter a medical record. If there is an error on the record, draw a single line through the error and make a note that it was an error, and why.
4. The record should be written in a timely manner. Events fade and memory can be challenged. Write the chart as soon as possible after the event. If there is some delay, note the reason.
5. Always be honest on the chart. Never record observations not made. Never try to cover up actions. (We can't always be right, but we must always be honest.) The record, your primary source of support, may be discredited if any of your observations are shown not to be accurate.

CALL: Injured party 10:15 AM

SCENE: Auto-pedestrian   Diagram:
    Single patient knocked down (not thrown
any distance) and pulled from the street prior
to arrival by bystanders. Patient laying on
sidewalk on arrival.

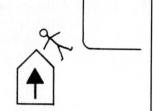

CC: Mid-teens male complaining of pain in the head and neck.

HISTORY:
    PATIENT: Denies loss of consciousness. Complains of head and
neck and left hip, but no other injuries. Denies pain in arms, legs, or
back.

    MOTHER: Bright red hair and lipstick—very excited—states
patient is "allergic to "everything," did not see accident.

    DRIVER: states patient stepped out and knocked down—not
thrown—and not knocked out.

PMH: PATIENT: No medial problems, no medications or surgery, and
never been hospitalized. Thinks he is allergic to penicillin and codeine.

EXAM: Alert male, scared but not confused.
     BP 110/70   P 98
HEAD—Hematoma right occiput, face nontender pupils equal reactive
NECK—Tender right side C-collar and placed on backboard
CHEST—nontender breath sounds equal
ABD—nontender soft
BACK—0
UP/LOW EXT—00   + Distal pulse and movement

Patient transported Code I to City General with C-collar and backboard.

10:25 en route—alert Rept VS: BP 118/70   P 70

10:30 arrived—patient alert, VS unchanged, moving all extremities

IMPRESSION: Auto-pedestrian with injuries head and left hip, and pain
in neck. No loss of consciousness.

Figure B-4   Example of Completed Narrative Report.

6. Always make any changes or additions to the chart clearly distinguished, timed, and dated. Changes after the fact may be used against you if the appearance is that you were trying to alter the record in your favor. Such alterations give the appearance of lying.

7. What do you do if there is a complication or bad result and you did not record pertinent information on the run report? The best method is to sit down immediately and write, as accurately as possible, the sequence of events using whatever records are available and the best of your memory. This is not as useful as a document transcribed at the time, but an accurate record even after the fact can be useful later in reconstructing the events.

An example of a completed narrative report is shown in Figure B–4.

Appendix C

Role of the EMS Helicopter

Larry Alred, R.N., C.E.N., EMT-P

The role of the EMS helicopter as a component of the emergency medical services system is well established. Hospital-based aeromedical helicopters have been transporting trauma patients directly from the scene of accidents since 1972. Intended as a secondary responder, the helicopter serves to complement existing ground EMS systems. The helicopter can be categorized as an adjunct to the EMT in the same sense as extrication tools, fire protection, and backup units. These provisions are not necessary on each call but must be available when needed to enhance the treatment of the patient.

In rural areas, many times the only means to keep the patient within the realm of the "golden hour" lies with the proper utilization of the EMS helicopter. Studies show that when helicopters are used to transport seriously injured trauma patients in rural areas, the expected mortality rates drop as much as 24 to 52%.

The ground units' medical control should have a major role in determining the need of the helicopter. Some factors that influence the decision to use the helicopter include type of injury, number of injured victims, time and distance from a definitive care hospital, level of EMTs, extrication, and weather. As a general rule, the EMT should consider air transport if the helicopter can transfer the seriously injured trauma patient to a hospital capable of definitive care for the patient's specific injuries more rapidly than can the ground ambulance.

No two aeromedical services are identical; therefore, it is recommended that the EMT consult the aeromedical service in their local area. Most aeromedical crews are capable of performing the following procedures directly at the scene: needle or surgical cricothyroidotomy, chest tube insertion, pericardiocentesis, intraosseous infusion, and IV cutdown. With the advent of the EMS helicopter, certain lifesaving procedures that were once performed only in the emergency department can now be performed at the scene. The advantage to these procedures at the scene are vital when extrication prolongs the initiation of definitive care.

The following are general guidelines that may assist the EMT when considering helicopter transport for trauma patients. The mechanisms of injury are vital in determining the need for air transport in certain instances. A high index of suspicion is the basis for requesting the helicopter in these cases. Many of the following are associated with high mortality rates and often result in severe internal injuries that can rarely be diagnosed in the field. Because of excellent compensatory mechanisms, patients in this group may appear only slightly injured at first glance. A thorough list of criteria for candidates for helicopter transport is beyond the scope of this manual. It is suggested that the EMT consult his or her local aeromedical program for more specific criteria.

Any "Load and Go" Situation

MVA with structural intrustion into victim's space
MVA in which extrication time > 15 minutes
Pedestrian struck and thrown > 15 feet
MVA with patient ejected from vehicle
ALS team required during transport
Smooth rapid transport required
MVA with associated fatalities
Pediatric Trauma Score < 8
Glasgow Coma Score < 10
Fall from > 15 feet
Trauma Score < 12

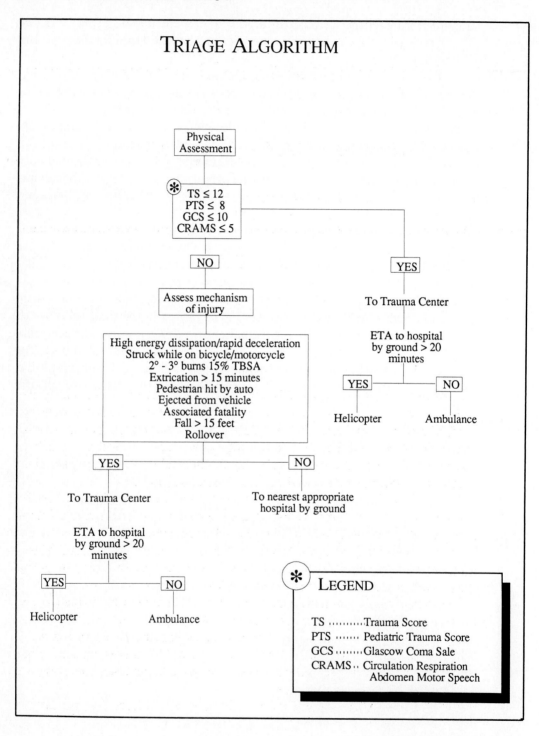

TRIAGE ALGORITHM

Physical
Assessment

TS ≤ 12
PTS ≤ 8
GCS ≤ 10
CRAMS ≤ 5

NO

Assess mechanism
of injury

High energy dissipation/rapid deceleration
Struck while on bicycle/motorcycle
2° - 3° burns 15% TBSA
Extrication > 15 minutes
Pedestrian hit by auto
Ejected from vehicle
Associated fatality
Fall > 15 feet
Rollover

YES

To Trauma Center

ETA to hospital
by ground > 20
minutes

YES   NO

Helicopter   Ambulance

NO

To nearest appropriate
hospital by ground

YES

To Trauma Center

ETA to hospital
by ground > 20
minutes

YES   NO

Helicopter   Ambulance

LEGEND

TS .... Trauma Score
PTS .... Pediatric Trauma Score
GCS .... Glascow Coma Sale
CRAMS .. Circulation Respiration
Abdomen Motor Speech

Appendix D

Trauma Scoring Systems

Diane Threadgill, R.N.
Dan Sayers, M.D.

To analyze medical information, you must make the data similar for all patients. Injury severity is very subjective and therefore varies from one observer or EMS system to another. This fact led physicians to develop trauma scoring systems which convert the degree of severity (how badly injured?) into numbers that can be fed into a computer. Having numbers allows us to compare large numbers of injured victims and to define standards of care.

In the 1970s, simple scoring systems in which numbers were assigned to specific abnormalities in the injured patient caught the imagination of the medical community. The scores were used for research and to determine which patients should be transported from the field directly to a trauma center. At the time of this document, the concept has been extensively tested and there is no convincing argument that scoring systems fail to work. They are here to stay.

Trauma scores are not specific and will not substitute for accurate field assessment by the EMT. However, determination of severity by the EMT's educated best estimate is not felt to be as reproducible as numerical trauma scores. A thorough primary survey, secondary survey, and MAST survey are still an absolute necessity, with injury identification and good communication being the cornerstone of good trauma care.

Most of the trauma scoring systems consider only factors that are easy to identify. Some scores are more useful on hospitalized patients, while others are easily applied in the prehospital setting. Decreased levels of consciousness, respiratory and circulatory abnormalities, and organ system injuries are scored in various ways. Mechanism of injury is used in some systems. We will focus on those which are useful in the field.

The Glasgow Coma Scale is accepted worldwide. Neurologic function is described by how well the patient responds to stimuli of increasing intensity. Ability to open the eyes, the clarity of speech patterns, and the movement of extremities on the best side are assigned numbers. More severe injuries generate lower scores.

The Champion Trauma Score grades respiratory rate, respiratory expansion, systolic blood pressure, and capillary return to describe the cardiopulmonary status. This is combined with a number that grades the Glasgow Coma Scale total. Again, lower numbers imply a more severely injured patient.

The CRAMS Scale combines systolic blood pressure with capillary refill for a number. It grades respiration for another number. Evidence for chest or abdomen injury generates a third number. Speech pattern and best motor response to pain are two additional factors that are scored. The five scores, all 0, 1, or 2, are added for a total. Here again, a lower total means that more severe injuries are present.

Table D-1 *Pediatric Trauma Scores*

	Score		
Component	+2	+1	−1
Size/weight	>20 kg	10–20 kg	<10 kg
Airway	Normal	Maintainable without invasive procedures	Requires invasive procedures
CNS	Alert, no history of loss of consciousness	Responds to verbal or painful stimuli	Unresponsive
Systolic BP	Pulse at wrist >90 mmHg	Carotid or femoral pulse palpable 50–90 mmHg	No palpable pulse <50 mmHg
Wounds	None	Minor	Major/penetrating
Fractures	None	Closed fracture	Open or multiple fractures

A system titled RPM (Respiratory/Pulse/Motor) utilizes respiratory rate, pulse, and best motor response. Another system, RSM (Respiratory/Systolic Pressure/Motor) grades respiratory rate, systolic pressure, and motor responses. These scales are very similar and are attempts to simplify the Trauma Score.

The Prehospital Index (PHI) grades systolic blood pressure, pulse, respiration, and consciousness. To these, a score for the presence or absence of penetrating chest or abdominal wounds is added. This scale gives a *higher* number to the more severly injured patient.

The Pediatric Trauma Score (PTS Table D.1) was developed as a physiologic and anatomic scoring system specific for pediatric patients. PTS uses +2, +1, −1 components which are added to create a total between −6 and +12. The child's size and weight are the first component, with 10 to 20 kg being the critical range. Airway is graded on the degree of maintenance. Invasive versus noninvasive procedures change the score. The third, CNS, is graded as awake, lethargic/obtunded or comatose/unresponsive. Systolic blood pressure is the fourth component and is probably best scored by palpating pulses since measured blood pressure is dependent on proper cuff size. Wounds and fractures are graded for the fifth and sixth components with minor ver-

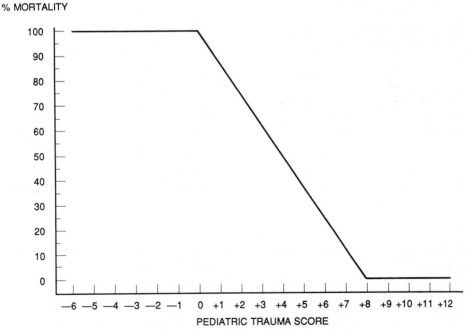

Figure D-1 Mortality Versus Pediatric Trauma Score

sus major/penetration and closed versus open/multiple being factors that increase severity.

This scoring system can be used as a rapid assessment protocol, identifying "load and go" situations, and predicting ultimate outcome (see Figure D-1). Any child with a PTS score of 8 or less is severly injured and requires the type of care available at major trauma centers. The pediatric trauma score may also be helpful in determining need for helicopter versus ground transport.

Most of these systems rate similar aspects of the patient's condition in different ways. The scores are not the same, but the information they convey is similar. They rate the severity of the patient's injuries and help estimate the patient's chances for survival. The scores help define the statistical probability that the patient will need trauma center care.

These scores are inadequate at defining such variables as prolonged out-of-hospital time and debilitating diseases which might significantly change the course of treatment. Except for the Pediatric Trauma Score, they are without discriminators for extremes of age. Most do not address the mechanism of injury. Even though the scores have these limitations, they are or will be in use in many EMS systems and you may use one or more of them as part of your trauma protocol. Remember that trauma scores are only a tool to help you make decisions about when and where to transport your patient; They do not take the place of careful patient assessment and management. *A patient's transport should never be delayed while you are trying to assign a number for severity of injury.*

——— Appendix E ———

Blood and Body Fluid Precautions in the Prehospital Setting

Richard N. Nelson, M.D.
Howard Werman, M.D.
Ronald Taylor, M.D.

EMTs have always incurred risks when carrying out their jobs. In the past, however, these have mostly involved highway hazards, fires, downed electrical wires, toxic substances, and scene security problems. Now the EMT must assume that he is also at risk of acquiring certain diseases from the patients he is treating. Fortunately, there are many precautions that the EMT may take which markedly reduces or eliminates this risk.

The spectrum of diseases to which the EMT is potentially exposed is beyond the scope of this book. However, two types of viral infections are particularly appropriate to discuss in conjunction with trauma management since their modes of transmission are primarily by blood and body fluids. In this chapter we discuss how you, as a prehospital provider, can protect yourself from the viruses that cause hepatitis B and acquired immunodeficiency syndrome (AIDS).

Hepatitis B

The term "viral hepatitis" is used to describe a group of infections involving the liver. At least four types of viruses are described: hepatitis A, hepatitis B, delta hepatitis, and non-A, non-B hepatitis. Because of their frequent contact with blood and needles, health care workers are considered at intermediate risk of becoming infected with hepatitis B virus. Fortunately, hepatitis B is the one form of hepatitis for which there is an effective vaccine. Delta hepatitis and non-A, non-B hepatitis, although spread through contact with infected serum, pose less of a risk to health care providers.

Hepatitis B virus (HVB) is a major cause of acute and chronic hepatitis, cirrhosis, and liver cancer. An estimated 200,000 persons are infected in the United States each year and between 500,000 and 1,000,000 persons are infectious carriers of the virus.

HVB is spread by blood or body fluids. Infection usually occurs from contaminated needle sticks or through sexual contact. Infection can also occur by contact of infectious secretions with skin lesions or mucosal surfaces. Routine testing of donor blood for HVB makes transmission from blood transfusion unlikely.

Although HVB infection is uncommon in the general population, members of certain groups are considered much more likely to harbor the virus. High-risk groups are immigrants from areas where HVB is prevalent, institutionalized persons, intravenous drug users, male homosexuals, hemophiliacs, household contacts of HVB patients, and hemodialysis patients.

Two types of products are available to protect against hepatitis B. The first, hepatitis B vaccine, produces active immunity against HVB infection. It is used both in routine immunization of high-risk persons and in persons recently exposed to HVB who wish to prevent infection. The second, hepatitis B immune globulin (IG and HBIG), contains antibodies to HVB and provides temporary, passive protection against HVB. HBIG and IG are used only when there has been significant exposure to HVB.

Acquired Immunodeficiency Syndrome

The acquired immunodeficiency syndrome (AIDS) is an infectious disease caused by human immunodeficiency virus (HIV). Patients with the disease develop a defect in their immune systems. This predisposes the AIDS patient to a variety of unusual infections that are not generally seen in healthy patients of a similar age. The disease has a uniformly high mortality and its incidence is increasing. At present, there is no effective vaccination or cure for the disease.

The AIDS virus appears to be transmitted in a manner similar to the hepatitis B virus. Although the virus has been cultured from a variety of body fluids (blood, semen, saliva, tears, breast milk, and urine), only blood, semen, and vaginal secretions have been implicated in transmission of the disease. There is no evidence to suggest that the HIV is transmitted by casual contact. Transmission to health care workers has been documented only after accidential parenteral exposure (needle stick) or exposure of mucous membranes and open wounds to large amounts of infected blood. The HIV appears to be different from the hepatitis B virus in two ways. The virus appears to be easily inactivated by common sterilization methods (EPA approved disinfectants, household bleach, alcohol) and the HIV is transmitted far less efficiently than the hepatitis B virus. Several studies have shown that there is less than a 1% rate of seroconversion (demonstrating antibodies to HIV) for health care workers who have experienced an accidental parenteral exposure.

Several groups have been identified as having a high risk of contacting AIDS. These include male homosexuals or bisexuals, intravenous drug abusers, patients who have received blood transfusions or pooled-plasma products (e.g., hemophiliacs), and heterosexual contacts of AIDS patients. However, because of the difficulty in identifying AIDS patients, all contacts with blood and/or body fluids should be considered a potential AIDS exposure.

Precautions for Prevention of Hepatitis B and AIDS Transmission

A. *General considerations*
  1. All emergency medical service personnel should be knowledgeable about hepatitis B and AIDS, including their etiologies, epidemiologies, and routes of transmission.
  2. Personnel who have open or weeping lesions should take special precautions to prevent exposure of these areas to blood or body fluids. If these lesions cannot be adequately protected, invasive procedures, other direct patient care activities, or handling of equipment used for patient care should be avoided.
  3. Routine handwashing should be performed before and after all patient contacts. Hands should be washed as soon as possible following exposure to blood or body fuilds.
  4. All EMS personnel are encouraged to be immunized against hepatitis B.

B. *Barrier precautions during patient exposures*
  1. Gloves should be worn if exposure to blood or other body fluids is anticipated. This precaution should be taken when performing an invasive procedure or handling any item soiled with blood or body fluid.

2. Disposable gowns, masks, and eye coverings are necessary only when extensive contact with blood or body fluids is anticipated. These precautions should be taken when aerosolization of blood or body fluids is likely (i.e., endotracheal intubation, EGTA insertion, vaginal deliveries, etc.)

3. Masks should be worn for any patient with respiratory complaints to prevent the possible transmission of respiratory infection (such as tuberculosis) to health care workers.

4. Direct mouth-to-mouth ventilation of patients during CPR is to be discouraged. Disposable mouthpieces should be utilized when mouth-to-mouth ventilation is indicated.

C. *Handling of items exposed to blood or body fluids*
1. Any sharp instrument should be considered potentially infective after patient use. Disposable syringes, needles, scalpel blades, and so on, should be placed directly in puncture-resistant containers. Needles should not be recapped, bent, or otherwise manipulated following use.

2. Any disposable equipment, such as masks, gowns, gloves, mouthpieces, and airways that have been contaminated by blood or body fluids, should be collected in an impervious plastic bag. These plastic bags should then be disposed of in proper waste containers available in the hospital emergency departments.

3. Any surface spills or nondisposable equipment not usually coming in contact with skin or mucous membranes should be washed with a low-sudsing detergent with a neutral pH. It should then be wet down or soaked for 10 minutes in a 1:10 dilution of household bleach (or 70% isopropyl alcohol). Bleach should not be used on metal objects because it causes corrosion.

4. Nondisposable medical devices that will frequently contact skin or mucous membranes should be washed thoroughly using a low-sudsing detergent with a neutral pH. They should then be soaked for 30 minutes or more in 2% alkaline glutaraldehyde (e.g., Cidex).

D. *Procedure after accidental exposure to blood or body fluids.*
1. The receiving facility should be notified at the time of the incident of the possible exposure and should be asked to cooperate in determining the serologic status of the individual. The name of the institution and the person notified should be recorded on a report form (see Figure E-1).

2. A complete written report of the incident should be completed as soon as possible. The trip sheet may be used to supplement, but not

REPORT OF SIGNIFICANT EXPOSURE
TO BLOOD OR BODY FLUID

NAME(S) OF EMS PERSONNEL: _____

NAME OF EMS SERVICE: _____

ADDRESS OF EMS SERVICE: _____

_____

PHONE NUMBER (WORK): _____ (HOME): _____

UNIT NUMBER: _____

DATE OF EXPOSURE: _____TIME OF EXPOSURE: _____

ADDRESS OF EXPOSURE: _____

_____

NAME OF PATIENT: _____

PATIENT'S ADDRESS: _____

_____

ROUTE OF EXPOSURE:

        parental exposure (needle stick)   ( )

        blood exposure to mucous membrane or open skin   ( )

        other body fluid to mucous membrane or open skin ( )

        other (please describe) _____ ( )

        _____

PRECAUTIONS TAKEN DURING TREATMENT:

        gloves   ( )

        mask   ( )

Figure E-1 Sample report form.

gown ( )

eye coverings ( )

other (please describe) _____

_____

PLEASE GIVE A COMPLETE DESCRIPTION OF THE CIRCUMSTANCES SURROUNDING THE EXPOSURE, INCLUDING MEASURES TAKEN AFTER EXPOSURE: _____

_____

_____

_____

_____

_____

_____

_____

_____

_____

INSTITUTION NOTIFIED: _____

DATE OF NOTIFICATION: _____ TIME OF NOTIFICATION: _____

NAME OF ATTENDING PHYSICIAN

NOTIFIED: _____

_____   _____
NAME OF PERSON FILING REPORT   DATE
        (please print)

_____
        SIGNATURE

Figure E–1 (continued)

```
SEROLOGIC DATA:

  PATIENT INFORMATION:

HIV antibody                              pos (   )              neg (   )

HBsAg                                     pos (   )              neg (   )


  PERSONNEL INFORMATION:

HIV antibody                              pos (   )              neg (   )
     NOTE: must be repeated at 6 weeks, 3 months, 6 months, and 1 year

HBsAg                                     pos (   )              neg (   )

HBsAb                                     pos ( ·)               neg (   )

Hepatitis B vaccination                   yes (   )              no  (   )
```

Figure E–1 (continued)

replace, this written report. A copy of this report should be forwarded to the EMS coordinator, the medical director, and the infection control committee (or equivalent body) of the receiving facility.

3. Any person who has had a significant exposure (i.e., needle stick or mucous membrane or skin-cut contact with blood or secretion) with an HIV or HBV patient, or with a patient whose serologic status is unknown, should undergo an HIV serology determination at the time of the incident. This should be repeated at 6 weeks, 3 months, 6 months, and 1 year following the exposure. If not already immunized, he should also receive HVB vaccine. Need for administration of hepatitis B immune globulin should be determined by the medical director.

4. In the case where an EMS provider is found to have a positive HVB or HIV serology, future actions should be determined by the EMS coordinator and medical director.

Summary

Prehospital providers, like most health care workers, are at risk of exposure to many contagious diseases. Because of the frequent presence of blood and secretions in the trauma victim, the EMT must take extra precautions to avoid exposure to the viruses that cause hepatitis B and AIDS. Knowledge of the modes of transmission of these viruses, as well as appropriate precautions, make it extremely unlikely that the EMT will contact any of these infections.

Appendix F

Drowning, Barotrauma, and Decompression Injury

James H. Creel, M.D.
John E. Campbell, M.D.

Drowning

Approximately 7000 people drown annually, making drowning the third leading cause of accidental death in the United States. Freshwater drownings are more common than saltwater drownings. There are more pool immersion accidents than accidents in lakes, ponds, and rivers. The peak incidence occurs in the warm months and involves mostly teenage victims. Children under the age of 4 are also common drowning victims.

Drowning is death from suffocation after submersion in the water. There are two basic mechanisms:

1. Breath holding, which leads to aspiration of water and wet lungs
2. Laryngospasm with glottic closure and dry lungs

Both lead to profound hypoxia and death. With the aspiration of at least 22 cc per kilogram of seawater (which is hypertonic to the plasma), fluid is drawn into the alveoli from the circulation. Aspiration of at least 22 cc per kilogram of fresh water (which is hypotonic to the plasma) causes fluid to be absorbed across the alveoli into the circulation. These are of no concern in the prehospital phase. Survival of the victim depends on the EMT's rapid evaluation and management of the ABCs.

Prehospital management must be initiated as soon as possible. Be aware of surfing/diving mechanisms which indicate potential occult C-spine injury. Protect the cervical spine during rescue of the victim. In water, CPR is generally ineffective. Remove the victim to a stable surface as soon as possible; then initiate CPR and appropriate protocol. An important factor to recognize is that while hypothermia may have been responsible for the near-drowning, it appears to provide the brain, heart, and lungs some degree of protection (diving reflex) by slowing of metabolism and preferential shunting of blood. Therefore, no one is dead until he is warm and dead; do not stop CPR.

Barotrauma

Barotrauma refers to injuries due to the mechanical effects of pressure on the body. We all live "under pressure" since the weight of the air in which we live exerts force on our body. At sea level the weight of air pressing on the body equals 14.7 pounds per square inch (psi). Since solids and liquids are not compressible, they are usually not affected by pressure changes. The study of barotrauma is the study of the effect of pressure on gas-filled organs of the body. Gas-filled organs are ears, sinuses, upper and lower airways, stomach, and intestines.

To understand the effects of pressure changes, one must know some properties of gases. Boyle's law states that the volume of a gas is inversely proportional to the pressure applied to it. This simply means that if you double the pressure on gas, the volume of the gas will decrease by one-half. If you halve the pressure on a gas, the volume will double. The pressure at sea level is called 1 atmosphere absolute (ATA). If you go up in an airplane (or climb a mountain) you have less atmosphere above you; thus the presence decreases and the gas inside the body expands. Most commercial airliners fly at about 35,000 feet elevation ($\frac{1}{5}$ ATA or gas volume five times normal) but are pressurized to a cabin pressure equal to 5000 to 8000 feet elevation ($\frac{2}{3}$ to $\frac{3}{4}$ ATA) so that gas expands to only about 1.2 to 1.4 times its original volume. Airline passengers notice no change except for "popping" of the ears as the expanding gas in the middle ears vents off through the eustachian tubes into the pharynx.

Water is much heavier than air. When one descends into salt water there is a change of 1 atmosphere for every 33 feet of depth (34 feet for fresh water). This means that at 33 feet of depth the body is subjected to 2 ATA and gas in the body has been compressed to one-half of its original volume. Because of the pressures involved, divers are exposed to certain potential injuries during both descent and ascent.

Trauma of Descent: "Middle Ear Squeeze"

Since there is a large pressure change during the first few feet of a dive, skin divers and snorkelers as well as scuba divers are subjected to this type of injury. If one takes a breath and descends rapidly to a depth of 33 feet, all of the gas in the body will decrease in volume by one-half. This includes gas in the lungs, intestines, stomach, sinuses, and middle ears. The elastic lungs, intestines, and stomach will simply decrease in size to match the volume of gas. Problems develop with the middle ears and sinuses if the pressure cannot be equalized. The sinuses (air pockets in the bones of the face and skull) each have an opening through which air from the pharynx can enter to equalize the pressure. If the openings are blocked, the diver will experience pain in the sinuses and may even develop bleeding and inflammation (barosinusitis). Other than the discomfort, this causes no serious problem. Each middle ear has an opening, the eustachian tube, through which air from the pharynx can enter to equalize pressure. If the eustachian tube is blocked (mucosal conjestion from allergy, infection, etc.) the pressure will push in on the eardrum and cause intense pain. This begins to be noticeable at a depth of 4 to 5 feet. If the diver cannot equalize the middle ear pressure and yet continues to descend, the pressure will eventually rupture the eardrum and flood the middle ear with cold water (even the warm waters of the Caribbean are 20° below body temperature). Cold water in the middle ear causes dizziness, nausea, vomiting, and disorientation ("twirly bends"). The result can be panic and drowning or near-drowning. The diver may surface rapidly and develop air embolism or neurologic decompression sickness. Vomiting under water can cause aspiration and drowning.

Barotitis media (middle ear squeeze) requires no field treatment. The pressure is relieved when the diver returns to the surface. If there is hearing loss or continued ear pain, the diver should see a physician for treatment of ruptured eardrum or bleeding into the middle ear. The conditions that EMTs are more likely to have to manage are the near-drowning cases caused by the disorientation from water in the middle ears.

Trauma of Ascent

Injuries from expanding gas can occur as divers ascend. These injuries are much more common in scuba divers since such injuries usually either require some time to develop (longer than a skin diver can hold his breath) or require the breathing of compressed air.

1. Reverse Middle Ear Squeeze: If a eustachian tube becomes blocked during a dive, the gas in the middle ear will expand and cause pain during ascent. If there is enough expansion, the eardrum can rupture, with all of the symptoms and dangers mentioned previously.

2. Gastrointestinal Barotrauma: If the diver swallows air while breathing compressed air or if the diver has previously eaten gas-forming foods (e.g., beans), he may accumulate a significant amount of stomach or intestinal gas during a dive. If he was at a depth of 66 feet the gas will expand to three times its original volume during ascent. If he is unable to expel this gas, he will develop abdominal pain and occasionally even collapse and develop a shocklike state.

3. Pulmonary Overpressurization Syndromes (Burst Lung):   These occur only in divers who have been breathing compressed air. During a dive the lungs are completely filled with air, which is at a pressure equal to the depth at which the diver is swimming. If a diver panics and surfaces without exhaling, the rapidly expanding gas will overinflate the lungs and cause one of the three overpressurization syndromes. Remember, the total volume of the lungs is about 6 L. An ascent from 33 feet would cause expansion to 12 L; 66 feet, 18 L; and 100 feet, 24 L. It is easy to see how delicate alveoli can be ruptured by this expansion. The expanding air will dissect into the interstitial space, pleural space, pulmonary venules, or a combination of the three.

   a. *Air in the interstitial space.* This is the most common form of pulmonary overpressurization syndrome. As millions of tiny air bubbles escape into the interstitial tissue, they may dissect into the mediastinum and up into the subcutaneous tissue of the neck. Symptoms may develop immediately upon surfacing or may not develop for several hours. The diver may have increasing hoarseness, chest pain, subcutaneous emphysema in the neck, and difficulty breathing and swallowing. Any diver with these symptoms should get oxygen (no positive pressure ventilations unless the diver is apneic) and transport to the hospital. While interstitial air does not require treatment with a recompression chamber (hyperbaric chamber), these victims often develop air embolism or decompression sickness. They should be observed in a facility that is capable of providing recompression treatment if necessary.

   b. *Air in the pleural space.* If the alveoli rupture into the pleural space a pneumothorax and possibly a hemothorax will develop. The amount of pneumothorax will depend on how much air escaped into the pleural space and how far the diver surfaced after the air entered the pleural space. A 10% pneumothorax at 33 feet will be a 20% pneumothorax at the surface. A 20 to 30% pneumothorax at 33 feet may be a tension pneumothorax at the surface. The symptoms will be the same as for interstitial air except that the diver will now have decreased breath sounds and hyperresonance to percussion on the affected side (may be on both sides). A tension pneumothorax will also have distended neck veins and shock (and possibly tracheal deviation—a late sign). These patients may require a needle decompression if they have a tension pneumothorax. Otherwise, give 100% oxygen and transport immediately.

c. *Air embolism.* The most serious syndrome of overpressurization is pulmonary air embolism. If the overdistended alveoli rupture into the pulmonary venules, the millions of tiny air bubbles can return to the left side of the heart and then up the carotid arteries to the small arterioles of the brain. These bubbles, composed mostly of nitrogen, obstruct the arterioles and produce symptoms similar to a stroke. The symptoms produced depend on which vessels are obstructed. There will usually be loss of consciousness and focal neurological signs. The symptoms almost always occur *immediately* when the diver surfaces. This is a very important point in differentiating air embolism from decompression sickness (which usually takes hours to develop). The patient should be placed in Trendelenburg's position (30° head down) on the left side, given 100% oxygen, and transported to a facility that can provide recompression treatment. The left side, head down position prevents further embolism of air to the brain and helps distend the vessels, thus allowing small bubbles to pass through and return to the lungs, where they can be eliminated. This is one instance where you should not hyperventilate or give positive pressure ventilations. Hyperventilation causes vasoconstriction, which will trap the bubbles. Positive pressure ventilation may force more air into the veins, worsening the injury (if the patient is not breathing, you must give positive pressure ventilation). This patient must have immediate recompression in a recompression chamber no matter how much time has passed since the injury and no matter how far away the recompression chamber may be. In a recompression chamber the pressure is raised to 6 ATA, which will decrease the size of the bubbles to one-sixth of their previous volume. This may allow them to pass through the capillaries back to the lungs to be expelled. Air embolism may rarely affect the coronary arteries, causing myocardial infarction, dysrhythmias, or cardiac arrest.

Decompression Illness

Decompression illness is caused by another property of gases. Henry's law states that the amount of gas dissolved in a liquid is directly porportional to the pressure applied. This means that twice as much gas would be dissolved in a liquid at 33 feet as at sea level. It also means that gas dissolved in a liquid at 33 feet will come out of solution as that liquid ascends. This is analogous to a sealed bottle of carbonated beverage, which has no bubbles as long as it is sealed but bubbles the instant the cap is removed and the pressure is released.

Nitrogen, which accounts for about 80% of the volume of inspired air, is an inert gas that dissolves in blood and fat. When a diver is under water, nitrogen dissolves in his blood and fat tissue. This nitrogen is released as he surfaces, so he must surface slowly enough to allow this nitrogen to be expelled through the lungs. The U.S. Navy has developed a set of tables of no-decompression limits which give general guidelines about how long one can stay at a certain depth without going through stage decompression during ascent. There are also standard air decompression tables for those dives that exceed the no-decompression limit. Theoretically, if one follows the recommendations of the tables, nitrogen bubbles will not form in the blood during ascent. This may not always be true because the tables were developed from studying U.S. Navy divers, who are uniformly young, healthy, well-conditioned men who were diving in salt water. There are now 3 million recreational scuba divers, and 300,000 new divers are certified each year. Sport divers are not uniformly young, healthy, and conditioned. They are often older, poorly conditioned, and not always healthy. A special problem is obesity. Fat absorbs about five times as much nitrogen as blood or other tissue, so obese divers require longer decompression times or shorter dives. Sport divers should be *very* conservative when using diving tables, especially when diving in fresh water or in lakes above sea level. The greatest danger occurs when a diver who has been submerged for a significant period of time has a diving accident, panics, and surfaces rapidly. Nitrogen bubbles will form in his blood and tissue just as carbon dioxide bubbles form in champagne. This is a different injury from barotrauma or pulmonary overpressurization syndrome and may exist along with any of the barotrauma syndromes. It is frequently seen in divers in near-drowning situations. The symptoms are almost always delayed for minutes to hours after a dive. As a general rule, symptoms that develop within 10 minutes of surfacing are caused by air embolism until proved otherwise. Symptoms developing after 10 minutes are decompression illness until proved otherwise.

A special case is that of the vacationing diver who is asymptomatic after a deep dive and then catches a plane home the same day. This diver may develop symptoms during flight since the cabin pressure is only $\frac{2}{3}$ or $\frac{3}{4}$ ATA. These symptoms may not appear until the diver has returned home far inland from the site of the dive. All emergency providers should have some knowledge of diving injuries.

Type I Decompression Illness

1. Cutaneous ("skin bends"):   Millions of tiny nitrogen bubbles may form in the micovasculature of the skin. This causes a generalized itching rash that may be red and inflamed or mottled with a central purple discoloration. It is called "marbleized skin." This condition requires no treatment but may be an early sign of more serious decompression sickness, so the patient must be observed. Give the patient 100% oxygen and transport to a facility capable of recompression therapy.

2. Musculoskeletal ("Bends" or "Pain-Only Bends"):   This is the most common presentation of decompression sickness. Over 85% of victims of decompression sickness will present with pain in the joints. The shoulders or knees are affected most commonly, but any joint may be affected. The pain is usually deep and aching, and there may be vague numbness around the affected joint. Characteristically, there are no physical findings and the pain may be eased by pressure such as inflating a blood pressure cuff. These patients require recompression therapy no matter how long it has been since the symptoms started and no matter how far the nearest recompression chamber may be.

B. Type II Decompression Illness

These syndromes are more serious and may be life threatening. They are emergencies that require rapid diagnosis and treatment.

1. Pulmonary ("Chokes"):   Nitrogen bubbles forming in the vasculature of the lungs cause symptoms like the interstitial pulmonary overpressurization syndrome. The patient will develop cough, chest pain, difficulty breathing, and sometimes hemoptysis. These symptoms usually develop within an hour of surfacing (50%) but may be delayed for up to 6 hours and even rarely for 24 to 48 hours. Pulmonary overpressurization syndrome usually appears within a few minutes of surfacing. In either case the patient requires oxygen and recompression therapy. Here again, be careful of positive pressure ventilation, as it may cause gas bubble emboli to the brain.

2. Neurologic: Nitrogen bubbles in the nervous system may present with any symptom from personality changes to specific localized neurologic changes. By far the most common symptoms involve the lower spinal cord and often produce weakness or paralysis of the legs and urinary bladder. Bladder problems are so common that historically, urinary catheters were considered essential equipment for divers. These patients must have recompression therapy or irreversible paralysis will occur.

Management of Diving Injuries

History

1. Type of diving and equipment used. This is very important. Remember that skin divers and snorkelers cannot get overpressurization syndrome or decompression sickness, but all divers can drown. The treatment for near-drowning is very different from that of decompression sickness or air embolism.

2. History of the dive. You need to know where the dive occurred, at what depth, how many dives, how long on the bottom, and any in-water decompression. This information is also needed for dives during the preceding 2 days.

3. Past medical history. Pulmonary problems that predispose to air trapping (asthma or obstructive lung disease) are frequently associated with overpressurization syndrome.

4. Exactly when the symptoms first occurred. This may be helpful in differentiating air embolism and decompression illness.

5. Complications of the dive. Did the diver run out of air? Was there an attack by marine animals? Did a diving accident occur?

6. Travel after the dive. Traveling at higher altitudes may precipitate decompression sickness.

Initial Management

1. Follow standard patient assessment protocol. Primary survey, transport decision, secondary survey.

2. If any chance of overpressurization syndrome or decompression illness, do not hyperventilate or give positive pressure ventilation. You will have to give positive pressure ventilation to apneic patients.

3. Check for hypothermia in all diving-accident victims.

4. Patients with air embolism or neurologic decompression sickness should be placed on their left side in the head-down position.

5. All diving accident victims should get oxygen.

6. Shock and other injuries are treated by routine protocols.

7. If a recompression facility is needed and you need information about the one nearest your facility, you may obtain assistance 24 hours a day through the National Diving Alert Network at Duke University (919-684-8111).

Appendix G

Useful Tables

Normal Respiratory Rates in Children

    Newborn: 40 to 60 per minute
    Infants: 20 to 30 per minute
    Older child: 12 to 20 per minute

Hypotensive Values

    Newborn: less than 50 mmHg
    Infant: less than 60 mmHg
    Child (up to age 6): less than 70 mmHg
    Child (older than 6): less than 90 mmHg

Tachycardia Values in Children

    Newborn: over 200
    Infant: over 180
    Child: over 150
    Adolescent: over 120

Size of Endotracheal Tube to use in a Child

$$\frac{16 \ + \ \text{age in years}}{4} = \text{size of tube (mm)}$$

Pediatric Trauma Score

Component	Score		
	+2	+1	−1
Size/weight	>20 kg	10–20 kg	<10 kg
Airway	Normal	Maintainable without invasive procedures	Requires invasive procedures
CNS	Alert, no history of loss of consciousness	Responds to verbal or painful stimuli	Unresponsive
Systolic BP	Pulse at wrist	Carotid or femoral pulse palpable	No palpable pulse
	>90 mmHg	50–90 mmHg	<50 mmHg
Wounds	None	Minor	Major/penetrating
Fractures	None	Closed fracture	Open or multiple fractures

Average Weights for Children

Age	Weight [lb (kg)]		Length [in. (cm)]	First fluid bolus (cc)
Neonate (term)	75	(3.5)	20 (51)	70
6 mo	17	(8)	26 (66)	160
1 yr	22	(10)	30 (75)	200
2 yr	28	(13)	35 (90)	260
3 yr	33	(15)	38 (100)	300
4 yr	37	(17)	41 (105)	340
5 yr	40	(20)	43 (110)	360
6 yr	48	(22)	46 (120)	440
8 yr	60	(27)	51 (130)	540
10 yr	73	(30)	55 (140)	660
12 yr	84	(38)	60 (150)	760
14 yr	110	(50)	64 (165)	1000

Pediatric Drugs and Dosages

Weight [kg (lb)]	Epinephrine (1:10,000)		Atropine (0.1 mg/mL)		Dextrose 50% (dilute the volume 1:1 with sterile water for injection)		Naloxone (0.4 mg/cc)	
	Dose (mg)	Volume (cc)	Dose (mg)	Volume (cc)	Dose (G)	Volume (cc)	Dose (mg)	Volume (cc)
1 (2.2)	0.01	0.1	0.1	1.0	0.5	1.0	0.01	0.025
5 (11)	0.05	0.5	0.1	1.0	2.5	5.0	0.05	0.125
7.5 (16)	0.075	0.75	0.1	1.0	3.75	7.5	0.075	0.19
10 (22)	0.1	1.0	0.1	1.0	5.0	10.0	0.1	0.25
12.5 (27)	0.12	1.25	0.12	1.25	6.25	12.5	0.12	0.3
15 (33)	0.15	1.5	0.15	1.5	7.5	15.0	0.15	0.38
20 (44)	0.2	2.0	0.2	2.0	10.0	20.0	0.2	0.5
25 (55)	0.25	2.5	0.25	2.5	12.5	25.0	0.25	0.62
30 (66)	0.3	3.0	0.3	3.0	15.0	30.0	0.3	0.75
35 (77)	0.35	3.5	0.35	3.5	17.5	35.0	0.35	0.9
40 (88)	0.4	4.0	0.4	4.0	20.0	40.0	0.4	1.0
50 (110)	0.5	5.0	0.5	5.0	25.0	50.0	0.4	1.0

Glasgow Coma Scale: The victim should be scored by the best response. This is a dynamic score and can be calculated multiple times during resuscitation and transport of a victim.

Eye opening	
Spontaneous	4
To voice	3
To pain	2
None	1

Motor response	
Obeys	6
Localizes	5
Withdraws	4
Flexion (decorticate)	3
Extension (decerebrate)	2
None	1

Verbal response	
Oriented	5
Confused	4
Inappropriate	3
Incomprehensible	2
None	1
Total	3 to 15

Pediatric Glasgow Coma Scale

		> 1 Year	*< 1 Year*
EYES OPENING	4	spontaneously	spontaneously
	3	to verbal command	to shout
	2	to pain	to pain
	1	no response	no response

		> 1 Year	*< 1 Year*
BEST MOTOR RESPONSE	6	Obeys	
	5	Localizes pain	Localizes pain
	4	Flexion-withdrawal	Flexion-normal
	3	Flexion-abnormal (Decorticate Rigidity)	Flexion-abnormal (Decorticate Rgidity)
	2	Extension (Decerebrate Rigidity)	Extension (Decerebrate Rigidity)
	1	No Response	No Response

		> 5 Years	< 2-5 Years	0-23 Months
BEST VERBAL RESPONSE	5	Oriented and converses	Appropriate words and phrases	Smiles, coos, cries appropriately
	4	Disoriented and converses	Inappropriate words	Cries
	3	Inappropriate words	Cried and/or screams	Inappropriate crying and/or screaming
	2	Incomprehensible sounds	Grunts	Grunts
	1	No Respose	No Response	No Response

Glossary

ABRUPTIO PLACENTA—early separation of the placenta from the uterus.

ACIDOSIS—condition caused by accumulation of acid or loss of base from the body.

ADVENTITIA—layer of loose connective tissue forming the outermost coating of an organ.

AEROBIC—requiring oxygen.

ALKALOSIS—pathologic condition resulting from accumulation of base or loss of acid in the body.

ANAEROBIC—lacking oxygen.

ANOXIA—absence of oxygen supply to the tissue.

ASPHYXIA—condition due to lack of oxygen, suffocation.

ASPIRATE—taking foreign matter into the lungs during inhalation.

ASSESSMENT—to evaluate the condition of a patient.

AVPU—description of the level of consciousness (i.e., A, alert; V, responds to verbal stimuli; P, responds to pain; U, unresponsive).

AVULSION—injury in which a piece of a structure is torn away.

AXIAL LOADING—compression forces applied along the long axis of the body. *Example:* A fall in which a victim lands on his feet and force is transferred up his legs to his back, causing a compression fracture of a lumbar vertebra.

BATTLE'S SIGN—Swelling and discoloration behind the ear caused by a fracture of the base of the skull.

BRONCHOSPASM—contraction of the smooth muscle of the bronchi.

BVM (BAG–VALVE–MASK)—system of artificial ventilation in which the oxygen inflow fills a bag that is attached to a mask by a one-way valve.

CAPILLARY BLANCH OR REFILL-TEST FOR IMPAIRMENT OF CIRCULATION—pressure on tip of the nail will cause the bed to turn white, if it does not turn pink again by the time it takes to say "capillary refill," the circulation is impaired.

CARBONACEOUS SPUTUM—sputum that is "sooty" or black.

CARINA—lowest part of the trachea, where the trachea divides to form the two mainstem bronchi.

CATECHOLAMINES—group of chemicals of similar structure that act to increase heart rate and blood pressure.

CENTRAL CORD SYNDROME—injury to the spinal cord that produces more loss of sensory and motor function in the arms than the legs.

CEREBRAL PERFUSION—blood flow to the brain.

CNS—central nervous system, the brain and spinal cord.

CONCUSSION—jarring injury to the brain resulting in disturbance of brain function.

CONSTRICTED—to shrink or contract.

CONTRACOUP—injury to the brain on the opposite side of the original blow.

CONTRALATERAL—situated or affecting the opposite side.

CONTUSION—bruising; the reaction of soft tissue to a direct blow.

COPIOUS—large amount.

COUP—injury to the brain on the same side as the original blow.

CREPITATION—feeling of crackling; the sensation of fragments of broken bones rubbing together.

CUSHING REFLEX—reflex whereby the body reacts to increased pressure on the brain by raising the blood pressure.

DECELERATION—to come to a sudden stop, decreasing speed.

DECUBENT POSITION—position assumed when lying down.

DENATURED—to destroy the usual nature of a substance.

DERMIS—inner layer of the skin, containing hair follicles, sweat glands, sebaceous glands, nerve endings, and blood vessels.

DIAPHORESIS—to perspire profusely.

DIURETIC—agent that promotes the excretion of urine.

DOLL'S EYES—oculocephalic reflex; a test of brainstem function that is never performed in the prehospital setting.

DURA—tough fibrous membrane forming the outermost of the three coverings of the brain.

EGTA—esophageal gastric tube airway; an improved EOA.

EOA—esophageal obturator airway.

EPIDERMIS—outermost layer of skin.

EPIDURAL—outside the dura; between the dura and the skull.

ETIOLOGY—cause of a particular disease.

ET TUBE—edotracheal tube.

EVISERATION—protruding of internal organs through a wound.

EXPEDITIOUS—quick, speedy.

EXSANGUINATE—to bleed to death.

FULL THICKNESS—third-degree burn.

GENIOGLOSSUS—muscle that pulls the tongue out of the mouth.

GRUNTING—deep, gutteral noise made in breathing; a sign of respiratory distress in small children.

HARE SPLINT—type of traction splint.

HEIMLICH MANEUVER—method of dislodging food or other material from the throat of a choking victim.

HEMIPARESIS—partial paralysis affecting one side of the body.

HEMOPTYSIS—to spit up blood or blood-stained sputum.

HEMOTHORAX—presence of blood in the chest cavity within the pleural space, outside the lung.

HYPERCARBIA—high blood carbon dioxide level.

HYPERESONANT—giving an increased vibrant sound on percussion, tympanic.

HYPERTYMPANY—hyperesonant.

HYPERVENTILATION—increased amount of air entering the lungs, >24 breaths per minute.

HYPOVOLEMIC SHOCK—hemmorrhagic shock; shock caused by insufficient blood or fluid within the body.

HYPOXIA—deficiency of oxygen reaching the tissues of the body.

INTRAABDOMINAL—within the abdomen.

INTRACRANIAL—within the skull.

INTRATHORACTIC—within the chest.

IPSALATERAL—situated on or affecting the same side.

JVD—jugular vein distention.

KINEMATICS—term that refers to possible motions of the body.

KLIPPEL SPLINT—type of traction splint.

LABIAL ANGLE—corner of the mouth.

LATERAL DECUBITUS POSITION—position assumed when lying on one's side.

LESION—injury or abnormal condition of a part.

LOC—level of consciousness. Also used to mean loss of consciousness.

MAP—mean arterial blood pressure.

MEAN ARTERIAL BLOOD PRESSURE—diastolic blood pressure plus one-half (systolic minus the diastolic blood pressure).

MEDIAL—toward the middle.

MORTALITY—frequency of death or death rate.

MVA—motor vehicle accident.

NECROSIS—death of tissue.

NEONATE—newborn infant.

NP AIRWAY—nasopharyngeal airway; an artificial airway positioned in the nasal cavity.

OCCULT INJURIES—hidden or concealed from view injuries.

OSTOMYELITIS—inflammation or infection or a bone or bones.

PALLOR—paleness, absence of skin color.

PALPATE—to examine by touch.

PARENCHYMAL—essential elements of an organ.

PARADOXICAL MOTION—motion of the injured segment of a flail chest, opposite to the normal motion of the chest wall.

PATENT—open.

PATHOPHYSIOLOGY—basic process of a disease.

PARESIS—slight or incomplete paralysis.

PARTIAL-THICKNESS BURN—burn that does not injure the full thickness of the skin. A first-degree burn involves only the epidermal layer. A second-degree burn involves the epidermis and part of the dermis.

PERFUSION—passage of blood or fluid through the vessels of an organ.

PIA MATER—innermost of the three layers of tissue that envelop the brain.

PLACENTA PREVIA—an abnormal location of the placenta, so that it covers the opening of the uterus (cervical os).

PNEUMOTHORAX—presence of air within the chest cavity in the pleural space, but outside the lung (collapsed lung).

POTENTIAL SPACE—space that does not exist except under abnormal circumstances. *Example:* Normally, the lungs completely fill the chest cavity, so that the pleural space (between the lungs and the chest wall) is only a potential space. If the pleural space contains blood, it is a hemothorax.

PULSE PRESSURE—sensation given by the heart contraction to the palpating finger.

RACCOON EYES—swelling and discoloration around both eyes; a late sign of basilar skull fracture.

RESPIRATORY RESERVE—lung tissue over and above the body's need to provide oxygenation for the body.

RTSS—radio telephone switch station; a type of radio that accesses the telephone lines.

SAGER SPLINT—type of traction splint.

SCAPHOID—shaped like a boat. When used to describe the abdomen, "scaphoid" means "sunken in."

SCUBA DIVER—diver who is able to remain under water by breathing compressed air from a breathing apparatus needing no connection with the surface. s(elf)-c(ontained) u(nderwater) b(reathing) a(pparatus).

SHEARING FORCES—forces that occur in such a direction to cause tearing of an organ.

SIBLING—brother or sister.

SKIN DIVER—diver who holds his breath when swimming under water. He uses no artificial breathing methods.

SNORING—to breathe in a hoarse, rough noise, usually with the mouth open.

SNORKELER—diver who uses a short tube (snorkel) in order to float on the surface and observe underwater life. When diving, a snorkeler must hold his breath.

SPONTANEOUS PNEMOTHORAX—collapsed lung caused by the rupture of a congentially weak area on the surface of the lung.

STRIDOR—breathing that has a high-pitched, harsh noise; a sign of impending airway obstruction.

STROKE VOLUME—amount of blood pumped by the heart in one beat.

SUBCUTANEOUS EMPHYSEMA—presence of air in soft tissue, giving a very characteristic crackling sensation on palpation; the "rice krispies" feeling.

TACHYPNEA—respiratory rate of 24 or more.

TAMPONADE—compression of a part of the anatomy, as the compression of heart by pericardial fluid.

TENSION PNEUMOTHORAX—condition in which air continuously leaks out of the lung into the pleural space, increasing pressure within the space with every breath the patient takes.

THOMAS SPLINT—type of traction splint.

TIDAL VOLUME—amount of air that is inspired and expired during one respiratory cycle.

TRACTION—action of drawing or pulling on an object.

TRAJECTORY—direction a missile takes in flight or in a body.

TRANSECTED—to cut transversely.

TRENDELENBURG POSITION—patient supine with lower body elevated about 30°.

VALLECULA—space between the base of the tongue and the epiglottis.

VASOMOTOR—affecting the size of a blood vessel.

VENOUS PRESSURE—pressure of the blood in the veins.

VISCERA—any large interior organ in any one of the three great cavities of the body, especially the abdomen.

VOLATILE—substance that evaporates rapidly at room temperature when exposed to air.

WHEEZING—whistling sounds made in breathing; a sign of spasm or narrowing of the bronchi.

Index